Asthma

Guest Editor

PASCAL CHANEZ, MD, PhD

CLINICS IN
CHEST MEDICINE

www.chestmed.theclinics.com

September 2012 • Volume 33 • Number 3

SAUNDERS an imprint of ELSEVIER, Inc.

W.B. SAUNDERS COMPANY

A Division of Elsevier Inc.

1600 John F. Kennedy Boulevard • Suite 1800 • Philadelphia, Pennsylvania 19103

http://www.theclinics.com

CLINICS IN CHEST MEDICINE Volume 33, Number 3
September 2012 ISSN 0272-5231, ISBN-13: 978-1-4557-4904-1

Editor: Katie Hartner
Developmental Editor: Donald E. Mumford

Clinics in Chest Medicine (ISSN 0272-5231) is published quarterly by Elsevier Inc., 360 Park Avenue South, New York, NY 10010-1710. Months of issue are March, June, September, and December. Periodicals postage paid at New York, NY and additional mailing offices. Subscription prices are $316.00 per year (domestic individuals), $506.00 per year (domestic institutions), $151.00 per year (domestic students/residents), $347.00 per year (Canadian individuals), $621.00 per year (Canadian institutions), $431.00 per year (international individuals), $621.00 per year (international institutions), and $211.00 per year (international and Canadian students/residents). International air speed delivery is included in all Clinics subscription prices. All prices are subject to change without notice. **POSTMASTER:** Send address changes to Clinics in Chest Medicine, Elsevier Health Sciences Division, Subscription Customer Service, 3251 Riverport Lane, Maryland Heights, MO 63043. **Customer Service: Telephone: 1-800-654-2452** (U.S. and Canada); **1-314-447-8871** (outside U.S. and Canada). **Fax: 1-314-447-8029. E-mail: journalscustomerservice-usa@elsevier.com** (for print support); **journalsonlinesupport-usa@elsevier.com** (for online support).

Reprints. For copies of 100 or more of articles in this publication, please contact the Commercial Reprints Department, Elsevier Inc., 360 Park Avenue South, New York, NY 10010-1710. Tel.: 212-633-3812; Fax: 212-462-1935; E-mail: reprints@elsevier.com.

Clinics in Chest Medicine is covered in *MEDLINE/PubMed (Index Medicus), Current Contents/Clinical Medicine, EMBASE/ Excerpta Medica, Science Citation Index,* and *ISI/BIOMED.*

Printed and bound by CPI Group (UK) Ltd, Croydon, CR0 4YY

Transferred to Digital Print 2012

Contributors

GUEST EDITOR

PASCAL CHANEZ, MD, PhD
Professor of Medicine, Département des
Maladies Respiratoires, AP-HM, Laboratoire
d'immunologie INSERM CNRS U 600,
UMR6212, Aix Marseille Université, Marseille,
France

AUTHORS

JACQUES AMEILLE, MD
Professor of Occupational Medicine, AP-HP,
Unité de pathologie professionnelle, Hôpital
Raymond Poincaré, Université de Versailles,
Garches, France

**ISABELLA ANNESI-MAESANO, MD,
PhD, DSc**
INSERM; UPMC Univ Paris 6, UMR S 707,
EPAR, Paris, France

NOUR BAÏZ, MSc
INSERM; UPMC Univ Paris 6, UMR S 707,
EPAR, Paris, France

AUDREESH BANERJEE, MD
Pulmonary, Allergy and Critical Care Division,
Department of Medicine, Perelman School of
Medicine, University of Pennsylvania, Airways
Biology Initiative, Philadelphia, Pennsylvania

P.J. BARNES, MD, PhD
Professor and Head of Respiratory Medicine,
Imperial College London, Airway Disease
Section, National Heart and Lung Institute,
London, United Kingdom

ELISABETH H. BEL, MD, PhD
Professor and Head of Respiratory Medicine,
Department of Pulmonology, Academic
Medical Centre, Amsterdam, The Netherlands

PATRICK BERGER, MD, PhD
Professor, Centre de Recherche Cardio-
thoracique de Bordeaux, Univ. Bordeaux;
INSERM, U1045, CIC 0005, Bordeaux,
France; Service d'Exploration Fonctionnelle
Respiratoire, CHU de Bordeaux, CIC 0005,
Pessac, France

JUDITH L. BLACK, MD, PhD
Professor, Pharmacology, University of
Sydney, Discipline of Pharmacology and
Woolcock Institute of Medical Research,
University of Sydney, Sydney, New South
Wales, Australia

EUGENE R. BLEECKER, MD
Professor of Genomics and Director, Center for
Genomics and Personalized Medicine, Wake
Forest School of Medicine, Winston Salem,
North Carolina

PIERA BOSCHETTO, MD, PhD
Associate Professor of Occupational
Medicine, Department of Clinical and
Experimental Medicine, University of Ferrara,
Ferrara, Italy

**LOUIS-PHILIPPE BOULET, MD,
FRCPC, FCCP**
Institut universitaire de cardiologie et de
pneumologie de Québec, Université Laval,
Québec, Canada

ARNAUD BOURDIN, MD, PhD
Professor, Doctor in Medicine, Department of Respiratory Disease, Hôpital Arnaud de Villeneuve, CHU Montpellier; INSERM U1046 Physiologie et Médecine expérimentale du coeur et des muscles, Université Montpellier 1 et 2, CHU Arnaud de Villeneuve, Montpellier, France

CHRISTOPHER E. BRIGHTLING, MD, PhD, FRCP
Infection and Inflammation Institute, Glenfield Hospital, University of Leicester, Leicester, United Kingdom

GAETANO CARAMORI, MD, PhD
Section of Respiratory Diseases, Department of Medical Sciences, Centro per lo Studio delle Malattie Infiammatorie Croniche delle Vie Aeree e Patologie Fumo Correlate dell'Apparato Respiratorio (CEMICEF), University of Ferrara, Ferrara, Italy

PASCAL CHANEZ, MD, PhD
Professor of Medicine, Département des Maladies Respiratoires, AP-HM, Laboratoire d'immunologie INSERM CNRS U 600, UMR6212, Aix Marseille Université, Marseille, France

KIAN FAN CHUNG, MD, DSc, FRCP
National Heart and Lung Institute, Imperial College and NIHR Biomedical Research Unit, Royal Brompton Hospital, London, United Kingdom

MARCO CONTOLI, MD, PhD
Section of Respiratory Diseases, Department of Medical Sciences, Centro per lo Studio delle Malattie Infiammatorie Croniche delle Vie Aeree e Patologie Fumo Correlate dell'Apparato Respiratorio (CEMICEF), University of Ferrara, Ferrara, Italy

ANGIRA DASGUPTA, MD, MRCP (UK)
Department of Medicine, St Joseph's Healthcare, McMaster University, Hamilton, Ontario, Canada

JACQUES DE BLIC, MD
Professor of Pediatry, Service de pneumologie et allergologie pédiatriques, Centre de référence des maladies respiratoires rares, Hôpital Necker Enfants Malades, Assistance Publique des Hôpitaux de Paris, Université Paris Descartes, Paris, France

ANTOINE DESCHILDRE, MD
INSERM U 1019 Lung Infection and Innate Immunity, Institut Pasteur, Université de Lille 2, Lille Cedex; Unité de pneumopédiatrie, Centre de compétence des maladies respiratoires rares, Université Lille 2 et CHRU, Hôpital Jeanne de Flandre, Lille, France

SERPIL C. ERZURUM, MD
Professor and Chair, Department of Pathobiology, Lerner Research Institute, Respiratory Institute, Cleveland, Ohio

GIACOMO FORINI, MD
Section of Respiratory Diseases, Department of Medical Sciences, Centro per lo Studio delle Malattie Infiammatorie Croniche delle Vie Aeree e Patologie Fumo Correlate dell'Apparato Respiratorio (CEMICEF), University of Ferrara, Ferrara, Italy

JULIET M. FOSTER, PhD
Clinical Management, Woolcock Institute of Medical Research, University of Sydney, New South Wales, Australia

MINA GAGA, MD, PhD
Director, 7th Respiratory Department and Asthma Centre, Athens Chest Hospital, Athens, Greece

BENJAMIN M. GASTON, MD
Professor, Department of Pediatric Pulmonary Medicine, University of Virginia School of Medicine, Charlottesville, Virginia

PHILIPPE GOSSET, PhD
INSERM U 1019 Lung Infection and Innate Immunity, Université de Lille 2, Institut Pasteur, Lille Cedex, France

GREGORY A. HAWKINS, PhD
Associate Professor of Genomics, Center for Genomics and Personalized Medicine, Wake Forest School of Medicine, Winston Salem, North Carolina

MARC HUMBERT, MD, PhD
Professor of Medicine, Director, INSERM U999, Pulmonary Hypertension: Pathophysiology and Novel Therapies, Professor of Respiratory Medicine, Service de Pneumologie et Réanimation Respiratoire, Centre National de Référence de l'Hypertension Pulmonaire Sévère, Hôpital Antoine Béclère Assistance Publique Hôpitaux de Paris, Université Paris-Sud 11, Clamart, France

SEBASTIAN L. JOHNSTON, MD, PhD
MRC and Asthma UK Centre in Allergic Mechanisms of Asthma, Centre for Respiratory Infection, Imperial College London, National Heart and Lung Institute, London, United Kingdom

MANON LABRECQUE, MD, MSc
Associate Professor, Chest Department, Sacré-Coeur Hospital, Université de Montréal, Montreal, Quebec, Canada

CATHERINE LEMIERE, MD, MSc
Professor of Medicine, Chest Department, Sacré-Coeur Hospital, Montreal, Quebec, Canada

BRUCE D. LEVY, MD
Associate Professor of Medicine, Harvard Medical School; Affiliate Member, Department of Anesthesiology, Perioperative and Pain Medicine, Center for Experimental Therapeutics and Reperfusion Injury, Brigham and Women's Hospital, Boston, Massachusetts

XINGNAN LI, PhD, MS
Assistant Professor of Genomics, Center for Genomics and Personalized Medicine, Wake Forest School of Medicine, Winston Salem, North Carolina

R. LOUIS, MD, PhD
Professor of Respiratory Medicine, Liege University, Head of Respiratory Medicine Department, CHU Liege, Belgium

YVES MAGAR, MD
Groupe Hospitalier Paris Saint-Joseph, rue Raymond Losserand, Paris, France

BRUNILDA MARKU, MD, PhD
Section of Respiratory Diseases, Department of Medical Sciences, Centro per lo Studio delle Malattie Infiammatorie Croniche delle Vie Aeree e Patologie Fumo Correlate dell'Apparato Respiratorio (CEMICEF), University of Ferrara, Ferrara, Italy

DEBORAH A. MEYERS, PhD
Professor of Genomics and Co-Director, Center for Genomics and Personalized Medicine, Wake Forest School of Medicine, Winston Salem, North Carolina

PARAMESWARAN NAIR, MD, PhD, FRCP, FRCPC
Department of Medicine, St Joseph's Healthcare, McMaster University, Hamilton, Ontario, Canada

REYNOLD A. PANETTIERI JR, MD
Professor, Pulmonary, Allergy and Critical Care Division, Department of Medicine, Perelman School of Medicine, University of Pennsylvania, Airways Biology Initiative, Philadelphia, Pennsylvania

NIKOS PAPADOPOULOS, MD, PhD
Allergy Department, 2nd Paediatric Clinic, University of Athens, Athens, Greece

ALBERTO PAPI, MD
Section of Respiratory Diseases, Department of Medical Sciences, Centro per lo Studio delle Malattie Infiammatorie Croniche delle Vie Aeree e Patologie Fumo Correlate dell'Apparato Respiratorio (CEMICEF), University of Ferrara, Ferrara, Italy

ALESSIA PAULETTI, MD
Section of Respiratory Diseases, Department of Medical Sciences, Centro per lo Studio delle Malattie Infiammatorie Croniche delle Vie Aeree e Patologie Fumo Correlate dell'Apparato Respiratorio (CEMICEF), University of Ferrara, Ferrara, Italy

DIRKJE S. POSTMA, MD, PhD
Professor of Pulmonology, Department of Pulmonary Medicine, University Medical Center Groningen, University of Groningen, Groningen, The Netherlands

JACQUES-ANDRÉ PRALONG, MD, MSc
Research Fellow, Research Center, Sacré-Coeur Hospital, Université de Montréal, Montreal, Quebec, Canada

HELEN K. REDDEL, MB, BS, PhD, FRACP
Research Leader, Clinical Management Group, Woolcock Institute of Medical Research, Clinical Associate Professor, University of Sydney, New South Wales, Australia

KONSTANTINOS SAMITAS, MD, PhD
Resident Pulmonologist, 7th Respiratory Department and Asthma Centre, Athens Chest Hospital, Athens, Greece

F. SCHLEICH MD
Head of Clinic, Department of Respiratory Medicine, CHU Liege, Belgium

CHARLES N. SERHAN, PhD
Simon Gelman Professor of Anesthesia, Harvard Medical School; Director, Department of Anesthesiology, Perioperative and Pain Medicine, Center for Experimental Therapeutics and Reperfusion Injury, Brigham and Women's Hospital, Boston, Massachusetts

REBECCA E. SLAGER, PhD, MS
Assistant Professor of Genomics, Center for Genomics and Personalized Medicine, Wake Forest School of Medicine, Winston Salem, North Carolina

ISABELLE TILLIE-LEBLOND, MD, PhD
Professor of Pulmonology, Pulmonary Department, University Hospital, Centre de Compétence des Maladies Respiratoires Rares Medical University of Lille, Hôpital Calmette, Lille Cedex, France; INSERM U 1019 Lung Infection and Innate Immunity, Université de Lille 2, Institut Pasteur, Lille Cedex, France

ISABELLE VACHIER, PhD
Respiratory Disease Department, Arnaud de Villeneuve Hospital, Montpellier, France

DANIEL VERVLOET, MD
Aix Marseille University, Marseille, France

ELEFTHERIOS ZERVAS, MD
Consultant Pulmonologist, 7th Respiratory Department and Asthma Centre, Athens Chest Hospital, Athens, Greece

Contents

This review discusses the diagnosis and phenotyping of asthma, with a special emphasis on phenotyping based on the nature of cellular inflammation and radiological imaging and how this could be used to direct the treatment of asthma and, in the future, to apply specifically directed therapies to specific phenotypes.

Diagnosis and treatment of asthma are currently based on assessment of patient symptoms and physiologic tests of airway reactivity. Research over the past decade has identified an array of biochemical and cellular biomarkers, which reflect the heterogeneous and multiple mechanistic pathways that may lead to asthma. These mechanistic biomarkers offer hope for optimal design of therapies targeting the specific pathways that lead to inflammation. This article provides an overview of blood, urine, and airway biomarkers; summarizes the pathologic pathways that they signify; and begins to describe the utility of biomarkers in the future care of patients with asthma.

There are increasing data to support the "hygiene" and "microbiota" hypotheses of a protective role of infections in modulating the risk of subsequent development of asthma. There is less evidence that respiratory infections can actually cause the development of asthma. There is some evidence that rhinovirus respiratory infections are associated with the development of asthma, particularly in childhood, whereas these infections in later life seem to have a weaker association with the development of asthma. The role of bacterial infections in chronic asthma remains unclear. This article reviews the available evidence indicating that asthma may be considered as a chronic infectious disease.

Diagnosis and management of severe asthma implies the definition of different entities, that is, difficult asthma and refractory severe asthma, but also the different phenotypes included in the term refractory severe asthma. A complete evaluation by a physician expert in asthma is necessary, adapted for each child. Identification of mechanisms involved in different phenotypes in refractory severe asthma may improve the therapeutic approach. The quality of care and monitoring of children with severe asthma is as important as the prescription drug, and is also crucial for differentiating between severe asthma and difficult asthma, whereby expertise is required.

Control-based asthma management has been incorporated in asthma guidelines for many years. This article reviews the evidence for its utility in adults, describes its strengths and limitations in real life, and proposes areas for further research, particularly about incorporation of future risk and identification of patients for whom phenotype-guided treatment would be effective and efficient. The strengths of control-based management include its simplicity and feasibility for primary care, and its limitations include the nonspecific nature of asthma symptoms, the complex role of β_2-agonist use, barriers to stepping down treatment, and the underlying assumptions about asthma pathophysiology and treatment responses.

CLINICS IN CHEST MEDICINE

Preface

Asthma is still a challenging disease in 2012. It is the most frequent chronic respiratory disorder nowadays. Despite major progress in the understanding of the mechanisms and the use of new strategies of treatment, asthma remains a potential life-long disorder. The crucial problems are clearly a better compliance to current treatments in patients with a mild persistent disease and an urgent need for innovative treatments to better control severe persistent asthma. The obvious heterogeneity of asthma makes it difficult to expect a single unified mechanism or trigger to explain its chronicity and severity. Overall, our challenge will be to find a way to interfere with the natural history of asthma. In the present issue of *Clinics in Chest Medicine*, international experts, working in the forefront of asthma, discuss the most recent burning questions raised by the disease.

We deliberately begin with a discussion of the role of compliance in asthma by Dr Boulet and colleagues, who point to the problem of nonadherence, resulting in increased severity, poor control, and high costs. Their main message is that adherence should be regularly reassessed by every single health care provider, incorporating patients' wishes to a very pragmatic aim of shared efficacy.

Today, the epidemiology of asthma is questionable and the global world in which we are living brings some changes in the overall prevalence. Baïz and Annesi-Maesano answer positively to the potential increase, particularly in low-income countries, or in some ethnic groups. This increased prevalence of asthma depends on exposure to various environmental factors but also favors the involvement of host susceptibility. In particular, gene–environment interactions starting in early life, perhaps before birth, using the epigenetic approach should be explored.

As in many polygenic diseases, the genetics of asthma is a complex and often discouraging area for researchers and clinicians in the real world. Slager and colleagues provide a comprehensive and modern view of this aspect of the condition with a special input, bringing together new phenotypes and understanding with findings in genome-wide studies of asthma susceptibility. They try to integrate lung function and biomarkers with these new findings to better understand the mechanisms of asthma progression. They believe that linking

the functional biology of the potential new variants discovered through genome-wide sequencing associated with well-defined phenotypes is the only way toward real personalized medicine in asthma.

The diagnosis of asthma is still a matter of debate. In daily practice, it is non–evidence-based and the definition remains very descriptive and relies on patient recall and perception of symptoms. Nair and colleagues recommend objective measurements of variable airflow obstruction, airway hyperresponsiveness, and airway inflammation for a secured diagnosis. Phenotyping of asthma is paramount but complex, new statistical approaches such as the unsupervised hierarchical cluster analysis has been used increasingly and is promising to identify phenotypes in an unbiased approach. Their potential value to assess future risks and to better manage patients requires further validation.

Objective biomarkers are "a holy grail" in chronic diseases and asthma does not escape this physician's quest. Erzurum and Gaston review the current state of the art of the potential biomarkers and their pathophysiological relevance. Based on the different clinical phenotypes and the potential underlying mechanisms, they report the need of a combined approach integrating clinical findings with the available biomarkers. This combined approach will certainly provide a way to control the most severe asthmatic patients better and to treat them accordingly.

Asthma pathobiology is an important area of research and it represents an integrated network of various mechanisms leading to chronic airway inflammation and structural changes of the bronchi. Airway smooth muscle (ASM) is a key player in most of the outcomes in asthma from bronchoconstriction to permanent airway hyperresponsiveness and decline in lung function. Black, Panettieri, Banerjee, and Berger address the importance of ASM to contribute to permanent airway abnormalities. It not only is an important target for bronchodilators but also has an important role to play in airway wall inflammation and remodeling. Thus, ASM may be a good candidate to target for innovative drugs.

Inflammation of the bronchi has been extensively described in asthma. Most of the inflammatory cells are recruited and activated and survive in

Clin Chest Med 33 (2012) xiii–xv
http://dx.doi.org/10.1016/j.ccm.2012.07.005

the airway wall leading to the persistency of the clinical expression of the disease. Uncontrolled asthma is associated with a potential defect of the resolution of inflammation as shown by Levy, Vachier, and Serhan. It is a finely regulated mechanism involving specialized pro-resolution mediators, often enzymatically issued from the arachidonic acid metabolism, such as LXA4 and PD1, in response to bronchial injuries. Bioactive stable analogue mimetics may represent original and innovative therapeutic ways for asthma and airway inflammation treatments.

Asthma is always a syndrome and the search for direct etiologies is often unfruitful. Microorganisms such as bacteria and viruses are in potential constant close contact with airway epithelium, which is largely abnormal in asthma. As in the analogy of the *Helicobacter* success story in the gastrointestinal tract, infection is presented as a potential factor able to create, induce loss of control, or maintain and sustain asthma. Papi and colleagues revisit asthma as a potential infectious disease. This is still a controversial area but new findings on the microbiota and exposure to infectious agents plead for a role increasing or inhibiting the development of the disease and modulating the degree of asthma control and severity.

Occupational asthma (OA) is heterogenous in clinical presentation and can be considered as asthma directly induced by work or aggravated by the contact to a deleterious agent at the work place. Lemiere and colleagues describe the changes in the presentation of OA and the constant emergence of new causative agents. They emphasize the need for a real detailed diagnosis to help workers and implement specific and efficient interventions on working sites.

Difficult asthma remains a major challenge in 2012. It is defined as an absence of control despite real effort including best pharmacotherapy for an optimal control. It requires a step-by-step assessment and Tillie-Leblond and colleagues point out the importance of investigating the diversity of difficult asthma in children. They discuss the need for early recognition and specific management. Various mechanisms are interacting to create this specific entity called severe asthma, which may benefit from new interventions. In adults, the phenotypes of severe asthma are different from those observed in childhood asthma. Gaga and colleagues bring evidence from recent cohorts studies that phenotypes of severe asthma are numerous and diverse. Severe asthma fits most of the requirement to be considered as an orphan disease, which can allow more money for research and a huge effort to develop new and effective therapies. Most of the international and national guidelines plead for a management of asthma based on control. This approach is pragmatic in essence and allows a wide spread of efficient and safe medications in primary and secondary care. Reddel reports that the control of asthma is difficult to assess based on objective measurements. Management based on control is an easy way to cope with asthma, but the limitations are obvious such as the variability in perception of symptoms. The current use of treatments is not homogenous with some concerns with bronchodilators use and the various barriers to step down according to the improved control. The use of control in the management of asthma in the real world is possible but may improve further through an increased use of tailor-made management in specific phenotypes of asthmatic patients. Inhaled corticosteroids (ICS) are the ultimate treatment of asthma. Louis, Schleich, and Barnes discuss the present and the future of ICS in asthma. This treatment has been shown to affect most of the major asthma outcomes including death and bronchial hyperresponsiveness in a positive way. ICS are particularly effective in combating Th2-driven inflammation featuring mast cell and eosinophilic airway infiltration, the so-called coherent form of the disease phenotype. Their effect on innate immunity and neutrophilic inflammation is rather poor and their ability to prevent airway remodeling and accelerated lung decline is highly controversial. Our current drugs and strategies have been able to change the daily control of asthma in most of our patients. The management is still symptomatic and no strategy at present aims to cure the disease. Bourdin and colleagues review the potential for immunological targeted therapies to better control severe asthma. These treatments should be investigated in other forms of the disease to know how they can really interfere with the natural history of the disease. The next evaluations will certainly question the advantages and drawbacks between efficacy and safety for their future. Overall, we are facing a fascinating new chapter of the knowledge of asthma: the discovery of phenotypes based on different parameters including genetic parameters will promote a real new personalized management to the benefit of our patients.

I do hope this issue of the *Clinics in Chest Medicine* will contribute to the knowledge in the field and will provoke new questions and potential studies for the interest of researchers, physicians, and patients.

As guest editor, I would like to thank all our colleagues for their outstanding contributions. I was honored to bring this adventure to a happy completion and thank Elsevier and in particular Katie Saunders and Sarah Barth, editors, *Clinics in Chest Medicine*, for their constant help and support.

DEDICATION

This issue is dedicated to Dr Pierre Aubas, who introduced me to chest diseases and the *Clinics in Chest Medicine* (see issue 25[3]), a long time ago, and to my family, Elsa, Brice, and Marie Joëlle Parayre-Chanez, for their infinite patience with me.

Pascal Chanez, MD, PhD
Département des Maladies Respiratoires
AP-HM, INSERM CNRS U 1067
UMR7733, AIX Marseille Université
Marseille, France

E-mail address:
pascal.chanez@univmed.fr

Adherence: The Goal to Control Asthma

Louis-Philippe Boulet, MD, FRCPC, FCCP[a],*,
Daniel Vervloet, MD[b], Yves Magar, MD[c],
Juliet M. Foster, PhD[d]

KEYWORDS

- Adherence • Compliance • Asthma control

KEY POINTS

- Asthma management requires adequate adherence to many recommendations, including therapy, monitoring of asthma control, avoidance of environmental triggers, and attending follow-up appointments.
- Poor adherence is common in patients with asthma and is often associated with increased health care use, morbidity, and mortality.
- Interventions to improve adherence demand tailoring to the individual by including patient-specific education, addressing patient fears and misconceptions, monitoring adherence, and developing a shared decision process.

INTRODUCTION

Asthma is a chronic condition that requires sufficient adherence to preventative and therapeutic interventions to achieve adequate control of the disease.[1] Control of asthma can be defined as minimal or no symptoms, optimal pulmonary function, few/no exacerbations, and the ability to enjoy normal activities.[2] Asthma control is the main goal of asthma therapy, but in order to achieve this it is crucial that the patient agrees with the diagnosis and is willing to follow the recommendations provided. This situation is particularly true for patients with severe asthma requiring polypharmacology, sometimes with potentially significant side effects.[3]

Optimal medication adherence (ie, taking medication as prescribed by the physician) is important to optimize the benefits of therapy. Timely modulation of dose strength by the physician according to

Disclosure: LPB: Advisory Boards: AstraZeneca, GlaxoSmithKline, Merck, and Novartis. Lecture fees: 3M, AstraZeneca, GlaxoSmithKline, Merck, and Novartis. Sponsorship for investigator-generated research: AstraZeneca, GSK, Merck, and Schering. Research funding for participating in multicenter studies: Altair, Asmacure, AstraZeneca, Boehringer-Ingelheim, Genentech, GlaxoSmithKline, Pharmaxis, Schering, Wyeth. Support for the production of educational materials: AstraZeneca, GlaxoSmithKline, and Merck Frosst. Governmental: Adviser for the Quebec INNESS. Organizational: Chair of the Canadian Thoracic Society Respiratory Guideline Committee and chair of GINA Guidelines Dissemination and Implementation Committee. Laval University Chair on Knowledge Translation, Prevention and Education in Respiratory and Cardiovascular Health. Member Knowledge Translation Canada (Canadian Institutes of Health Research). DV: GlaxoSmithKline, AstraZeneca, Stallergenes, ALK, MundiPharma. YM: Lecture or training sessions fees: AstraZeneca, GlaxoSmithKline, MSD. JMF: Research funding: AstraZeneca and Nycomed. Lecture fees: AstraZeneca, Pharmaceutical Society of Australia and GlaxoSmithKline.

[a] Institut universitaire de cardiologie et de pneumologie de Québec, Université Laval, 2725 chemin Ste-Foy, Québec, QC G1V 4G5, Canada; [b] Clinical Management, Aix Marseille University, La croix du sud villa 21, 68 ch Vallon de Toulouse, Marseille 13009, France; [c] Groupe Hospitalier Paris Saint-Joseph, 185 rue Raymond Losserand, Paris 75014, France; [d] Woolcock Institute of Medical Research, University of Sydney, PO Box M77, Missenden Road, New South Wales 2050, Australia
* Corresponding author.
E-mail address: lpboulet@med.ulaval.ca

Clin Chest Med 33 (2012) 405–417
http://dx.doi.org/10.1016/j.ccm.2012.06.002
0272-5231/12/$ – see front matter © 2012 Published by Elsevier Inc

the severity and variability of the disease is needed to ensure that asthma control is maintained. The treatment can be adjusted by the patient or caregiver with the guidance of an agreed written asthma action plan, but poor adherence can also apply to the use of written asthma action plans as well as environmental recommendations (eg, allergen avoidance) and follow-up visits. Poor inhaler technique is also a common form of unintentional poor adherence.[4]

This article focuses on medication adherence. The criteria proposed to define medication adherence and its various patterns are discussed, current research on adherence in asthma and its effects on asthma control is reviewed, and determinants and predictors of poor adherence are identified. Available methods of assessing adherence are reviewed, as well as interventions that could improve it. Future perspectives and research needs are discussed.

DEFINITION OF ADHERENCE TO ASTHMA THERAPY

Adherence, a term sometimes used interchangeably with compliance, observance, or concordance, describes the extent to which patients' medication-taking behavior is in keeping with the prescription provided.[5] Adherence includes 3 specific components: (1) acceptance of the recommendation (the patient agrees to take the medication/follow the recommendation), (2) observance of the prescription (the patient uses the treatment as suggested by the physician), and (3) persistence (the extent to which the patient follows the prescription over time). Adherence is often considered a dichotomous variable in studies, with a specific cutoff (eg, 60%, 80%), but in reality it is a continuum, expressed in different degrees and patterns. There is no formal consensus on the cutoff used to define poor and good adherence; it usually ranges from less than 60% to less than 100% of prescribed doses.[6] In asthma, the concept of poor adherence is mostly applied to underuse of daily maintenance (preventative) therapy, but overuse of preventative therapy and as-needed reliever therapy (fast-acting β_2-agonists), can also be problematic.

Current Data on Adherence to Asthma Therapy and its Effect on Asthma Control

Since the introduction of inhaled corticosteroids (ICS; also referred to as controller) more than 30 years ago, numerous studies have been published to assess the extent of poor adherence to preventative treatment in asthma and its impact on asthma control.

Several forms of poor adherence have been described: (1) taking less than the daily prescribed dose (suboptimal/poor adherence), (2) therapeutic gaps of variable duration (eg, periods of optimal/good adherence followed by short/long periods of zero use) (erratic poor adherence) (3) failure to refill the prescription after an initial adherent period (nonpersistence) and (4) failure to fill the first prescription provided (primary poor adherence).

The average rate of adherence in asthma is believed to be between 30% and 70%[7–11] and a World Health Organization report in 2003 based on key studies in adults and children showed that mean adherence was around 50%.[5] However, adherence rates are dependent on the accuracy of the measurement method, and a review of studies using electronic monitoring in the 1990s showed that patients took prescribed doses of ICS on only 20% to 73% of days and only 46% to 59% of patients had correct inhalation technique, reducing the effectiveness of inhaled treatment.[12]

STUDIES OF LARGE ASTHMATIC POPULATIONS

Studies in large Health Maintenance Organization (HMO) populations confirm high rates of nonadherence in asthma, although the data are limited to dispensed prescriptions and do not take into account prescribing that deviates from current guidelines. Williams and colleagues[13] studied 405 adults aged 18 to 50 years, in an HMO in Michigan over a period of 3 years. Adherence to ICS, calculated as a percentage of days covered between 2 prescription refills, was approximately 50%. Poor adherence was related to a greater number of emergency room visits, filled prescriptions of oral steroids, and total number of days of treatment with oral steroids. The investigators estimated that more than half of the 80 asthma-related hospitalizations recorded during the monitoring period could have been avoided with optimal adherence. In a more recent study of 1064 patients with asthma aged 5 to 56 years from the same HMO, 8% of patients displayed primary poor adherence (ie, did not fill the first controller prescription provided)[14] and mean adherence was even lower than the mean adherence (30%) in other large studies.[15,16]

In a study of 351 participants with current asthma from the Tasmanian Longitudinal Health Study cohort, only 26% used an adequate amount of controller medication (defined as the minimally adequate amount recommended by national asthma guidelines for a given severity [mild, moderate, severe]). Lung function was significantly lower for the group with inadequate treatment compared with the adequately treated group, suggesting that proper use of controller medication could protect against the progressive decline in lung function associated with increasing severity.[17]

In a study of 5504 patients with asthma listed in a pharmaceutical company database in the United States, more than 50% who filled an initial prescription for fluticasone propionate/salmeterol did not fill a second prescription in the next 12 months. Patients who were the most likely to be adherent were men older than 35 years, those with comorbidities, a lower copayment, and moderate to severe asthma symptoms.[18]

POOR ADHERENCE IN CHILDHOOD ASTHMA

A review of 10 studies in pediatric asthma reported a mean adherence rate of 48% for controller medication,[19] and more recently, a survey study[20] found that only 55% of children with persistent asthma reported using daily preventative medication. In a cohort study involving 42 primary care practices in 3 regions of the United States and 638 children (mean age 9.4 years), one-third of children prescribed daily controllers used them 4 days or fewer per week.[21] Children with suboptimally controlled asthma reported using controllers less than recommended or not receiving controller medication at all. In a cross-sectional, 1-month follow-up study using electronic monitoring in 75 children aged 8 to 16 in the United States,[22] adherence with controller medications was 46% (median) of the prescribed dose. Low adherence is important in children because it can be a predictor for difficult asthma, along with other factors such as home environment and corticosteroid responsiveness.[23] Perception of the severity of the disease or vulnerability of the patient can influence adherence. Parents who consider their child more vulnerable to illness may be more likely to use regular preventive medications, seek medical advice, and keep the schoolchildren at home.[24]

POOR ADHERENCE WITH ORAL CORTICOSTEROIDS

Adherence with oral corticosteroids is also suboptimal. Cooper and Hickson[25] found that of 6035 children under the care of Medicaid, who attended the emergency department or were hospitalized for an exacerbation of asthma, only about half were supplied with oral corticosteroids in the days after the event, and this was even lower in black children (47%) compared with 64% in other populations.

POOR ADHERENCE IN DIFFICULT-TO-CONTROL ASTHMA AND AFTER ACUTE ASTHMA

Poor adherence to oral and inhaled corticosteroid therapy seems to be a common reason for poor asthma control in difficult asthma, although patients may be reluctant to admit it. Gamble and colleagues[26] found that despite initial denial, 35% of patients with difficult asthma (63 of 188) filled 50% or fewer prescriptions of controller medication. Patients who filled 50% or fewer prescriptions had significantly lower asthma quality-of-life (QoL) scores and 25% of these patients had 3 or more admissions in the previous year, compared with only 10% of patients who filled more than half of their prescriptions. Furthermore, 23 of 51 patients (45%) tested for blood plasma cortisol and blood plasma prednisolone were found to be nonadherent to oral corticosteroids; this was corroborated by a similar rate in another study.[26] When Krishnan and colleagues[27] followed up 60 patients hospitalized for an exacerbation of asthma, they found that use of controllers and oral corticosteroids decreased to 50% of the prescribed dose at 7 days after hospital discharge and that poor adherence was significantly associated with worse asthma control.

The link between poor adherence and worse asthma control is further supported by an epidemiologic study of administrative claims from more than 20 managed care plans located throughout the United States.[28] Of 12,636 patients who had used the emergency department for acute asthma, 75% had not received ICS in the year preceding the event, and in those for whom ICS was prescribed, the average supply was 3 canisters per year, representing about half of the minimum required. In contrast, more than 50% of patients received an average of 4.11 short-acting-agonist canisters in 12 months, indicating dependence on short-acting β_2-agonists in preference to ICS use. Prescriptions dispensed for controller therapy increased 2.6-fold in the month after the emergency department event, but returned to the initial numbers. Thus, neither suboptimal chronic asthma nor severe acute asthma seems a sufficient incentive to improve treatment adherence. Many patients may prefer to take controller medications only during symptomatic periods instead of taking regular preventative therapy.

The problem of poor adherence is not specific to asthma, but affects all chronic diseases. For example, only 45% of patients with osteoporosis continue to take their treatment after a year, and 21% of diabetic patients have treatment interruptions for more than 20% of the year in hypoglycemic agents, antihypertensive drugs, and statins.[29]

Patterns, Determinants, and Prediction of Adherence/Poor Adherence

Predicting poor adherence is difficult because there is no typical nonadherent patient. Predicting poor adherence usually results from various patients' characteristics and external influences.[30] The optimal method for identifying the determinants of poor adherence in a given individual remains to be further studied, but a patient-report questionnaire can be a useful starting point.[31]

Types of poor adherence

Unintentional poor adherence Unintentional poor adherence usually occurs when there are misconceptions about how or when to take the treatment. Patients may forget the physician's instructions[32] and the difference between on-demand rescue medication and regular daily preventative medication is often misunderstood. In qualitative research in Australia, 128 parents of children with asthma were interviewed about their knowledge about the disease, attitudes, beliefs, and knowledge of asthma medications, and only 42% of parents had a basic understanding of the mode of action of β-agonists, and 0% for inhaled corticosteroids.[33] Erratic poor adherence is common and usually results from forgetfulness or a busy lifestyle, despite patient understanding and agreement to take the medication as prescribed.[5]

In asthma, modifying the regimen according to the level of control of asthma, guided by a written asthma action plan, is an important aspect of disease management. Patients may not have received clear instructions or they may have forgotten instructions or perhaps lost or never received a written action plan. They may have difficulty remembering the asthma control criteria that trigger the need to change the dose regimen. If they received a plan, they may not use it or misunderstand it.

Intentional poor adherence Intentional poor adherence occurs when a patient makes a conscious decision to deviate from the prescription, for example by deliberately not filling the prescription, modifying the treatment regimen, or discontinuing treatment.[34] Patients may believe that the treatment is not necessary, use alternative or complementary therapies,[35] be concerned about side effects or unpleasant taste, so that real or perceived disadvantages outweigh the benefits of the medication. In some instances, this choice is appropriate and does not result in

a loss of asthma control, although the opposite often occurs. Patients have the right to decide about their therapy, but they should understand how to adequately monitor asthma control, how to appropriately adjust treatment, and be aware of the consequences of any treatment changes.[36]

Patient-related or external-related drivers of adherence

Poor adherence may be driven by factors related to the patient or external to the patient, as shown in **Box 1**.

Patient factors Patients decide whether to take a medication according to their beliefs and attitudes, perceived benefits versus risks or side effects (safety), past health experiences, practical issues, self-efficacy, and the influence of their peers.[5,37,38] Adherence is influenced by patient understanding, perceptions, culture, comorbidities, and treatment complexity. Patients may forget to take their medications, misunderstand how to use them, or have an inadequate perception of asthma control.[39] In a telephone survey in Canada of more than 600 adults with asthma,[40] more than 40% of patients did not know how ICS worked, 46% indicated that they were reluctant to take ICS regularly, and only 25% discussed their fears and concerns about ICS with their primary care provider. The main concerns reported by patients in this study were weight gain caused by taking ICS and loss of treatment effectiveness with long-term use.

Different patients use different coping strategies to deal with asthma diagnosis and management. In a qualitative study of adults with asthma,[41] 3 main coping mechanisms influenced adherence to preventive asthma therapy: the asthma deniers/distancers, the asthma accepters, and the pragmatics. The investigators suggested that an asthmatic patient's self-perception of the disease could influence adherence to preventive asthma therapy.

In asthma, psychological comorbidity may affect adherence and lead to poor asthma management,[38,42] and mood disorders such as depression and anxiety have been associated with poor adherence after hospitalization.[43,44] Although levels of psychological comorbidity are higher in asthma than in the general population, they do not necessarily differ between milder or more severe disease.[6]

Factors external to the patient External factors influencing poor adherence include access to health care services, socioeconomic factors (eg, cost of treatment), side effects of therapy, and relationships with health care providers.[45] Health

Box 1
Factors influencing adherence to therapy

Unintentional poor adherence

- Misunderstand treatment
- Forgetfulness, busy schedules, lifestyle
- Do not realize the need for adherence
- Forget physician's instructions
- Do not remember asthma control criteria indicating that the medication should be changed

Intentional poor adherence

- Patients believe that they do not need the treatment
- Decide to use another type of nonmedical therapy
- Fear of side effects or simply not liking the taste
- Patients believe that real or perceived disadvantages outweigh the benefits

Patient-related drivers of poor adherence

- Beliefs and attitudes, cultural background
- Perceived benefits versus risk or side effects (safety)
- Patients' lack of perception of their own vulnerability to illness
- Past health experiences
- Practical issues
- Self-efficacy
- Influence of their peers

Factors external to the patient

- Access to health care services and medication
- Socioeconomic factors, poverty, inner-city environment
- Therapy (eg, side effects, or those related to health care providers)
- Short consultations, no education provided

Treatment characteristics

- Too complex
- Not adapted
- Associated with significant side effects
- Cost of medication
- Polypharmacology
- Bad taste

care providers may not provide enough information or fail to discuss patients' misconceptions or concerns about therapy. In busy clinics in which time is limited, self-management support such as this could be delivered by an asthma nurse or asthma educator when available. Skilled allied health care professionals may be able to facilitate behavior change and provide shared decision making, which may be difficult to deliver in short consultations with the doctor.[46]

Participation in decision making around treatment is likely to enhance adherence. The treatment regimen may be too complex, or fit poorly into the patient's lifestyle.[42] Venables and colleagues[47] found that 61% of patients prefer a once-a-day treatment, 12% a twice-a-day treatment, and 27% expressed no preference. The high cost of medication and the use of multiple medications can be a barrier to adherence.

How to Assess Adherence (eg, in Research, at the Clinic)

Common adherence assessment methods include patient self-report, canister weighing, prescription refills, and electronic monitoring.[48–50] Self-report and prescription refill are around only 60% and 70% accurate, respectively,[48] and canister weighing is not feasible for all types of inhaler devices. Electronic monitoring is usually considered the gold standard because the time and date of every inhaler actuation are recorded, allowing detailed assessment of adherence patterns, but it is relatively expensive. New-generation electronic monitoring devices also provide reminders for missed doses, remote data uploads, and feedback on controller use (**Fig. 1**), which can be accessed by both patients and doctors.[51]

Some key points to consider when choosing a method of adherence assessment for a particular context are listed in the decision chart (**Table 1**). These points include data fidelity requirements (ie, accuracy of adherence data), cost weighting (eg, does adherence monitoring outweigh treatment costs?) and capacity (eg, justification for staff time for adherence monitoring). For example, in the hospital clinic, the aim may be to rule out poor adherence to inhaled corticosteroids in severe asthma before starting an expensive add-on treatment such as omalizumab. The potential cost savings inherent in distinguishing poor adherence from poor treatment response to inhaled corticosteroids, as well as the avoidance of side effects of unnecessary therapy, justify the purchase of adherence monitoring devices, staff time, and training.

However, in the primary care clinic, self-report may be the only method available because of

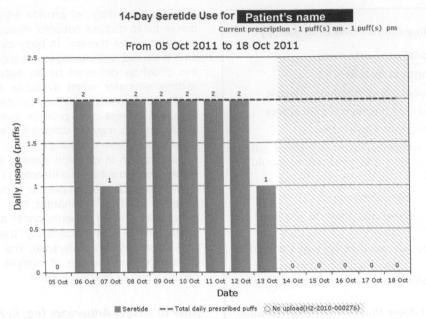

Fig. 1. An example of controller use feedback from SmartTrack live. (*Reproduced* with the permission of Nexus6 Ltd, Auckland, New Zealand.)

scare resources. Although self-report is less accurate than more objective methods, it can provide a reasonable picture of patients' adherence. Different methods of self-report can provide strikingly different results. For example, when Foster and colleagues[31] compared electronically recorded adherence with a series of 3 short questions about controller inhaler use in the last 4 weeks versus the Morisky adherence self-report score (**Fig. 2**), they found that the 3 short questions correlated more strongly with electronically recorded adherence ($r = 0.62$; $P<.0001$) than the Morisky score ($r = -0.45$; $P<.0001$). For patients self-reporting less than 100% adherence in response to the 3 short questions, the correlation with objective adherence was even stronger ($r = 0.82$, $P<.0001$), suggesting that self-reports of suboptimal adherence are more accurate than self-reports of optimal adherence.

How to Improve Adherence to Asthma Treatment

A review of randomized controlled trials of interventions to promote adherence to pharmacologic treatment in chronic diseases[52] reported that more than half of the interventions resulted in significant but mostly modest improvements in adherence. Successful interventions were complex, multifaceted and included more than 1 intervention, such as counseling, education, more convenient care, self-monitoring, reinforcement, reminders, and other forms of additional follow-

up (**Box 2**). However, as described in the next section, relatively simple strategies can also be effective.

STRATEGIES TO IMPROVE ADHERENCE
Education

Providing the patient and family with a rationale for treatment recommendations, benefits versus potential side effects, and side effect management tools can promote adherence. Asthma education can include[53–57] the delivery of written materials by a health care professional, teaching self-management skills, telephone follow-up, individual versus educational group sessions, involvement of support groups, medication adherence monitoring and feedback, counseling, and inhaler technique training.

Patient education, particularly when it addresses adherence to treatment and understanding of the role of medications, can improve asthma control[58–60] and may improve adherence,[30,54,61,62] although few studies have used objective adherence measurement. A recent 24-week, randomized controlled trial investigated the effect of self-management education, which included self-management intervention sessions, education on asthma facts, and medication actions, as well as individualized components such as verbal and graphic interpretation of spirometric results, peak flow trends, metered dose inhaler technique errors, and results of allergen skin testing, along with specific strategies for control of personally relevant

Table 1
Adherence assessment method decision chart

Setting	Context	Fidelity Requirements of Adherence Data	Cost Weighting	Justification/ Capacity (Expertise and Time)	Adherence Measurement Method Recommended
Clinic	Secondary care	High fidelity: adherence data direct critical clinical decisions (eg, patients' eligibility for add-on therapy)	Cost/risk of treatment outweighs cost of objective adherence measurement	Cost savings gleaned from objective adherence measurement and avoidance of side effects of unnecessary add-on therapy could justify the purchase of adherence monitoring devices, staff training and time	Electronic monitoring
	Primary care	Medium to high fidelity: adherence data contribute to clinical decisions (eg, stepping up treatment or referral)	Cost of objective adherence measurement outweighs cost/risk of treatment	Difficult to justify the purchase of adherence monitoring devices, staff training and time	Self-report Prescription refill data are rarely available but, if time allows, use date of last script to estimate the average number of puffs taken per day[a]
Research	Adherence is a key measure	High fidelity: adherence data determine research outcomes	Study aims outweigh cost of objective adherence measurement	Research question justifies cost of objective adherence measurement	Electronic monitoring
	Adherence is a minor measure	Medium to high fidelity: adherence data contribute to research findings	Cost of objective adherence measurement outweighs study aims	Research question does not justify cost of objective adherence measurement	Prescription refill data if the budget allows, otherwise use self-report

[a] This method is less reliable if the patient has more than 1 GP or shares the inhaler with family members.

environmental exposures on long-term adherence to ICS and markers of asthma control. Compared with control individuals, participants randomized to the intervention showed a 9-fold greater odds of more than 60% adherence to the prescribed dose at the end of the intervention and maintained a 3-fold greater odds of more than 60% adherence at 24 weeks; perceived control of asthma improved, night-time awakenings decreased, and inhaled β-agonist use decreased in intervention participants compared with control individuals.[30]

However, the resources and expertise needed to offer these kinds of interventions are often not available in real-world practice.[63]

Behavioral strategies such as reminders, contracting, and reinforcement can be used to promote adherence behaviors.[64] Behavioral interventions that consider patient's preferences seem most effective. For example, 612 adults with poorly controlled asthma randomized to shared decision making (ie, clinicians and patients negotiated a treatment regimen that accommodated patient

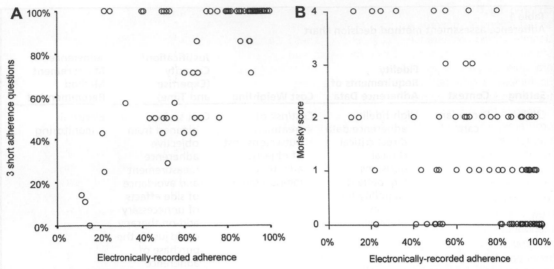

Fig. 2. Relative strength of association between electronically recorded adherence and 3 short adherence questions (*A*: r = 0.62; *P*<.0001) versus Morisky score questionnaire (*B*: r = –0.45; *P*<.0001). The 3 short questions were: "Lots of people don't take their inhaler exactly as prescribed. In the last 4 weeks: 1. How many days per week have you been taking your [name of controller] inhaler? 2. How many times per day? 3. How many puffs do you take each time?" (*From* Foster JM, Smith L, Bosnic-Anticevich SZ, et al. Identifying patient-specific beliefs and behaviors for conversations about adherence in asthma. Intern Med J 2012;42(6):e139; with permission.)

goals and preferences) had significantly better controller adherence, higher cumulative controller medication dose, and significantly improved clinical outcomes such as asthma-related QoL, health care use, rescue medication use, and lung function at 1 year, compared with patients randomized to usual care (which including traditional asthma education).[62]

Adherence with environmental interventions remains a difficult issue. Although commonly considered to play a role in the difficult-to-control

asthma, environmental control is complex and adherence to current recommendations on allergen and tobacco avoidance, for example, seem far from optimal.[65,66] After a 1-year educational intervention, adherence to house-dust mite reduction measures was 70%, and removal of a domestic animal was implemented by less than 20% at 1 year.[67] A 6-month individualized educational intervention program based on the Prochaska transtheoretic model, in a population of adult patients with asthma living with domestic animals to which they were sensitized, resulted in improved knowledge of the effects of asthma and the influence of allergens in the intervention group.[68] However, only 29% of the intervention group and 21% of the control group removed their pets within 6 months. Successful environmental interventions require more careful development and may need to be implemented over a longer period.

Van der Meer and colleagues[69] looked at adherence to daily electronic peak expiratory flow (PEF) monitoring using the Internet or SMS (Short Message Service), over a 4-week period, in a group of 97 asthmatic adolescents aged 12 to 17 years. Adherence (83%) and reliability of home PEF measurements was high during the study period, although feedback on monitoring was not provided. Long-term results remain uncertain and the investigators speculate that the lack of feedback could reduce compliance over time. Daily home spirometry with teletransmission to an expert medical center over 12 months in

---

Box 2
Interventions to improve adherence

- Education: clear instructions about treatment and disease management
- Multidisciplinary care with common message
- Monitoring adherence
- Closer follow-up
- Simplification of regimens
- Adaptation of treatment to patient's characteristics
- Shared decision process
- Self-management programs with educational and behavioral components
- Memory aids and reminders
- Incentives: reinforcements
- Multifaceted interventions

children aged 6 to 16 years did not result in a reduction of severe asthma exacerbations, despite good adherence (70%–90%). These studies show that teenagers are interested and are able to adhere to daily monitoring but its usefulness is doubtful unless monitoring reliably translates into improvements in asthma control.[70]

Despite the successes of individual educational programs for asthma sufferers, adherence to therapy remains suboptimal, similar to adherence in other chronic conditions.[71–73] Some explanations for this situation include insufficient tailoring of interventions to patients' needs and expectations, insufficient communication around patients' views of benefits, detrimental effects of recommendations (adopting a shared decision approach to consultations can improve this), and in some instances failure to incorporate patient choice in treatment decisions. Furthermore, repetition and reinforcement of interventions are important, so controlled studies looking at the provision of adherence feedback during consultations may show only modest and short-lived improvements in clinical outcomes and adherence. Dunbar and colleagues[64] suggested that the most powerful reinforcer of patient behavior is the clinician's time and attention to the patient. The length of time a patient spends with the clinician is positively correlated with adherence rates.[74,75] Assessing patients' knowledge, understanding, and beliefs toward the recommendation and initiating a clear, empathic, and motivating communication with patients, addressing the possible causes of poor adherence, may help.[76]

Simplification of the Treatment Regimen

Simplifying the regimen (eg, reducing the number of inhalers and doses per day) and using a low-cost treatment with no or minimal side effects may be useful.[77] Promoting regular habits (eg, taking the medication before cleaning teeth or at the same time every day) can also be beneficial.

Improved Communication Between Patient and Caregivers

Effective communication between patients and health care providers is imperative for promoting adherence.[74,78,79] Poor adherence can result from misunderstandings about treatment recommendations, so clear, consistent, and frequently reinforced information from physicians and allied health care professionals is needed. The cultural beliefs and background of the patient should also be taken into account when addressing adherence to self-management recommendations, including medications.

Medication Reminders

In a 24-week randomized controlled study of adult/adolescent patients with asthma, twice-daily reminders for missed doses improved controller adherence by 18% in favor of reminders, although there were no significant differences in clinical outcomes.[80] In adults with asthma, automated interactive voice response telephone calls that enquired about symptoms, delivered education, and encouraged prescriptions refills resulted in a 32% improvement in controller adherence compared with the control group, but no differences in clinical outcomes were found.[81]

Reminders maintain adherence in asthmatic children,[82] as does feedback to patients on their adherence to medication. When patients are aware that their adherence is being monitored, it improves in the short-term (eg, 4 months) but studies of long-term monitoring and feedback are needed[83,84]

Supervised Medication Taking

In pediatric asthma, good results were reported after a once-daily at-school controller supervision program, with a small improvement in asthma control and adherence close to 100% in the supervised group compared with 38% in the usual care group.[85] However, the provision of asthma education and free controller in both groups likely reduced the differences observed.

Pharmacy-Based Programs

A 6-month pharmacy-based asthma program resulted in improved adherence (prescription refill/self-report) and clinical outcomes compared with patients in control pharmacies.[86,87] A 16-week study of metered dose inhaler technique instruction led to improvement in inhaler technique, with enhanced improvement seen in the group receiving a physical demonstration in addition to oral/written instructions.[4]

PERSPECTIVES AND FUTURE RESEARCH

The design and methodology of future studies can be improved, and the measurement of clinical outcomes and objective adherence rates should be included in all new research. The dichotomy of good adherence/poor adherence using arbitrary cut points may be insensitive to variations over time and proportionally large changes may be misinterpreted; for example, an intervention may be considered effective if a patient doubles adherence from 10% to 20%. Although short-term improvements are beneficial, interventions should be designed to improve long-term asthma control and reduce the risk of future events such as asthma exacerbations. Adherence can fluctuate over time, so repeated prospective assessments, such as those provided by electronic monitoring, will provide a better picture of temporal treatment use.

Simple, tailored interventions promoting patient involvement in their own care can be beneficial. A wide range of different barriers and facilitators to adherence may occur in the same patient, which may further differ depending on the type of poor adherence. For example forgetfulness might be improved with reminders and intentional underuse by discussion/education around the patient's concerns or beliefs. Interventions require step-by-step management and support of patients and caregivers, but barriers may also need to be addressed at the health care systems level, at which resources are often scarce.

In clinical practice, a partnership should be established with the patient, based on empathy and trust. Clinicians should enquire as regularly as possible about the patient's agreement with and adherence to current recommendations. Individual barriers and facilitators to adherence should be discussed, and incentives to adherence should be part of current interventions, such as developing a contract with the physician or educator to try to achieve a specific goal, involving another member of the family or other reinforcement methods. Improved communication between the patient/caregiver and health care professionals and provision of consistent health information could promote adherence. Methods such as coaching, reinforcement, and regular follow-up can encourage adherence and could be provided by allied health care professionals, including nurses, pharmacists, lay educators, and even peers. Interventions should take into account the cultural background, preferences, and beliefs of the patient, and acknowledge the patient's perspective on pros and cons of treatment, as in the shared decision model. If a partnership has been developed between patient and doctor, motivated, well-informed patients can take responsibility for their day-to-day self-management, discuss their goals and expectations, and access resources and support. How patients with asthma deal with their health problems, set priorities, and perceive treatment requires more research so that patients' involvement in their own health care can be optimized.

Support groups composed of well-informed individuals or guided by health professionals can also play a role in reinforcing appropriate self-management and resolving fears and misconceptions about the treatment.[88] Electronic communication such as online social networks, in addition to electronic monitoring and reminders, may offer an opportunity to promote adherence and require more research.[89,90]

Poor treatment adherence is a particularly important problem in severe asthma and it should be addressed seriously.[91] In a recent study in vulnerable, low-income adults with moderate to severe asthma, a problem-solving intervention was not better than standard asthma education in improving adherence; however, medication was provided for free and patients were aware of monitoring, so adherence was unusually high throughout the study (52%–61%) and led to an improvement in expiratory flows, QoL, and self-reported asthma control in both groups.[61] So, simple strategies such as provision of medication and adherence monitoring could be cost-effective in populations with the most troublesome disease and high health care use, although long-term effectiveness needs to be determined. The role of adherence in the severity or progression of asthma should also be further assessed.

SUMMARY

Poor adherence is a major problem and often results in inadequate use of treatments, insufficient control of the disease, and increased health care use and costs. It has many determinants, including suboptimal knowledge of the disease and its treatment, lack of self-management skills, and insufficient or ineffective interventions or communication. Despite extensive research on poor adherence, and many novel interventional approaches, a practical and definitive solution remains elusive and demands further research. In the meantime, adherence should be regularly monitored in clinical settings, ideally using objective measures, and interventions delivered that incorporate patient's preferences and perceptions and include elements of shared decision and common goals, because these are likely to be most effective. It might be pertinent to ask if good adherence in asthma is an achievable goal. We believe that it is, but with the proviso that behavior change usually takes time and requires multiple interventions, particularly tailored education in patients willing to receive it. Even modest improvements in adherence can lead to significant clinical improvements. Good communication between patients and health care providers is key to understanding and addressing patients' personal barriers to adherence.

REFERENCES

1. Bateman ED, Hurd SS, Barnes PJ, et al. Global strategy for asthma management and prevention: GINA executive summary. Eur Respir J 2008;31(1): 143–78.

2. Reddel HK, Taylor DR, Bateman ED, et al. An official American Thoracic Society/European Respiratory Society statement: asthma control and exacerbations: standardizing endpoints for clinical asthma trials and clinical practice. Am J Respir Crit Care Med 2009;180(1):59–99.

3. Chanez P, Wenzel SE, Anderson GP, et al. Severe asthma in adults: what are the important questions? J Allergy Clin Immunol 2007;119(6):1337–48.

4. Bosnic-Anticevich SZ, Sinha H, So S, et al. Metered-dose inhaler technique: the effect of two educational interventions delivered in community pharmacy over time. J Asthma 2010;47(3):251–6.

5. Bender B, Boulet LP, Chaustre I, et al. Asthma. In: Sabaté E, editor. Adherence to long-term therapies: evidence for action. Geneva (Switzerland): World Health Organization; 2003. p. 47–58.

6. Foster JM, Lavoie KL, Boulet LP. Treatment adherence and psychosocial factors. In: Chung KF, Bel EH, Wenzel SE, editors. Difficult-to-treat severe asthma. Sheffield (UK): The European Respiratory Society; 2011. p. 28–49.

7. Bender B, Milgrom H, Rand C. Nonadherence in asthmatic patients: is there a solution to the problem? Ann Allergy Asthma Immunol 1997;79(3):177–85.

8. Milgrom H, Bender B, Ackerson L, et al. Noncompliance and treatment failure in children with asthma. J Allergy Clin Immunol 1996;98(6 Pt 1):1051–7.

9. Horn CR, Clark TJ, Cochrane GM. Compliance with inhaled therapy and morbidity from asthma. Respir Med 1990;84(1):67–70.

10. Sockrider MM, Wolle JM. Helping patients better adhere to treatment regimen. J Respir Dis 1996;17:204–16.

11. Spector SL, Kinsman R, Mawhinney H, et al. Compliance of patients with asthma with an experimental aerosolized medication: implications for controlled clinical trials. J Allergy Clin Immunol 1986;77(1 Pt 1):65–70.

12. Cochrane MG, Bala MV, Downs KE, et al. Inhaled corticosteroids for asthma therapy: patient compliance, devices, and inhalation technique. Chest 2000;117(2):542–50.

13. Williams LK, Pladevall M, Xi H, et al. Relationship between adherence to inhaled corticosteroids and poor outcomes among adults with asthma. J Allergy Clin Immunol 2004;114(6):1288–93.

14. Williams LK, Joseph CL, Peterson EL, et al. Patients with asthma who do not fill their inhaled corticosteroids: a study of primary nonadherence. J Allergy Clin Immunol 2007;120(5):1153–9.

15. Watts RW, McLennan G, Bassham I, et al. Do patients with asthma fill their prescriptions? A primary compliance study. Aust Fam Physician 1997;26(Suppl 1):S4–6.

16. Bronstein JM, Santer L, Johnson V. The use of Medicaid claims as a supplementary source of information on quality of asthma care. J Healthc Qual 2000;22(6):13–8.

17. Kandane-Rathnayake RK, Matheson MC, Simpson JA, et al. Adherence to asthma management guidelines by middle-aged adults with current asthma. Thorax 2009;64(12):1025–31.

18. Bender BG, Pedan A, Varasteh LT. Adherence and persistence with fluticasone propionate/salmeterol combination therapy. J Allergy Clin Immunol 2006;118(4):899–904.

19. Creer TL. Medication compliance and childhood asthma. In: Krasneger NA, Epstein L, Johnson SB, et al, editors. Developmental aspects of health compliance behavior. Hillsdale (IN); New Jersey, Hove (Belgium), London: Lawrence Erlbaum Associates; 1993. p. 303–33.

20. Diette GB, Skinner EA, Markson LE, et al. Consistency of care with national guidelines for children with asthma in managed care. J Pediatr 2001;138(1):59–64.

21. Lozano P, Finkelstein JA, Hecht J, et al. Asthma medication use and disease burden in children in a primary care population. Arch Pediatr Adolesc Med 2003;157(1):81–8.

22. Walders N, Kopel SJ, Koinis-Mitchell D, et al. Patterns of quick-relief and long-term controller medication use in pediatric asthma. J Pediatr 2005;146(2):177–82.

23. Ranganathan SC, Payne DN, Jaffe A, et al. Difficult asthma: defining the problems. Pediatr Pulmonol 2001;31(2):114–20.

24. Spurrier NJ, Sawyer MG, Staugas R, et al. Association between parental perception of children's vulnerability to illness and management of children's asthma. Pediatr Pulmonol 2000;29(2):88–93.

25. Cooper WO, Hickson GB. Corticosteroid prescription filling for children covered by Medicaid following an emergency department visit or a hospitalization for asthma. Arch Pediatr Adolesc Med 2001;155(10):1111–5.

26. Gamble J, Stevenson M, McClean E, et al. The prevalence of nonadherence in difficult asthma. Am J Respir Crit Care Med 2009;180(9):817–22.

27. Krishnan JA, Riekert KA, McCoy JV, et al. Corticosteroid use after hospital discharge among high-risk adults with asthma. Am J Respir Crit Care Med 2004;170(12):1281–5.

28. Stempel DA, Roberts CS, Stanford RH. Treatment patterns in the months prior to and after asthma-related emergency department visit. Chest 2004;126(1):75–80.

29. Briesacher BA, Andrade SE, Fouayzi H, et al. Comparison of drug adherence rates among patients with seven different medical conditions. Pharmacotherapy 2008;28(4):437–43.

30. Janson SL, McGrath KW, Covington JK, et al. Individualized asthma self-management improves medication adherence and markers of asthma control. J Allergy Clin Immunol 2009;123(4):840–6.

31. Foster JM, Smith L, Bosnic-Anticevich SZ, et al. Identifying patient-specific beliefs and behaviours for conversations about adherence in asthma. Intern Med J 2012;42(6):e136–44.

32. DiMatteo MR. Enhancing patient adherence to medical recommendations. JAMA 1994;271(1):79–83.

33. Donnelly JE, Donnelly WJ, Thong YH. Inadequate parental understanding of asthma medications. Ann Allergy 1989;62(4):337–41.

34. Dekker FW, Dieleman FE, Kaptein AA, et al. Compliance with pulmonary medication in general practice. Eur Respir J 1993;6(6):886–90.

35. Slader CA, Reddel HK, Jenkins CR, et al. Complementary and alternative medicine use in asthma: who is using what? Respirology 2006;11(4):373–87.

36. Légaré F, Ratté S, Stacey D, et al. Interventions for improving the adoption of shared decision making by healthcare professionals. Cochrane Database Syst Rev 2010;5:CD006732.

37. Ponieman D, Wisnivesky JP, Leventhal H, et al. Impact of positive and negative beliefs about inhaled corticosteroids on adherence in inner-city asthmatic patients. Ann Allergy Asthma Immunol 2009;103(1):38–42.

38. Wamboldt M, Wamboldt F. Psychosocial aspects of severe asthma in children. In: Szefler S, Leung D, editors. Severe asthma: pathogenesis and clinical management. New York: Marcel Dekker; 1996. p. 465–96.

39. Boulet LP, Phillips R, O'Byrne P, et al. Evaluation of asthma control by physicians and patients: comparison with current guidelines. Can Respir J 2002;9(6): 417–23.

40. Boulet LP. Perception of the role and potential side effects of inhaled corticosteroids among asthmatic patients. Chest 1998;113(3):587–92.

41. Adams S, Pill R, Jones A. Medication, chronic illness and identity: the perspective of people with asthma. Soc Sci Med 1997;45(2):189–201.

42. Sackett DL. Compliance with therapeutic regimes. Baltimore (MD): Johns Hopkins University Press; 1976.

43. DiMarco F, Santus P, Centanni S. Anxiety and depression in asthma. Curr Opin Pulm Med 2011; 17(1):39–44.

44. DiMarco F, Verga M, Santus P, et al. Close correlation between anxiety, depression, and asthma control. Respir Med 2010;104(1):22–8.

45. Haynes RB, Taylor DW, Sackett DL. Compliance in health care. Baltimore (MD): Johns Hopkins University Press; 1979.

46. Dilorio C, McCarty F, Resnicow K, et al. Using motivational interviewing to promote adherence to antiretroviral medications: a randomized controlled study. AIDS Care 2008;20:273–83.

47. Venables T, Addlestone M, Smithers A, et al. A comparison of the efficacy and patient

acceptability of once daily budesonide via Turbohaler and once daily fluticasone propionate via disc-inhaler at an equal daily dose of 400µg in adult asthmatics. Br J Clin Res 1996;7:15–32.

48. Hansen RA, Kim MM, Song L, et al. Comparison of methods to assess medication adherence and classify nonadherence. Ann Pharmacother 2009;43(3):413–22.

49. Jentzsch NS, Camargos PA, Colosimo EA, et al. Monitoring adherence to beclomethasone in asthmatic children and adolescents through four different methods. Allergy 2009;64(10):1458–62.

50. Lacasse Y, Archibald H, Ernst P, et al. Patterns and determinants of compliance with inhaled steroids in adults with asthma. Can Respir J 2005;12(4):211–7.

51. Foster JM, Smith LS, Usherwood T, et al. Assessing the reliability and validity of the SmartTrack: an electronic adherence monitor for pressurized metered dose inhalers (PMDI) [abstract]. Am J Respir Crit Care Med 2011;183:A1442.

52. Haynes RB, Sackett DL, Gibson ES, et al. Improvement of medication compliance in uncontrolled hypertension. Lancet 1976;1(7972):1265–8.

53. Bailey WC, Richards JM Jr, Brooks CM, et al. A randomized trial to improve self-management practices of adults with asthma. Arch Intern Med 1990;150(8):1664–8.

54. Windsor RA, Bailey WC, Richards JM Jr, et al. Evaluation of the efficacy and cost effectiveness of health education methods to increase medication adherence among adults with asthma. Am J Public Health 1990;80(12):1519–21.

55. Gibson PG, Powell H, Wilson A, et al. Self-management education and regular practitioner review for adults with asthma. Cochrane Database Syst Rev 2009;3:CD001117.

56. Taitel MS, Kotses H, Bernstein IL, et al. A self-management program for adult asthma. Part II: cost-benefit analysis. J Allergy Clin Immunol 1995;95(3):672–6.

57. Boulet LP, Chapman KR, Green LW, et al. Asthma education. Chest 1994;106(Suppl 4):184S–96S.

58. Magar Y, Vervloet D, Steenhouwer F, et al. Assessment of a therapeutic education programme for asthma patients: "un souffle nouveau". Patient Educ Couns 2005;58(1):41–6.

59. Dalcin PT, Grutcki DM, Laporte PP, et al. Impact of a short-term educational intervention on adherence to asthma treatment and on asthma control. J Bras Pneumol 2011;37(1):19–27.

60. Boulet L, Gibson P. Role of asthma education. In: FitzGerald JM, Ernst P, Boulet LP, et al, editors. Evidence-based asthma management. Hamilton (Ontario): BC Dekker; 2001. p. 275–90.

61. Apter AJ, Wang X, Bogen DK, et al. Problem solving to improve adherence and asthma outcomes in urban adults with moderate or severe asthma: a randomized controlled trial. J Allergy Clin Immunol 2011;128(3):516–23.

62. Wilson SR, Strub P, Buist AS, et al. Shared treatment decision making improves adherence and outcomes in poorly controlled asthma. Am J Respir Crit Care Med 2010;181(6):566–77.

63. Robichaud P, Laberge A, Allen MF, et al. Evaluation of a program aimed at increasing referrals for asthma education of patients consulting at the emergency department for acute asthma. Chest 2004;126(5): 1495–501.

64. Dunbar J, Marshall G, Hovell M. Behavioral strategies for improving compliance. In: Haynes RB, editor. Compliance in health care. Baltimore (MD): John Hopkins University Press; 1979. p. 174–90.

65. De Boeck K, Moens M, Van Der Aa N, et al. 'Difficult asthma': can symptoms be controlled in a structured environment? Pediatr Pulmonol 2009;44(8):743–8.

66. FitzGerald JM, Shahidi N. Achieving asthma control in patients with moderate disease. J Allergy Clin Immunol 2010;125(2):307–11.

67. Cote J, Cartier A, Robichaud P, et al. Influence of asthma education on asthma severity, quality of life and environmental control. Can Respir J 2000;7(5): 395–400.

68. Hagan L, Valois P, Patenaude H, et al. Asthma counselling targeted to removal of domestic animals. Can Respir J 2008;15(1):33–8.

69. van der Meer V, Rikkers-Mutsaerts ER, Sterk PJ, et al. Compliance and reliability of electronic PEF monitoring in adolescents with asthma. Thorax 2006;61(5):457–8.

70. Deschildre A, Béghin L, Salleron J, et al. Home tele-monitoring (FEV1) in children with severe asthma does not reduce exacerbations. Eur Respir J 2012; 39(2):290–6.

71. Haynes RB, McKibbon KA, Kanani R. Systematic review of randomised trials of interventions to assist patients to follow prescriptions for medications. Lancet 1996;348(9024):383–6.

72. Haynes RB, McDonald H, Garg AX, et al. Interventions for helping patients to follow prescriptions for medications. Cochrane Database Syst Rev 2002;2:CD000011.

73. McDonald HP, Garg AX, Haynes RB. Interventions to enhance patient adherence to medication prescriptions: scientific review. JAMA 2002;288(22):2868–79.

74. Korsch BM, Negrete VF. Doctor-patient communication. Sci Am 1972;227(2):66–74.

75. Dunbar-Jacob J. Predictors of patient adherence: patient characteristics. In: Shumaker SL, editor. Handbook of health behavior change. New York: Springer; 1998.

76. Kreps GL, Villagran MM, Zhao X, et al. Development and validation of motivational messages to improve prescription medication adherence for patients with chronic health problems. Patient Educ Couns 2011;83(3):375–81.

77. Feldman R, Bacher M, Campbell N, et al. Adherence to pharmacologic management of hypertension. Can J Public Health 1998;89(5):I16–8.

78. Partridge MR. The asthma consultation: what is important? Curr Med Res Opin 2005;21(Suppl 4): S11–7.

79. Hukla B. Patient-clinician interaction and compliance. Baltimore (MD): John Hopkins University Press; 1979.

80. Charles T, Quinn D, Weatherall M, et al. An audiovisual reminder function improves adherence with inhaled corticosteroid therapy in asthma. J Allergy Clin Immunol 2007;119(4):811–6.

81. Bender BG, Apter A, Bogen DK, et al. Test of an interactive voice response intervention to improve adherence to controller medications in adults with asthma. J Am Board Fam Med 2010;23(2):159–65.

82. Weinstein AG. Clinical management strategies to maintain drug compliance in asthmatic children. Ann Allergy Asthma Immunol 1995;74(4):304–10.

83. Burgess SW, Sly PD, Devadason SG. Providing feedback on adherence increases use of preventive medication by asthmatic children. J Asthma 2010; 47(2):198–201.

84. Nides MA, Tashkin DP, Simmons MS, et al. Improving inhaler adherence in a clinical trial through the use of the nebulizer chronolog. Chest 1993;104(2):501–7.

85. Gerald LB, McClure LA, Mangan JM, et al. Increasing adherence to inhaled steroid therapy among schoolchildren: randomized, controlled trial of school-based supervised asthma therapy. Pediatrics 2009;123(2):466–74.

86. Apter AJ, Boston RC, George M, et al. Modifiable barriers to adherence to inhaled steroids among adults with asthma: it's not just black and white. J Allergy Clin Immunol 2003;111(6):1219–26.

87. Gamble J, Fitzsimons D, Lynes D, et al. Difficult asthma: people's perspectives on taking corticosteroid therapy. J Clin Nurs 2007;16(3A):59–67.

88. Janis IL, Rodin J. Attribution, control, and decision making: social psychology and health care. In: Stone GC, Cohen F, Adler NE, editors. Health psychology: a handbook. San Francisco (CA): Jossey-Bass; 1979. p. 487–521.

89. van Onzenoort HA, Verberk WJ, Kroon AA, et al. Electronic monitoring of adherence, treatment of hypertension, and blood pressure control. Am J Hypertens 2012;25(1):54–9.

90. Spaulding SA, Devine KA, Duncan CL, et al. Electronic monitoring and feedback to improve adherence in pediatric asthma. J Pediatr Psychol 2012; 37(1):64–74.

91. Heaney LG, Horne R. Non-adherence in difficult asthma: time to take it seriously. Thorax 2012; 67(3):268–70.

Is the Asthma Epidemic Still Ascending?

Nour Baïz, MSc[a,b],
Isabella Annesi-Maesano, MD, PhD, DSc[a,b,*]

KEYWORDS

• Asthma • Prevalence • Evolution • Air pollution • Passive smoking • Hygiene hypothesis • Lifestyle

KEY POINTS

- Asthma is one of the most prevalent chronic conditions affecting, approximately 300 million people worldwide, up to 1 in 10 adults and 1 in 3 children in some countries.
- Asthma is a complex disease that it still not fully understood. The type of asthma definition adopted has influenced knowledge about asthma distribution and etiology.
- In the case of asthma prevalence, accurate estimation has been hindered by varying definitions of asthma and methods of data collection, each combining to make data comparison across studies difficult, with the exception of International Study of Asthma and Allergy in Childhood and European Community Respiratory Health Survey, which unfortunately have not used biologic and clinical markers of the disease.
- Although treatment for asthma has improved substantially, the prevalence of asthma continues to increase, particularly in low and middle income countries, or in some ethnic groups in which prevalence was previously low.
- Observed spatio-temporal variations in the increased prevalence of asthma depend on exposure to environmental factors such as allergens (because of new conditions of exposure).

INTRODUCTION

Asthma is a phenotypically heterogeneous disorder of multifactorial origins resulting from complex interactions between genetic and environmental determinants. So far, several genes and environmental factors have been associated with an increased risk of developing asthma and may play a major role in asthma susceptibility. Evidence is strong for an increased risk of asthma associated with allergenic exposure, respiratory infections, air pollutants, tobacco smoke, and allergic rhinitis (AR).

Asthma is considered as a major public health problem in most countries, regardless of their level of development. According to the World Health Organization (WHO), globally there are at least 300 million people suffering from asthma and more than 250,000 asthma-related deaths each year.[1] In the United States, the annual cost of asthma is estimated to be nearly $18 billion. Direct costs account for nearly $10 billion (hospitalizations are the single largest portion of direct cost), and indirect costs account for $8 billion (lost earnings due to illness or death). This is the consequence of marked changes in asthma distribution and burden observed in the past decades. Asthma prevalence has been increasing since the early 1980s across all age, sex, and racial groups. Moreover, the asthma mortality rate has risen in some ethnic groups (African Americans in the United States) and individuals age 85 years and

[a] Institut National de la Santé et de la Recherche Médicale (INSERM) UMR S 707, Department of Epidemiology of Allergic and Respiratory Diseases, Paris F-75012, France; [b] Université Pierre et Marie Curie (UPMC), UPMC Univ Paris 6, UMR S 707, EPAR, Paris F-75012, France
* Corresponding author. Department of Epidemiology of Allergic and Respiratory Diseases, UMR-S 707 \INSERM & UPMC Paris 6, Medical School Saint Antoine, 27 rue Chaligny, 75571 Paris CEDEX 12, France.
E-mail address: isabella.annesi-maesano@inserm.fr

Clin Chest Med 33 (2012) 419–429
http://dx.doi.org/10.1016/j.ccm.2012.06.001
0272-5231/12/$ – see front matter © 2012 Elsevier Inc. All rights reserved.

older. This increase is of particular concern, because it comes at a time when mortality rates from most natural causes are on the decline in several countries and because asthma death is in principle avoidable. Rising numbers and rates of asthma-related hospitalizations, especially in children and in some ethnic groups (African Americans in the United States) are also alarming.

Despite the growing understanding of asthma pathophysiology, much remains to be learned about the exact causes responsible for asthma development and the ways to prevent this condition. This article reviews data on asthma prevalence trends and associated risk factors in the past decades, with emphasis on childhood asthma for which data are more abundant and for which misclassification is reduced. Important unanswered research questions are raised to explain the observed trends, and suggestions for future research are provided.

IN SEARCH OF AN ASTHMA DEFINITION

Asthma is characterized by varying degrees of allergic responses, airflow obstruction, and airway inflammation causing a range of symptoms including cough, wheezing, chest tightness, and shortness of breath. In spite of this diversity, the definitions that have been applied at the population level to count the number of asthmatics and follow its progression have been based uniquely on asthma-like symptoms and diagnosis. To date, most population-based studies have used self-administered questionnaires on symptoms to distinguish between asthmatic and nonasthmatic subjects. Indeed, this method represents clear advantages in terms of cost, convenience, and the resulting optimization of sample sizes and response rates. Most studies of asthma in children are based on the definitions of asthma (a doctor's diagnosis of asthma ever) and asthma-like symptoms based on the International Study of Asthma and Allergy in Childhood (ISAAC) validated questionnaire.[2] The epidemiologic study of asthma in adults presents additional difficulties, which include the duration of the disease, the type/duration of treatment, occupational exposure, environmental exposure, smoking, and comorbidities. Worldwide epidemiologic surveys on adult asthma have been mainly performed using the European Community Respiratory Health Survey (ECRHS) questionnaire, conceived to standardize the epidemiologic investigation of asthma and allergies in adults. Although standardized questionnaires allow prevalence comparisons and assessment of trends across studies worldwide, these symptom questionnaires have potential issues arising from subjective symptom recognition and because they are dependent on the interpretation and judgment of the person responding to the questionnaire.[3] Recently this problem has been overcome by the introduction of asthma phenotypes or endotypes based on several entities of the diseases.[4]

SPATIAL AND TEMPORAL DISTRIBUTION OF ASTHMA PREVALENCE AND RISK FACTORS
Spatial Distribution

Thanks to the multicentric epidemiologic studies based on the use of standardized and validated questionnaires and tools, an increasing amount of comparable data on asthma is available worldwide. The most up-to-date prevalence rates of childhood asthma worldwide can be obtained from the ISAAC study,[5] conducted in representative samples of adolescents aged 13 to 14 years old in 56 countries, and the ECRHS study,[6] conducted in representative samples of adults aged 20 to 44 years in 25 countries (mostly in Europe). Results show a great disparity in the prevalence of asthma across the world, between countries and within countries, with a trend toward more developed and westernized countries having higher rates of asthma,[5] with as high as a 20- to 60-fold difference. Asthma symptoms were most prevalent (as much as 20%) in the United Kingdom, Australia, New Zealand, and Republic of Ireland; they were lowest (as low as 2%–3%) in Eastern Europe, Indonesia, Taiwan, Greece, Uzbekistan, India, and Ethiopia. Among European countries, the United Kingdom had the highest current prevalence of self-reported asthma symptoms among children aged 13 to 14 years, higher than other comparable European countries, such as Germany (ranked 19th) and France (ranked 20th). In Europe, the lowest prevalence of wheeze or asthma was reported in what was previously East Germany, and in Eastern countries such as Albania, indicating the possibility that the Western lifestyle may be involved. Similar geographic variations in wheezing prevalence were observed in the last 12 months among children aged 6 to 7 years old surveyed in 28 of the 56 countries of the study. Asthma symptoms were more common in boys than girls. The comparison between the ISAAC and ECRHS study in the countries where this was possible showed a good overall agreement for the distribution of wheezing and asthma prevalence between the 2 surveys, with higher figures for both adults wheezing and asthma in English-speaking countries. Globally, there is more asthma in countries with Western lifestyle compared with others. Geographic variations in asthma prevalence certainly depend on variations in environmental risk factors. They may also in part reflect international differences in health care systems, as well as more specific differences in asthma recognition and diagnosis.

Temporal Distribution

The investigation of the sequential trends of asthma prevalence has been made possible through epidemiologic population-based studies, which employed the same methodology in similar samples, at different periods. It seems now established that the number of asthmatics, after having almost doubled over the last 30 to 40 years, might have reached a plateau in countries where asthma prevalence is the most important. However, recent data from the United States indicate a new increase in asthma prevalence.

Increase of asthma prevalence

Over the last decades, the increase in asthma prevalence has been well documented in several studies. Among them, two epidemiological studies of the Midspan Family Study Surveys were performed 20 years apart and used the same methods. They compared the prevalence of asthma in 1,708 parents and 1,124 offspring in the Renfrew and Paisley area of Scotland. At the time of assessment (1972–1976 and 1996), both populations were aged 45–54 years. The prevalence of asthma had more than doubled from 3% to 8.2% in the 20 years of survey, which was strictly independent of the genetic background because of the familial design of the study in pairs of the same sex. At least a doubling of the prevalence of asthma has also been reported in centers in Nordic countries, such as Finland and Sweden among both children[7] and adults.[8,9] A study undertaken by the Union Chimique Belge Institute of Allergy in Belgium concluded that the prevalence of asthma in Western Europe has doubled in the last 10 years.[10] In a population-based Swedish study performed in subjects followed for 10 years, the cumulative incidence of asthma was of 3.4% among men and 4.5% among women. In addition, the incidence of asthma was higher in children than in adults (1.1% and 0.8% per year). Similarly, 25 years ago, the incidence of asthma was 2% in the Swiss population; the incidence has increased and is currently 8%.[11]

Worldwide, rates of asthma also as assessed using national statistics and surveys have increased significantly between the 1960s and 2008.[12,13] Some 9% of US children had asthma in 2001, compared with just 3.6% in 1980. In the United States, data from several national surveys reveal the age-adjusted prevalence of asthma increased from 7.3 to 8.2% during the years 2001 through 2009.[14] WHO reports that 10% of the Swiss population suffers from asthma today (WHO, 2007), compared with just 2% 25 to 30 years ago. In France, 4.15 million people suffered from asthma in 2006 while 3.5 million had suffered in 1998).[15]

To sum up, asthma patterns vary throughout the world and considerable increases in the prevalence of asthma have occurred globally over recent decades.[16–18]

Stagnation or decrease of asthma prevalence

Nevertheless, the last comparison of data from phases 1 and 3 of ISAAC conducted according to the same standardized methodology suggests a stagnation of asthma prevalence in children living in high-income countries, where the prevalence of asthma was already very high (**Fig. 1**, **Table 1**). This is consistent with von Hertzen's and Haahtela's review of reviewed studies on time trends in asthma prevalence, published between 2000 and 2004.[19] Of the 20 identified investigations, 13 revealed a decreasing or stable trend for asthma or current wheeze at any time during the study period, both in adults and children. It has been emphasized in several European countries and elsewhere (eg, Australia, United States), that the rising trends in asthma prevalence among adults may have reached a plateau or may even be decreasing, following a steady increase for the past decades. In one study,[20] wheezing increased in the older children and decreased in the younger age group, and in another study,[21] the prevalence of asthma increased, whereas wheezing decreased. The authors suggest that in affluent Westernized societies, the increasing trend in asthma in adults and adolescents may have plateaued or even reversed, while the situation is more ambiguous in younger children.

The fact that the prevalence of allergic rhinitis and eczema is still increasing worldwide in all classes of age suggests a separation in the course of asthma and allergic asthma, which has not be investigated so far.[2]

The proportion of asthma attributable to atopy in children has been estimated to be 38%, but there is significant variation between studies, ranging from 25 to 63%.[22] In the ISAAC phase 2 study, it has been reported that the population fraction of asthma attributable to atopy differed greatly between countries according to economic growth, being 40.7% in study centers from high-income countries and 20.3% in centers from low-income countries.[23] A nonatopic phenotype was the most common presentation of childhood asthma in low-income populations.[23–25]

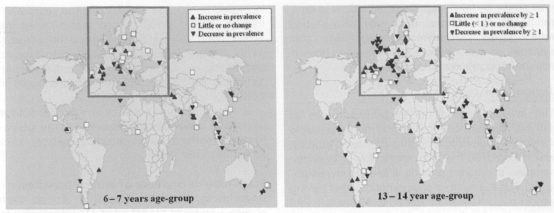

Fig. 1. World map showing direction of change in prevalence of asthma symptoms for 6- to 7-year age group and 13- to 14-year age group, on a follow-up period of 7 years (ISAAC phase 1 to phase 3). Each symbol represents a center. (*From* Asher MI, Montefort S, Bjorksten B, et al. Worldwide time trends in the prevalence of symptoms of asthma, allergic rhinoconjunctivitis, and eczema in childhood: ISAAC Phases One and Three repeat multicountry cross-sectional surveys. Lancet 2006;368:733; with permission.)

Table 1
Direction of change in prevalence of childhood asthma for 6- to 7-year age group and 13- to 14-year age group, on a follow-up period of 7 years (ISAAC phase 1 to phase 3).

Region	Asthma Symptoms		
	Increase	Decrease	Little or No Change
6 to 7-years age group			
English-speaking Africa	0	0	1
Asia-Pacific	2	5	5
Eastern Mediterranean	4	0	0
Indian subcontinent	2	2	2
Latin America	2	1	4
North America	1	0	1
Northern and eastern Europe	2	2	5
Oceania	1	2	2
Western Europe	11	2	7
Total	25	14	27
13- to 14-year age group			
Africa (English and French-speaking)	5	2	2
Asia-Pacific	6	4	5
Eastern Mediterranean	2	2	2
Indian subcontinent	2	4	2
Latin America	7	3	5
North America	1	0	1
Northern and eastern Europe	9	2	1
Oceania	0	3	2
Western Europe	10	20	4
Total	42	40	24

From Asher MI, Montefort S, Bjorksten B, et al. Worldwide time trends in the prevalence of symptoms of asthma, allergic rhinoconjunctivitis, and eczema in childhood: ISAAC Phases One and Three repeat multicountry cross-sectional surveys. Lancet 2006;368:733; with permission.

All together these findings indicate that international differences in asthma symptom prevalence have reduced, particularly in the 13- to 14-year age group, with decreases in prevalence in English-speaking countries and Western Europe and increases in prevalence in regions where prevalence was previously low. In addition, these findings suggest that, although asthma symptom prevalence is no longer increasing in most English-speaking and Western European countries, its global burden may continue to rise.[26]

Recent trends

Recently, the US Centers for Diseases Control and Prevention (CDC) reported that asthma prevalence increased from 7.3% in 2001 to 8.4% in 2010, when 25.7 million persons had asthma, and prevalence is now at its highest level in the United States. For the period 2008 to 2010, asthma prevalence was higher among children than adults, and among multiple-race, black, and American Indian or Alaska Native persons than white persons. People of multiple races had an incidence of 14.1%, while Asians had the lowest incidence (5.2%). Blacks had an incidence of 11.2%, while whites had an incidence of 7.7%. Hispanics of Puerto Rican descent had the highest prevalence, 16.1%. Children (9.5%) having a higher asthma prevalence than adults (7.7%) suggests that the disease will become a greater problem in the future. From 2001 to 2009, health care visits for asthma per 100 persons with asthma declined in primary care settings, while asthma emergency department (ED) visits and hospitalization rates were stable. For the period 2007 to 2009, black persons had higher rates for asthma ED visits and hospitalizations per 100 persons with asthma than white persons, and a higher asthma death rate per 1000 persons with asthma. Compared with adults, children had higher rates for asthma primary care and ED visits, similar hospitalization rates, and lower death rates. Obesity, which has increased dramatically in the United States in the past decades could explain the rise in asthma prevalence because of the well-known relationship between obesity and asthma. In this respect, it would be interesting to stratify the prevalence of asthma according to body mass index (BMI).

FACTORS RESPONSIBLE FOR TRENDS IN ASTHMA PREVALENCE
Factor Explaining Asthma Increase

Because the rise of asthma prevalence has been far too rapid to implicate any genetic basis for change and because of the great disparities in asthma prevalence and severity of the disease on a worldwide scale and between individuals with similar genetic background and living in different environments, the intervention of environmental and lifestyle factors that have shown marked changes in the past decades has been evoked for the asthma prevalence increase, among which the ones related to the so-called hygiene hypothesis (**Table 2**).[16]

Table 2
Factors responsible for increase or stagnation in asthma prevalence

Factors Responsible for an Increase	Factors Responsible for a Stagnation in High-Income Countries
Environmental factors • Allergens (because of new exposure conditions) • Parental smoking, since in utero life • Outdoor and indoor air pollution • Excess of hygiene • Diet • Stress Increased host susceptibility • Excess of hygiene • Decreased number of miscarriages and perinatal morbimortality • In utero events (maternal hormone and medication intake during pregnancy, fetal distress...)[a] • Prematurity, low birth weight • Diet • Stress	• Cohort effect: Western lifestyle more efficient in the 1960s than since the 2000s[a] • Efficiency of asthma treatments, resulting in a decrease of consultations for asthma and asthma prevalence[a] • Increased professional awareness of the disease[a] • No more people susceptible to develop asthma because of environmental influences (of the past decades)[a]

[a] Few or no data.

Environmental factors initially proposed to explain the increased global prevalence of asthma include increased prevalence of maternal smoking,[27,28] increased air pollution,[29,30] changed diet,[31-34] and stress.[35]

Passive smoking

Building upon previous findings from 79 prospective studies, a recent meta-analysis showed that exposure to passive smoking increases the incidence of wheeze and asthma in children and young people by at least 20% and that preventing parental smoking is crucially important to the prevention of asthma.[36] Exposure to pre- or post-natal passive smoke exposure was associated with a 30% to 70% increased risk of incident wheezing (strongest effect from postnatal maternal smoking on wheeze in children aged 2 years or younger, odds ratio [OR] = 1.70, 95% confidence interval [CI] = 1.24–2.35, 4 studies) and a 21% to 85% increase in incident asthma (strongest effect from prenatal maternal smoking on asthma in children aged 2 years or younger, OR = 1.85, 95% CI = 1.35–2.53, 5 studies).

Outdoor and indoor air pollution

Whereas it is well established that short-term exposure to air pollution is related to an increase in asthma hospitalization, visits and medication, data on the causal role of chemical air pollution in the development of asthma are considered by some authors as still insufficient. Long-term exposure to ozone may increase the prevalence of asthma and asthmatic symptoms.[37-39] Long-term exposure to outdoor residential nitrogen dioxide (NO_2) was associated with a history of doctor-diagnosed asthma in children in the 6 Cities Study[40] and adults In the Swiss Cohort Study on Air Pollution and Lung and Heart Diseases in Adults study.[41] A Japanese cohort study also reported an association between NO_2 levels and asthma incidence.[42] In contrast, a Norwegian study found no association between modeled NO_2 exposure at the birth address and doctor-diagnosed asthma in a large cohort of children.[43] There is evidence that living near high-traffic roads is associated with asthma (http://www.healtheffects.org/). First, McConnell and colleagues[38] observed that the incidence of new diagnoses of asthma in children is associated with physical exercise in areas with high concentrations of ozone and particulate matter. Since then, other prospective cohort studies have indicated that long-term exposure to traffic pollution could contribute to the development of asthma-like symptoms and allergic sensitization in children.[44] In the French Etude des Déterminants

pré et post-natal du développement et de la santé de l'ENfant birth cohort (http://eden.vjf.inserm.fr/), it was found that among modifiable environmental exposures, the impact of traffic-related air pollution was greater than that of passive smoking and molds.[45]

Fewer data concern exposure to indoor air and asthma. The most consistent finding for asthma induction in childhood is related as previously said to exposure to environmental tobacco smoke and to living in homes close to busy roads, and to exposure to dampness. In the case of measurement-based exposure assessments of chemical air pollutants, relationships have been found between fine particulate matter and several volatile organic compounds (VOCs).[46] Evident dampness or mold has consistent positive associations with asthma.[47] However, limited associations exist in the case of measured microbiologic agents or microbial VOCs as objective assessments of mold contamination.[48] These findings are critical, because indoor exposure to air pollutants has been assessed only for short periods. No robust data exist on temporal trends of aeroallergens, well-known risk factors of asthma and allergies, although individual exposure in indoor settings has been modified by modern lifestyle. The upsurge in the prevalence of allergies is observed as societies become more affluent and urbanized. In many low-income and middle-income countries, including rural areas in India, people rely on solid fuel (wood, cow dung, or crop residues) that they burn in simple stoves or open fires for domestic energy.[49] Secondhand smoke has become more common as parents become affluent enough to buy cigarettes. Together, these factors generate indoor air pollution that is estimated to be as much as 5 times as severe in poor countries as in rich ones.[50]

Climate change

Climate change provides an additional plausible explanation for both increasing asthma susceptibility and increasing severity observed over several decades.[51] There are many types of asthma, and climate change may explain the component of the increase that is allergic asthma, particularly pollen-induced asthma. Indeed climate change significantly affects plant distribution and pollination, as well as mold proliferation. This is likely to be a significant proportion of asthma cases. For example, Grossman[52] suggests that up to 78% of people with asthma also suffer from allergic rhinitis. Furthermore, although the hypothesis that trends in air pollution have been major determinants for the rise in prevalence of asthma and allergic disease in recent decades is now generally disproved,[53,54] air pollution is likely to have its own effects on pollen production.[55] Moreover, climate change, change in ambient temperatures, and changes in weather during pollen seasons can cause both biologic and chemical changes to pollens and have direct adverse consequences on human health by inducing disease exacerbations, especially in urban and polluted regions.

Diet

In the past 2 decades, increasing evidence has suggested that modern diets may contribute to the increase in the prevalence of asthma.[56] Modern diets in most westernized countries differ considerably from those of previous generations, in which asthma prevalence was lower. In contrast with traditional diets, which mainly consist of locally produced, fresh, seasonal and less processed food, modern diets predominantly consist of processed foods that have been modified, stored, and transported over long distances. In addition, because of changes in agricultural techniques and increased storage and transportation, nutritional content has changed. For example, it was reported that mineral content of vegetables, fruit, and meat has declined.[57] From the supplementation point of view, the available epidemiologic evidence is weak but nonetheless supportive with respect to the association between deficiencies of the nutrients selenium; zinc; vitamins A, C, D, and E and low fruit and vegetable intake and the development of asthma and allergic disorders as shown by a recent meta-analysis.[58] In addition, a Mediterranean diet has been proposed for the prevention of asthma. Experimental studies of these exposures, randomized–controlled trials in particular, are warranted.

Stress

Stress is also considered to affect the expression of asthma and thus its prevalence through multidimensional endocrine, neural, immune, and behavioral processes. There is observational evidence that severe negative life events may increase the risk of children's asthma attacks over subsequent weeks[35] and may be associated with asthma symptoms among adolescents.[59] The association between stressful life events and an increased risk of asthma has also been reported in retrospective studies[60–62] and in at least one prospective study[63] among adults.

Hygiene hypothesis

Further potential explanatory factors of the increase in asthma prevalence come under the hygiene hypothesis, which proposes that greater risk of atopy results from altered challenges to the immune system in early life, particularly reduced infections, and the consequent development of a bias toward

T-helper type 2 immune response over T-helper type 1.[64] Specific factors proposed under the hygiene hypothesis include changed immunization practices,[65,66] changed living conditions and increased exposure to indoor allergens,[67] increased use of antibiotics,[68–70] and reduced exposure to endotoxins.[71–73] Furthermore, studies examining the hygiene hypothesis have not been entirely consistent, with some showing no effects of these exposures on subsequent development of asthma.[74] Inconsistencies may result from different social trends that alter exposures in more than one direction. Although the hygiene hypothesis has been proposed as one explanation for the increases in symptom prevalence, it does not appear entirely to account for the time trends, since the increases have occurred for both nonatopic (noneosinophilic) and atopic (eosinophilic) asthma, whereas the hygiene hypothesis would only explain trends for atopic asthma.[75] The hygiene hypothesis is also unlikely to explain the considerably higher prevalence of asthma in many Latin American countries and in US inner cities, which are more consistent with changes in environmental exposures other than hygiene.[24,76,77] Although some trends may have reduced potentially protective exposures (increased urbanization, reduced family size, and increased maternal work stress during pregnancy), others (eg, greater use of formal child care) may increase the protective exposures. However, it is well established that respiratory infections are a risk factor for asthma exacerbations.

Other factors

Among the most recent factors proposed to explain asthma increase, there is the use of paracetamol during pregnancy, which has been associated with an increased risk of childhood asthma with a pooled OR for the risk of current wheeze in the children of women who were exposed to any paracetamol during any stage of pregnancy of 1.21 (95% CI 1.02–1.44).[78] This is consistent with the fact that asthma increase is paralleled by aspirin decrease. However, other studies are needed to better estimate this risk.

Host susceptibility

It has also been suggested that the increase in asthma could be due to a more susceptible population in the past decades (see **Table 2**). Susceptibility would have increased as the result of early life events. Indeed, there is epidemiologic evidence for multiple prenatal factors impacting early life respiratory morbidity.[79,80] In utero exposures including tobacco smoke exposure, dietary exposures including vitamin D, and prenatal infections and exposure to microbial products may modulate both atopy and respiratory disease. In addition, there is recent evidence that in utero exposures can affect the children's health through its impact on the newborn's immune system.[81]

Similarly, there exists significant association between asthma and the caesarean sections and other prenatal events such as the decreased number of miscarriages and prematurity and low birth weight.[82] Diet and stress could also contribute to individual susceptibility. The mechanisms of action of these factors need further investigation and may act via various pathways, including effects on lung development, allergic and nonallergic inflammation, and airway remodeling. It remains to be determined also if some of these early life factors that predispose to wheezing will all translate into increased risk of asthma. Indeed several studies have shown the existence of nontransient wheezing in early life.

Factor Explaining Asthma Prevalence Stagnation

Just as it is not known why prevalence has increased since the 1950s so far, it is not known why prevalence should now be decreasing.[21] The latest data on temporal trends in the prevalence of asthma are in favor of stagnation or decrease of the number of asthmatics in high-income countries due to the cessation of environmental influences. Perhaps the most striking finding is the apparent decline in symptom prevalence in English-speaking countries. This contrasts with the hygiene hypothesis, as it does not seem apparent that the English-speakinglanguage countries have become less hygienic in recent decades, although increases in infant and childhood infections could have occurred due to specific factors such as increased use of childcare facilities.[83] Other established asthma risk factors do not appear to explain the worldwide asthma prevalence patterns[31,70,84–86] or time trends, particularly the decline in English-speaking countries. It also seems unlikely that the decline in symptom prevalence is due to decreased recognition and labeling of asthma symptoms, given that the prevalence of asthma ever has increased. This could explain why, in some countries, symptom prevalence has not increased or has even declined, but the prevalence of asthma ever has increased. It should also be noted that the findings for asthma ever are to some extent reassuring with regard to the findings for current asthma symptoms, since they indicate that increased recognition and diagnosis of asthma have not been accompanied by an increase in reporting of asthma symptoms; such an increase would have been expected if the symptom

prevalence patterns were entirely due to differences in recognition and labeling of symptoms. Further results of population-based studies showed a stagnation of asthma prevalence combined with an increase in the use of inhaled corticosteroids (ICs) in industrialized countries.[87] Although the use of IC may explain the reduction of asthma-related symptoms and hospitalizations, it only influences the decrease in asthma prevalence to a negligible extent. Moreover, we observed a decline in the prevalence of allergic rhinitis and emphysema, for which ICs are not prescribed.

One plausible hypothesis that may explain this decrease is that genetic potential could not be further expressed in the absence of important environmental changes, as observed in industrialized countries (see **Table 2**). Indeed, environmental influences may have reached their maximum expression in inducing disease in susceptible individuals. However, it remains difficult to assess the validity of this hypothesis from the epidemiologic point of view. Additional factors that may explain the reversing trend prevalence of asthma are (see **Table 2**):

- An increased professional awareness of the disease, which can reduce overdiagnosis in children.
- The implementation of national and global asthma prevention and management guidelines that have led to earlier detection and improved treatment of asthmatics.
- Changes in disease severity may be one potential factor and as a result, asthma may have become milder, independent of increased use of inhaled corticosteroids, which may be reflected in changed trends of prevalence.

SUMMARY

Asthma is one of the most prevalent chronic conditions, affecting approximately 300 million people worldwide, up to 1 in 10 adults and 1 in 3 children in some countries. However, asthma is a complex disease that it still not fully understood. The type of asthma definition adopted has influenced knowledge on asthma distribution and etiology. In the case of asthma prevalence, accurate estimation has been hindered by varying definitions of asthma and methods of data collection, each combining to make data comparison across studies difficult, with the exception of ISAAC and ECRHS, which unfortunately have not used biologic and clinical markers of the disease. For instance, the use of incomplete definitions of asthma has led to an underestimation of asthma prevalence and resulted in gaps in the identification of asthma-related risk and protective factors.

Although treatment for asthma has improved substantially, the prevalence of asthma continues to increase, particularly in low- and middle-income countries, or in some ethnic groups in which prevalence was previously low. Observed spatio-temporal variations in the increased prevalence of asthma depend on exposure to environmental factors such as allergens (because of new conditions of exposure), parental smoking, air pollution, excess of hygiene, and more in general lifestyle. Recently, several arguments are also in favor of the involvement of host susceptibility and stress in the observed increase of asthma prevalence.

Further investigations are needed to better understand asthma development, mechanisms of exacerbation, and its evolution worldwide. In particular, gene–environment interactions starting in early life using the epigenetic approach should be explored to better understand asthma epidemiologic evolution.

REFERENCES

1. World Health Organization. Global surveillance, prevention and control of chronic respiratory diseases: a comprehensive approach. Geneva (Switzerland): World Health Organization; 2007.

2. Asher MI, Montefort S, Bjorksten B, et al. Worldwide time trends in the prevalence of symptoms of asthma, allergic rhinoconjunctivitis, and eczema in childhood: ISAAC phases one and three repeat multicountry cross-sectional surveys. Lancet 2006;368: 733.

3. Martinez FD. Trends in asthma prevalence, admission rates, and asthma deaths. Respir Care 2008; 53:561.

4. Agache I, Akdis C, Jutel M, et al. Untangling asthma phenotypes and endotypes. Allergy 2012;67(7): 835–46.

5. The International Study of Asthma and Allergies in Childhood (ISAAC) Steering Committee. Worldwide variation in prevalence of symptoms of asthma, allergic rhinoconjunctivitis, and atopic eczema: ISAAC. Lancet 1998;351:1225.

6. European Community Respiratory Health Survey. Variations in the prevalence of respiratory symptoms, self-reported asthma attacks, and use of asthma medication in the European Community Respiratory Health Survey (ECRHS). Eur Respir J 1996;9:687.

7. Aberg N, Hesselmar B, Aberg B, et al. Increase of asthma, allergic rhinitis and eczema in Swedish schoolchildren between 1979 and 1991. Clin Exp Allergy 1995;25:815.

8. Bjornsson E, Plaschke P, Norrman E, et al. Symptoms related to asthma and chronic bronchitis in three areas of Sweden. Eur Respir J 1994;7:2146.

9. Huovinen E, Kaprio J, Laitinen LA, et al. Incidence and prevalence of asthma among adult Finnish men and women of the Finnish Twin Cohort from 1975 to 1990, and their relation to hay fever and chronic bronchitis. Chest 1999;115:928.

10. UCB. European allergy white paper. Brussels (Belgium): The UCB Institute of Allergy; 1997.

11. Lundback B, Ronmark E, Jonsson E, et al. Incidence of physician-diagnosed asthma in adults—a real incidence or a result of increased awareness? Report from The Obstructive Lung Disease in Northern Sweden Studies. Respir Med 2001;95:685.

12. Anandan C, Nurmatov U, van Schayck OC, et al. Is the prevalence of asthma declining? Systematic review of epidemiological studies. Allergy 2010;65: 152.

13. Grant EN, Wagner R, Weiss KB. Observations on emerging patterns of asthma in our society. J Allergy Clin Immunol 1999;104:S1.

14. Vital signs: asthma prevalence, disease characteristics, and self-management education: United States, 2001–2009. MMWR Morb Mortal Wkly Rep 2011;60:547.

15. Delmas MC, Fuhrman C. Asthma in France: a review of descriptive epidemiological data. Rev Mal Respir 2010;27(2):151–9.

16. Bach JF. The effect of infections on susceptibility to autoimmune and allergic diseases. N Engl J Med 2002;347:911.

17. Isolauri E, Huurre A, Salminen S, et al. The allergy epidemic extends beyond the past few decades. Clin Exp Allergy 2004;34:1007.

18. Pearce N, Douwes J, Beasley R. The rise and rise of asthma: a new paradigm for the new millennium? J Epidemiol Biostat 2000;5:5.

19. von Hertzen L, Haahtela T. Signs of reversing trends in prevalence of asthma. Allergy 2005;60:283.

20. Wang XS, Tan TN, Shek LP, et al. The prevalence of asthma and allergies in Singapore; data from two ISAAC surveys seven years apart. Arch Dis Child 2004;89:423.

21. Anderson HR, Ruggles R, Strachan DP, et al. Trends in prevalence of symptoms of asthma, hay fever, and eczema in 12-14 year olds in the British Isles, 1995-2002: questionnaire survey. BMJ 2004;328:1052.

22. Pearce N, Pekkanen J, Beasley R. How much asthma is really attributable to atopy? Thorax 1999; 54:268.

23. Weinmayr G, Weiland SK, Bjorksten B, et al. Atopic sensitization and the international variation of asthma symptom prevalence in children. Am J Respir Crit Care Med 2007;176:565.

24. Penny ME, Murad S, Madrid SS, et al. Respiratory symptoms, asthma, exercise test spirometry, and

atopy in schoolchildren from a Lima shanty town. Thorax 2001;56:607.

25. Pereira MU, Sly PD, Pitrez PM, et al. Nonatopic asthma is associated with helminth infections and bronchiolitis in poor children. Eur Respir J 2007;29:1154.

26. Braman SS. The global burden of asthma. Chest 2006;130:4S.

27. Lodrup Carlsen KC. The environment and childhood asthma (ECA) study in Oslo: ECA-1 and ECA-2. Pediatr Allergy Immunol 2002;13(Suppl 15):29.

28. Ulrik CS, Backer V. Atopy in Danish children and adolescents: results from a longitudinal population study. Ann Allergy Asthma Immunol 2000;85:293.

29. D'Amato G, Liccardi G, D'Amato M. Environmental risk factors (outdoor air pollution and climatic changes) and increased trend of respiratory allergy. J Investig Allergol Clin Immunol 2000;10:123.

30. Rios JL, Boechat JL, Sant'Anna CC, et al. Atmospheric pollution and the prevalence of asthma: study among schoolchildren of 2 areas in Rio de Janeiro, Brazil. Ann Allergy Asthma Immunol 2004;92:629.

31. Ellwood P, Asher MI, Bjorksten B, et al. Diet and asthma, allergic rhinoconjunctivitis and atopic eczema symptom prevalence: an ecological analysis of the International Study of Asthma and Allergies in Childhood (ISAAC) data. ISAAC Phase One Study Group. Eur Respir J 2001;17:436.

32. Hijazi N, Abalkhail B, Seaton A. Diet and childhood asthma in a society in transition: a study in urban and rural Saudi Arabia. Thorax 2000;55:775.

33. Seaton A, Devereux G. Diet, infection and wheezy illness: lessons from adults. Pediatr Allergy Immunol 2000;11(Suppl 13):37.

34. Sigurs N, Hattevig G, Kjellman B. Maternal avoidance of eggs, cow's milk, and fish during lactation: effect on allergic manifestations, skin-prick tests, and specific IgE antibodies in children at age 4 years. Pediatrics 1992;89:735.

35. Sandberg S, Paton JY, Ahola S, et al. The role of acute and chronic stress in asthma attacks in children. Lancet 2000;356:982.

36. Burke H, Leonardi-Bee J, Hashim A, et al. Prenatal and passive smoke exposure and incidence of asthma and wheeze: systematic review and meta-analysis. Pediatrics 2012;129:735.

37. Jorres R, Nowak D, Magnussen H. The effect of ozone exposure on allergen responsiveness in subjects with asthma or rhinitis. Am J Respir Crit Care Med 1996;153:56.

38. McConnell R, Berhane K, Gilliland F, et al. Asthma in exercising children exposed to ozone: a cohort study. Lancet 2002;359:386.

39. Peden DB, Setzer RW Jr, Devlin RB. Ozone exposure has both a priming effect on allergen-induced responses and an intrinsic inflammatory action in the nasal airways of perennially allergic asthmatics. Am J Respir Crit Care Med 1995;151:1336.

40. Penard-Morand C, Raherison C, Charpin D, et al. Long-term exposure to close-proximity air pollution and asthma and allergies in urban children. Eur Respir J 2010;36:33.

41. Ackermann-Liebrich U, Leuenberger P, Schwartz J, et al. Lung function and long term exposure to air pollutants in Switzerland. Study on Air Pollution and Lung Diseases in Adults (SAPALDIA) Team. Am J Respir Crit Care Med 1997;155:122.

42. Shima M, Nitta Y, Ando M, et al. Effects of air pollution on the prevalence and incidence of asthma in children. Arch Environ Health 2002;57:529.

43. Oftedal B, Nystad W, Brunekreef B, et al. Long-term traffic-related exposures and asthma onset in schoolchildren in oslo, norway. Environ Health Perspect 2009;117:839.

44. Laumbach RJ, Kipen HM. Respiratory health effects of air pollution: update on biomass smoke and traffic pollution. J Allergy Clin Immunol 2012;129:3.

45. Zhou C, Baiz N, Zhang T. Annesi-Maesano I; EDEN Mother-Child Cohort Study Group. Modifiable environmental exposures related to asthma phenotypes in the first year of childhood in children of the EDEN mother–child cohort study. BMC Public Health 2012, in press.

46. Hulin M, Simoni M, Viegi G. Isabella Annesi-Maesano respiratory health and indoor air pollutants based on measurement exposure assessments. ERJ, in press.

47. Mendell MJ, Mirer AG, Cheung K, et al. Respiratory and allergic health effects of dampness, mold, and dampness-related agents: a review of the epidemiologic evidence. Environ Health Perspect 2011;119:748.

48. Hulin M, Moularat S, Kirchner S, et al. Positive associations between respiratory outcomes and fungal index in rural inhabitants of a representative sample of French dwellings. Int J Hyg Environ Health 2012. [Epub ahead of print].

49. Pawankar R, Canonica GW, Holgate ST, et al, editors. The WAO white book on allergy. World Allergy Organization; 2011.

50. Bousquet JKN, editor. Global surveillance, prevention and control of chronic respiratory diseases: a comprehensive, approach. Geneva (Switzerland): World Health Organization; 2007.

51. Ayres JG, Forsberg B, Annesi-Maesano I, et al. Climate change and respiratory disease: European Respiratory Society position statement. Eur Respir J 2009;34:295.

52. Grossman J. One airway, one disease. Chest 1997;111:11S.

53. Charpin D, Pascal L, Birnbaum J, et al. Gaseous air pollution and atopy. Clin Exp Allergy 1999;29:1474.

54. Strachan DP. The role of environmental factors in asthma. Br Med Bull 2000;56:865.

55. D'Amato G, Liccardi G, D'Amato M, et al. The role of outdoor air pollution and climatic changes on the rising trends in respiratory allergy. Respir Med 2001;95:606.

56. McKeever TM, Britton J. Diet and asthma. Am J Respir Crit Care Med 2004;170:725.

57. Thomas D. A study on the mineral depletion of the foods available to us as a nation over the period 1940 to 1991. Nutr Health 2003;17:85.

58. Nurmatov U, Devereux G, Sheikh A. Nutrients and foods for the primary prevention of asthma and allergy: systematic review and meta-analysis. J Allergy Clin Immunol 2011;127:724.

59. Turyk ME, Hernandez E, Wright RJ, et al. Stressful life events and asthma in adolescents. Pediatr Allergy Immunol 2008;19:255.

60. Kilpelainen M, Koskenvuo M, Helenius H, et al. Stressful life events promote the manifestation of asthma and atopic diseases. Clin Exp Allergy 2002;32:256.

61. Lefevre F, Moreau D, Semon E, et al. Maternal depression related to infant's wheezing. Pediatr Allergy Immunol 2011;22:608.

62. Levitan H. Onset of asthma during intense mourning. Psychosomatics 1985;26.939.

63. Loerbroks A, Apfelbacher CJ, Thayer JF, et al. Neuroticism, extraversion, stressful life events and asthma: a cohort study of middle-aged adults. Allergy 2009;64:1444.

64. Strachan DP. Family size, infection and atopy: the first decade of the "hygiene hypothesis. Thorax 2000;55(Suppl 1):S2.

65. Portengen L, Sigsgaard T, Omland O, et al. Low prevalence of atopy in young Danish farmers and farming students born and raised on a farm. Clin Exp Allergy 2002;32:247.

66. von Mutius E. The rising trends in asthma and allergic disease. Clin Exp Allergy 1998;28(Suppl 5):45.

67. Kaiser HB. Risk factors in allergy/asthma. Allergy Asthma Proc 2004;25:7.

68. Cohet C, Cheng S, MacDonald C, et al. Infections, medication use, and the prevalence of symptoms of asthma, rhinitis, and eczema in childhood. J Epidemiol Community Health 2004;58:852.

69. Droste JH, Wieringa MH, Weyler JJ, et al. Does the use of antibiotics in early childhood increase the risk of asthma and allergic disease? Clin Exp Allergy 2000;30:1547.

70. Foliaki S, Nielsen SK, Bjorksten B, et al. Antibiotic sales and the prevalence of symptoms of asthma, rhinitis, and eczema: the International Study of Asthma and Allergies in Childhood (ISAAC). Int J Epidemiol 2004;33:558.

71. Eder W, von Mutius E. Hygiene hypothesis and endotoxin: what is the evidence? Curr Opin Allergy Clin Immunol 2004;4:113.

72. Eduard W, Douwes J, Omenaas E, et al. Do farming exposures cause or prevent asthma? Results from a study of adult Norwegian farmers. Thorax 2004;59:381.

73. Gehring U, Bolte G, Borte M, et al. Exposure to endotoxin decreases the risk of atopic eczema in infancy: a cohort study. J Allergy Clin Immunol 2001;108:847.

74. von Hertzen LC, Haahtela T. Asthma and atopy—the price of affluence? Allergy 2004;59:124.

75. Douwes J, Pearce N. Asthma and the westernization 'package'. Int J Epidemiol 2002;31:1098.

76. Mallol J, Sole D, Asher I, et al. Prevalence of asthma symptoms in Latin America: the International Study of Asthma and Allergies in Childhood (ISAAC). Pediatr Pulmonol 2000;30:439.

77. Salvi SS, Babu KS, Holgate ST. Is asthma really due to a polarized T cell response toward a helper T cell type 2 phenotype? Am J Respir Crit Care Med 2001;164:1343.

78. Eyers S, Weatherall M, Jefferies S, et al. Paracetamol in pregnancy and the risk of wheezing in offspring: a systematic review and meta-analysis. Clin Exp Allergy 2011;41:482.

79. Kumar R. Prenatal factors and the development of asthma. Curr Opin Pediatr 2008;20:682.

80. Seaton A, Godden DJ, Brown K. Increase in asthma: a more toxic environment or a more susceptible population? Thorax 1994;49:171.

81. Baiz N, Slama R, Bene MC, et al. Maternal exposure to air pollution before and during pregnancy related to changes in newborn's cord blood lymphocyte subpopulations. The EDEN study cohort. BMC Pregnancy Childbirth 2011;11:87.

82. Annesi-Maesano I, Moreau D, Strachan D. In utero and perinatal complications preceding asthma. Allergy 2001;56:491.

83. Robertson CF, Roberts MF, Kappers JH. Asthma prevalence in Melbourne schoolchildren: have we reached the peak? Med J Aust 2004;180:273.

84. Anderson HR, Poloniecki JD, Strachan DP, et al. Immunization and symptoms of atopic disease in children: results from the International Study of Asthma and Allergies in Childhood. Am J Public Health 2001;91:1126.

85. Burr ML, Emberlin JC, Treu R, et al. Pollen counts in relation to the prevalence of allergic rhinoconjunctivitis, asthma and atopic eczema in the International Study of Asthma and Allergies in Childhood (ISAAC). Clin Exp Allergy 2003;33:1675.

86. von Mutius E, Pearce N, Beasley R, et al. International patterns of tuberculosis and the prevalence of symptoms of asthma, rhinitis, and eczema. Thorax 2000;55:449.

87. Annesi-Maesano I. L'obésité un nouveau facteur de risque d'asthme? In: Margaux O, editors. Répercussions respiratoires de l'obésité. Constats et prise en charge. Paris: JP Laaban Éditeur; 2005:37–48.

Genetics of Asthma Susceptibility and Severity

Rebecca E. Slager, PhD, MS[a], Gregory A. Hawkins, PhD[a],
Xingnan Li, PhD, MS[a], Dirkje S. Postma, MD, PhD[b],
Deborah A. Meyers, PhD[a], Eugene R. Bleecker, MD[a],*

KEYWORDS

- Asthma • Genetics • Susceptibility • Severity • Personalized medicine • Therapy • Lung function

KEY POINTS

- Genes and environmental exposures interact to influence risk of asthma susceptibility and severity.
- Two large meta-analyses of asthma susceptibility identified 4 chromosomal regions that were associated with asthma in individuals of different ethnic backgrounds: loci in the ORMDL3 region of 17q21, IL1RL/IL18R on chromosome 2q, TSLP on 5q22, and IL33 on chromosome 9p24.
- Genome-wide screens for asthma susceptibility in Asian populations identified genetic variants in the major histocompatibility complex gene region (human leukocyte antigen region) on chromosome 6p21 associated with asthma risk; this locus has been a significant predictor of asthma susceptibility in several genetic studies.
- Genes that are associated with asthma subphenotypes, such as lung function, biomarkers levels, and asthma therapeutic responses, can provide insight into mechanisms of asthma severity progression.
- A joint model of risk variants in lung function genes identified in the general population were highly associated with lower lung function and increased severity in asthma populations.
- A pharmacogenetic genome-wide screen identified 2 correlated genetic variants in the GLCCI1 gene related to response to inhaled glucocorticoids.
- Future genetic studies for asthma susceptibility and severity will incorporate exome or whole-genome sequencing in comprehensively phenotyped asthmatics, which will contribute to personalized asthma therapy.

INTRODUCTION

Asthma is a heterogeneous disease with a complex cause. The interaction of genes and environmental exposures influences the development of asthma and determines the expression or progression of the disease (**Fig. 1**).[1] An overall aim of genetic studies in a complex disease such as asthma is to identify a group of genetic variants that will predict risk for development (susceptibility) or progression (severity) of asthma. Genetic factors related to asthma susceptibility and severity are not limited to a single gene but are caused by several gene variants that each contribute to the risk architecture.

There has been major progress in determining the genetic factors that are associated with asthma susceptibility, using genome-wide association study

Financial disclosure: This work was funded by NHLBI grants HL69167 and HL101487. RES was supported by HL089992 and HL101487.

[a] Center for Genomics and Personalized Medicine, Wake Forest School of Medicine, Medical Center Boulevard, Winston-Salem, NC 27157, USA; [b] Department of Pulmonary Medicine, University Medical Center Groningen, University of Groningen, Hanzeplein 1, 9713 GZ Groningen, The Netherlands

* Corresponding author. Wake Forest University Health Sciences, Medical Center Boulevard, Winston-Salem, NC 27157.

E-mail address: ebleeck@wakehealth.edu

Clin Chest Med 33 (2012) 431–443
http://dx.doi.org/10.1016/j.ccm.2012.05.005
0272-5231/12/$ – see front matter © 2012 Elsevier Inc. All rights reserved.

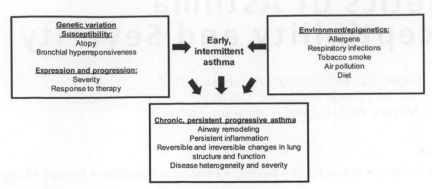

Fig. 1. Gene-environment interactions in asthma susceptibility and severity.

(GWAS) approaches.[2–11] GWAS genes such as interleukin (IL) 13, IL33, its receptor IL1 receptorlike 1 isoform 1 (IL1RL1), and thymic stromal lymphopoietin (TSLP) have been linked to asthma and several other allergic phenotypes, suggesting dysregulation of shared inflammatory pathways. In addition, the major histocompatibility complex (MHC) region, which was one of the first asthma susceptibility loci identified,[12] seems to contribute to asthma and allergen sensitization.[2] Regulatory T cell signaling may also play a role in asthma, because the SMAD family member 3 (SMAD3) gene, which encodes a transcriptional modulator related to transforming growth factor β, has also been identified in several genome-wide screens for asthma. Several of these susceptibility genes and their biologic pathways have been replicated in some, but often not all, asthma populations, suggesting that there may be heterogeneity in the genetic risk in

populations of different ethnic backgrounds.[7,13] Results from major GWAS studies of asthma are reviewed in this article and are summarized in **Table 1**.

Many of the large genome-wide screens that have identified genes important to asthma susceptibility were based on a clinical diagnosis of asthma rather than more comprehensive phenotypes that would also evaluate the mechanisms of disease progression and severity. Current studies are now using more extensive characterization to investigate the progression of asthma. Thus, asthma severity may be related to specific subphenotypes, some of which are discussed in this article and summarized in **Table 2**: (1) genes related to pulmonary function; (2) biomarkers related to asthma progression and risk of exacerbations; (3) pharmacogenetic interactions in which an individual may have reduced responsiveness, or be resistant, to a specific asthma

Table 1
Significant asthma susceptibility GWAS variants from meta-analyses or replicated studies

Gene(s)	Chromosomal Region	Ethnic Background(s)	References
ORMDL3/GSDML	17q21	All	Moffatt et al,[3,8] 2010, 2007; Torgersen et al,[11] 2011
IL1RL1/IL18R1	2q11	All	Moffatt et al,[3] 2010; Torgerson et al,[11] 2011
TSLP	5q22	All	Moffatt et al,[3] 2010; Torgerson et al,[11] 2011; Hirota et al,[30] 2011
IL33	9p24	All	Moffatt et al,[3] 2010; Torgerson et al,[11] 2011
SMAD3	15q23	European	Moffatt et al,[3] 2010
RORA	15q22	European	Moffatt et al,[3] 2010
HLA-DQ/DR	6p21	All	Moffatt et al,[3] 2010; Li et al,[2] 2010; Hirota et al,[30] 2011; Noguchi et al,[31] 2011
IL13	5q31	European	Moffatt et al,[3] 2010; Li et al,[2] 2010
PYHIN1	1q23	African	Torgerson et al,[11] 2011

Table 2
Selected GWAS associations for asthma severity and related traits

Trait	Gene(s)	References
Lung function measures (FEV$_1$/FVC or FEV$_1$)		
General population	HHIP, GPR126, ADAM19, AGER/PPT2, FAM13A, PTCH1, PID1, HTR4, GSTCD, TNS1, NOTCH4/AGER/PPT2, THSD4l, NTS12/GSTCD/NPNT, MFAP2, TGFB2, HDAC4, RARB, MECOM, SPATA9, ARMC2, NCR3, ZKSCAN3, CDC123, C10orf11, LRP1, CCDC38, MMP15, CFDP1, and KCNE2	Repapi et al,[42] 2010; Hancock et al,[41] 2010; Soler Artigas et al,[47] 2011
Asthma populations	HHIP, IL6R	Li et al,[43] 2011; Hawkins et al,[61] 2012
Total serum/plasma IgE levels		
General population	STAT6, FCER1A, IL13/RAD50	Weidinger et al,[75] 2008; Granada et al,[76] 2012
Asthma populations	HLA-DR, STAT6, FCER1A, IL13/RAD50, C11orf30-LRRC32	Moffatt et al,[3] 2010; Li et al,[43] 2011
Eosinophil levels		
General population	IL1RL1, IKZF2, IL5, SH2B3	Gudbjartsson et al,[81] 2009
Atopic conditions	TSLP/WDR36 (eosinophilic esophagitis) WDR36, IL33, MYB (eosinophil levels and atopic asthma)	Rothenberg et al,[82] 2010; Gudbjartsson et al,[81] 2009
Response to asthma therapy		
Inhaled corticosteroids	GLCCI1	Tantisira et al,[88] 2011

Abbreviations: FEV$_1$, forced expiratory volume in 1 second; FVC, forced vital capacity; IgE, immunoglobulin E.

therapy; or (4) specific gene-by-environment interactions.

GENOME-WIDE ASSOCIATION STUDIES OF ASTHMA SUSCEPTIBILITY

Before 2007, candidate genes in known asthma and allergy biologic pathways were tested for association with asthma susceptibility,[7] and family studies and positional cloning techniques identified several putative chromosomal loci related to asthma.[6,14–17] For example, the T helper 2 (TH2) immunologic pathway is one of the most replicated pathways in human and animal asthma studies.[7,18–22] However, many of the other positive genetic associations from candidate pathways and family studies have not been consistently replicated, possibly because of small sample sizes, population stratification, inconsistent phenotype definitions, and lack of adequate gene coverage.[7] Following the transition to GWAS, risk variants discovered in these genome-wide screens were more likely to be replicated, at least in populations of similar ethnic background. This article highlights some of the newer studies and meta-analyses of asthma susceptibility and severity, including GWAS in multiple ethnic groups.

GWAS of Asthma Susceptibility in Multiple Ethnic Groups

Based on a doctor's diagnosis of asthma, the first asthma susceptibility GWAS was published by Moffatt and colleagues,[8] representing the European a multidisciplinary study to identify the genetic and environmental causes of asthma in the European Community (GABRIEL) consortium in 2007. This report identified genetic markers in ORMDL3 (ORM1-like 3) on chromosome 17q12-21 as predictors of childhood asthma susceptibility. A large follow-up study in the same European cohort verified this finding, because single-nucleotide polymorphisms (SNPs) spanning approximately 380 kb in the ORMDL3 genomic region were associated with asthma.[3] Several subsequent GWAS have also confirmed this result, and this is one of the most highly replicated susceptibility loci in genome-wide screens for asthma.[9,11,23,24] However, because of the high degree of linkage disequilibrium (LD) in this region that spans several genes, it is still not clear whether

ORMDL3 or a nearby gene is the risk gene with the causative variant(s).[25] A splice-site mutation that is in strong LD with ORMDL3 but located the adjacent gasderminlike B (GSDMB) gene was recently identified by the 1000 Genomes Project, indicating that this may be a causal risk variant for asthma.[26] This example highlights the importance of new genetic sequencing projects and how these technologies continue to facilitate understanding of the genetics of asthma.

Although many of the initial asthma GWAS studies were performed in non-Hispanic white discovery cohorts, there is a need to investigate the genetic pathways that play a role in asthma in individuals of different ethnic backgrounds, especially because minority groups such as African Americans are more likely to experience higher asthma morbidity and mortality than white people.[27,28] Populations of different ancestry also have different patterns of gene variation and LD that can alter the gene-specific risk variants. Although the GABRIEL consortium consisted of European individuals with asthma and unaffected controls, the EVE meta-analysis was established in North America to identify genetic factors that contribute to asthma susceptibility in multiple ethnic groups. Five major susceptibility loci were identified in 5416 asthma cases and replication was performed in an additional 12,649 individuals of European American, African American or African Caribbean, and Latino ancestry. Four of the chromosomal regions that reached genome-wide significance in EVE had been previously identified in GABRIEL or other studies: loci in the ORMDL3 region of 17q21, the IL1RL/IL18R (IL18 receptor) loci on chromosome 2q, the TSLP gene region on 5q22, and IL33 on chromosome 9p24.[11] These loci are associated with asthma development in all 3 ethnic groups, whereas a novel susceptibility locus in individuals of African descent was identified near at the pyrin and HIN domain family, member 1 (PYHIN1) gene on chromosome 1q23.[11] Before the EVE analysis, one of the only asthma GWAS performed in populations of African ancestry was performed in African American asthma cases and controls from the United States and African Caribbean individuals from Barbados. Adjusting for racial admixture, this study identified polymorphisms in the α-1B-adrenergic receptor (ADRA1B) on chromosome 5q33, prion-related protein (PRNP) on chromosome 20pter-p12, and dipeptidyl peptidase 10 (DPP10) on chromosome 2q12.3-q14.2 as predictors of asthma.[29] Although DPP10 had been identified in earlier positional cloning studies of asthma,[14] many of these associations seem to be limited to individuals of African ancestry.

GWAS of Asthma in Asian Populations

Genome-wide screens for asthma susceptibility in Asian adults and children were published in 2011 and both identified genetic variants in the HLA gene region on chromosome 6p21 as highly associated with asthma risk. In the Japanese population, 7171 adult asthma cases and 27,912 unaffected individuals were genotyped in the discovery and replication cohorts, identifying 5 loci associated with susceptibility to adult asthma, 2 of which had previously been reported: the HLA region and the TSLP/WD repeat domain 36 (WDR36) locus. Three additional genomic regions were also significant at the genome-wide significance level: the ubiquitin specific peptidase 38 (USP38)/GRB2-associated binding protein 1 (GAB1) locus on chromosome 4q31, loci on chromosome 10p14, and a region of chromosome 12q13.[30] In a separate GWAS of childhood asthma in 938 Japanese pediatric patients with asthma and 2376 controls, SNPs were tested for association with asthma susceptibility and highly significant associations were tested for replication in independent Japanese samples and in Korean samples. This analysis determined that genetic variants in the HLA-DP locus were associated with the risk of pediatric asthma across Asian populations.[31]

Furthermore, a replication study in 710 asthma cases and 656 unaffected controls in the Chinese Han population tested specific variants in the ORMDL3/GSDMB region of chromosome 17q21, providing further evidence that this locus was associated with adult-onset asthma risk in multiple ethnic groups.[23]

The specific role and functional biology of novel GWAS loci such as ORMDL3 in the pathogenesis of asthma is still unknown. However, there is strong evidence from asthma GWAS of the biologic importance of pathways that communicate epithelial damage to the adaptive immune system, ultimately leading to airway inflammation. Moreover, cytokines derived from epithelial cells such as TSLP and IL33 may promote the TH2 response through activation of receptors such as IL1RL1 on cell types such as mast cells, TH2 cells, and regulatory T cells.

GENETIC STUDIES OF ASTHMA SEVERITY AND RELATED PHENOTYPES

Because initial GWAS focused primarily on childhood-onset asthma and asthma susceptibility, it is uncertain whether the same genes that contribute to asthma predisposition also play a role in the progression and severity of disease. In addition, population-based studies often rely on limited phenotypes such as a physician's diagnosis to accommodate large sample sizes. However, comprehensive studies of asthma severity require more intense, time-consuming, and costly phenotyping that can result in smaller cohort sizes. Asthma severity studies also require different comparison groups than susceptibility studies. Instead of unaffected individuals, subjects with severe asthma should be compared with individuals with mild asthma, which can be an additional complexity for subject recruiting. Analysis of asthma severity can include intermediate phenotypes such as measures of pulmonary function, bronchial hyperresponsiveness (BHR), biomarkers, and response to asthma therapy.

GWAS of Severe, Persistent Asthma

Li and colleagues[2] performed a GWAS for asthma susceptibility and severity in a comprehensively phenotyped, longitudinal cohort of 473 non-Hispanic white adult cases in The Epidemiology and Natural History of Asthma: Outcomes and Treatment Regimens (TENOR) study,[32,33] compared with Illumina general population controls. In this analysis, several variants in the RAD50/IL13 region of chromosome 5q31.1 were identified as predictors of asthma susceptibility. An SNP in intron 2 of RAD50 (adjacent to IL13) was one of the most highly associated with asthma, although strong correlation between variants in this LD block makes it difficult to identify the causal variant.[2] However, this is an important example of a genome-wide study identifying a biologically relevant gene (IL13) that had been observed in several candidate gene studies.[7,34] IL13 is an important regulator of allergen-induced asthma in mice[35,36] and also seems to contribute to asthma in this severe allergic cohort. This study also identified variants in the HLA-DR/DQ region on chromosome 6p21.3 associated with asthma, a genomic region that has been replicated in many candidate genes studies[37,38] and GWAS,[3,30,31] as discussed earlier.

Lung Function

Extensive phenotypic characterization in the National Heart, Lung, and Blood Institute (NHLBI)—sponsored Severe Asthma Research Program (SARP) cohort indicates that one of the primary determinants of asthma severity is lung function.[39,40] Identifying the genetic determinants of pulmonary function, a statistically powerful objective measure, therefore represents a relevant approach to defining genes that contribute to asthma severity.

There are currently no GWAS powered to test the progression of asthma severity and longitudinal lung function decline. However, 2 large meta-analyses for normal lung function have been performed in the European general population. The cohorts for heart and aging research in genomic epidemiology (CHARGE) and SpiroMeta consortiums both identified the hedgehog interacting protein (HHIP) gene associated with the lung function measures forced expiratory volume in 1 second (FEV_1) or the FEV_1/forced vital capacity (FVC) ratio,[41,42] along with 11 other genomic regions for normal pulmonary function (see **Table 2**). To better understand whether these genetic variants also play a role in asthma populations, Li and colleagues[43] tested 14 SNPs in these candidate genes for association with pulmonary function measures in a meta-analysis of 3 independent asthma cohorts (n = 1441): the NHLBI–sponsored SARP[39,40] and Collaborative Studies on the Genetics of Asthma (CSGA) studies[44]; and the TENOR study.[32,33] This analysis identified the HHIP/rs1512288 variant as a significant predictor of FEV_1 and FVC in asthma. In a joint model, an increasing number of risk variants in these lung function genes were highly associated with lower FEV_1 and increased asthma severity,[43] showing the close relationship between pulmonary function and asthma severity. This additive approach has been used successfully to predict prostate cancer risk[45,46] and may have important clinical applications to personalized medicine in the future.

In a large (approximately 90,000 European individuals in the discovery and replication cohorts) follow-up meta-analysis from the CHARGE and SpiroMeta consortia, an additional 16 loci for normal lung function were identified at the genome-wide significance level (see **Table 2**).[47] These genes are related to several different physiologic pathways including cell growth, signaling, and migration. It remains to be determined whether these genes or pathways also contribute to lung function variation in individuals with asthma; however, a region of 6p21.33 that contains a nonsynonymous SNP in lymphotoxin α (LTA) and a correlated SNP in the promoter region of tumor necrosis factor α (TNFA), were identified in this lung function analysis.[47] These genes have previously been linked to asthma susceptibility.[48,49] Other plausible asthma-related mechanisms include TGF-β signaling, which can induce mucin expression in bronchial epithelial cells.[50]

IL6 is a cytokine that becomes systemically or locally increased during inflammatory processes.[51] Increased IL6 expression has been observed with lung inflammation and injury[52] and increased serum IL6 levels have been reported in subjects with asthma,[53] chronic obstructive pulmonary disease (COPD),[54–58] and, more recently, in a small severe asthma study.[59] For IL6 to have a role in inflammatory lung disease, the IL6 receptor must also be involved, which seems to be the case. In a genome-wide association study of 57,800 subjects, the IL6R gene was identified as an asthma susceptibility gene,[60] and, more recently, the common IL6R coding variation rs2228145 (Asp358Ala) was identified as a potential genetic modifier of lung function in asthma and as a novel genetic marker of asthma.[61] In this last study, subjects of European ancestry with asthma who inherited the minor C allele of rs2228145 (Ala358) had the lowest mean percent predicted FEV_1, FEV_1/FVC, and the highest mean levels of methacholine responsiveness (PC20). The frequency of the rs2228145 C allele was significantly higher in phenotypic asthma clusters consisting of subjects with more severe asthma,[40] and high serum levels of the soluble form of the IL6 receptor (sIL6R) were associated with lower lung function.[61] In cells that do not possess the membrane-bound IL6 receptor, the active IL6/sIL6R complex can bind the membrane-bound coreceptor glycoprotein 130 (gp130) and initiate the IL6 signaling cascade, resulting in phosphorylation and activation of signal transducer and activator of transcription 3 (STAT3) protein, a transcription factor that has been linked to airway inflammation and changes in lung function.[62–65] This extracellular process is termed IL6 transsignaling and has been associated with a range of inflammatory diseases,[51,66] including rheumatoid arthritis,[67] Crohn disease,[68] and inflammatory bowel disease.[69] Long-term exposure to IL6 transsignaling may induce morphologic changes in smooth muscle structure and may be an important component in long-term development of airway remodeling in obstructive lung disease. Anti-IL6R therapy is currently being used to control disease progression in inflammatory diseases such as rheumatoid arthritis,[70–74] and thus there is the possibility that anti-IL6R therapy could also be important in the treatment of airway diseases such as asthma.

Biomarkers

Biomarkers such as serum immunoglobulin (Ig) E levels and blood or sputum eosinophil levels may be important predictors of asthma severity or risk of exacerbations. Therefore, many asthma cohorts, as well as large population-based studies, have evaluated genetic factors related to these biomarkers (see **Table 2**). The GABRIEL cohort performed a genome-wide study for genetic factors associated with total serum IgE levels in 7087 subjects with asthma and 7667 controls, and identified 1 novel locus in the class II region of MHC which was significant at the genome-wide level.[3] This study also observed several genetic variants associated with IgE levels in the Fc fragment of IgE, high affinity I (FCER1A), IL13, and signal transducer and activator of transcription (STAT6) genes. These regions were also reported in previous GWAS for IgE in the general population,[75] including a recent analysis by the Framingham cohort.[76] In GABRIEL, genes that were associated with asthma susceptibility generally did not overlap with those associated with IgE. The investigators therefore concluded that loci strongly associated with IgE levels may not play an important role in the development of asthma but may contribute to severity or progression of the disease.[3] To identify additional genes associated with IgE levels in non-Hispanic white asthma populations, Li and colleagues[43] tested SNPs on chromosome 11q13.5 between the open reading frame 30 (C11orf30) and leucine-rich repeat containing 32 (LRRC32) genes, which had previously been identified in genetic analyses of related inflammatory conditions such as atopic dermatitis,[77] childhood eczema,[78] and Crohn disease.[79] Four SNPs in this region were significantly associated with total serum IgE levels after adjustment for multiple testing, suggesting a common genetic regulation for IgE levels in atopic diseases.[80]

Asthma genes identified through GWAS have also been identified as predictors of blood eosinophil levels, an inflammatory biomarker likely related to asthma pathogenesis and progression. For example, a large population-based GWAS of 9392 Icelanders identified an IL1RL1 variant that was associated with eosinophil counts and asthma, and SNPs in WDR36, IL33, and MYB that were nominally associated with eosinophil counts and atopic asthma.[81] The 5q22 genomic region spanning TSLP and WDR36 genes, which has been associated with asthma in several reports,[3,11] is also associated with pediatric eosinophilic esophagitis, an allergic disorder characterized by excess eosinophils in the esophagus. Based on expression studies, the investigators concluded that TSLP is the most likely causative gene in this region.[82]

ASTHMA THERAPY

Another genetic mechanism that can produce asthma that is more severe or difficult to manage is response to asthma therapy. New developments in pharmacogenetics research (see **Table 2**) are discussed later.

Corticosteroid (Glucocorticoid) Pathway

Glucocorticoid (GCs) steroids are currently the most common antiinflammatory asthma therapy.

Regular use of steroids is generally effective and reduces mortality caused by asthma.[83] However, chronic steroid use can result in side effects that may be alleviated by targeted, inhaled drug delivery to the lung. There is a subset of patients with severe asthma who require high doses of inhaled and oral steroids to control symptoms and asthma exacerbations.[39,40] However, there is also considerable variability in response to corticosteroids, with a significant number of patients who have no response. Little is known about the pharmacogenetic interactions of this complex pathway,[84,85] although there is likely a genetic component to the variability in corticosteroid responses in childhood and adult asthma.[86]

The Hop protein (encoded by the STIP1 gene) is involved in activation of the glucocorticoid receptor and is a novel therapeutic target in the glucocorticoid pathway. In a pharmacogenetic analysis, STIP1 single-nucleotide and haplotypic variation was related to changes in FEV$_1$ in response to treatment with inhaled corticosteroids (ICS). There was a heterogeneous response to steroids; approximately half of STIP1 haplotypes were associated with reduced corticosteroid response and the other half with greater sensitivity to ICS.[87]

A recent genome-wide study by Tantisira and colleagues[88] evaluated 4 asthma populations (n = 935) to identify pharmacogenetic associations related to response to inhaled glucocorticoids. A significant, replicated association was found in 2 correlated SNPs, rs37972 and rs37973, in the glucocorticoid-induced transcript 1 (GLCCI1) gene, which confer a lung function response to inhaled glucocorticoids and are also associated with reduced GLCCI1 expression and luciferase reporter activity. Using data pooled from all treatment trials, the overall mean (±standard error) increase in FEV$_1$ for ICS-treated subjects homozygous for the rs37973 variant allele was significantly less than for subjects homozygous for the common allele (3.2 ± 1.6% vs 9.4 ± 1.1% respectively). In this analysis, genotype was estimated to account for 6.6% of inhaled glucocorticoid response variability, which is an example of a replicated pharmacogenetic analysis with functional verification.[88] In addition, Tantisira and colleagues[86] also showed that variation in the corticotrophin-releasing hormone receptor 1 gene (CRHR1) is associated with improved lung function response to corticosteroids in 3 asthma clinical trial populations.

β2-Adrenergic Pathway

β-Adrenergic receptor agonists, or β-agonists, are commonly prescribed medications for relief of bronchoconstriction and long-term symptom treatment in asthma. Short-acting β-agonists (SABA) and long-acting β-agonists (LABA) target β2-adrenergic receptors on the surface of airway smooth muscle cells and other lung or inflammatory cells.[83] Many pharmacogenetic studies have explored whether β2 adrenergic receptor (ADRB2) gene variation could explain differences in bronchodilator response among patients with asthma or identify a subgroup of patients with reduced response.[83,89] Many of these studies focused on the common, functionally nonsynonymous Gly16Arg and Gln27Glu mutations.[90,91] For example, reduced pharmacologic responses to use of SABA but not to LABA in individuals homozygous for the ADBR2 Arg16 variant have been reported.[92–96] However, there are additional rare variants in ADRB2 that may also play a role in response to therapy. Extensive resequencing of the ADRB2 locus in African Americans and non-Hispanic white people with asthma revealed 4 rare ADRβ2 polymorphisms that were analyzed for association with asthma severity outcomes: 25bp insertion-deletion at nucleotide -376, Asn15Ser (rs33973603), Thr164Ile (rs1800888, also identified by Liggett and colleagues[97]), and Ser220Cys (rs3729943).[98] African American cases with rare ADRB2 alleles treated with LABA showed a greater percentage of sputum eosinophils compared with African American cases with common alleles (28% vs 7%; P = .02) or those with rare alleles not treated with LABA (28% vs 0.4%; P = .01).[99] In addition, non-Hispanic white asthma cases with rare alleles treated with LABA showed a significantly increased number of urgent care and emergency department visits for asthma in the past year compared with patients with asthma with ADRB2 common alleles.[99] These analyses suggest that rare and common gene variation may modulate response to asthma therapy.

T-Helper 2 Pathway

There are several novel therapies currently under development targeting molecules in the T-helper 2 (TH2) pathway. Two recent clinical trials of these biologics identified specific population subgroups with improved therapeutic responses based on biomarker levels or specific genotypes. Corren and colleagues[100] hypothesized that anti–IL13 therapy would benefit patients with asthma with a baseline profile consistent with IL13 activity. In a randomized, double-blind, placebo-controlled study of lebrikizumab, a monoclonal antibody to IL13, patient subgroups were prespecified according to TH2 status (based on total IgE level and blood eosinophil counts) and serum periostin level. After 12 weeks, the mean increase in FEV$_1$

was 5.5 percentage points higher in the anti-IL13 group compared with the placebo group in the overall trial ($P = .02$). However, among patients in the high-periostin or high fraction of exhaled nitric oxide subgroup, the increase from baseline FEV_1 was 8.2 percentage points higher in the anti-IL13 group than placebo.[100]

In addition, Wenzel and colleagues[101] reported results from a clinical trial of the anti-IL4 receptor antagonist pitrakinra. In an ICS-withdrawal, double-blind, randomized, placebo-controlled, multicenter trial in 534 patients with uncontrolled, moderate to severe asthma, participants were randomized to 1 mg (n = 132), 3 mg (n = 137), or 10 mg (n = 128) pitrakinra or placebo (n = 137) twice daily for a 12-week treatment period. In the overall study population, efficacy was not shown; however, statistically significant efficacy was observed in prespecified subpopulations including (1) subjects with increased blood eosinophil levels (peripheral blood count >350 cells/mm^3, n = 125), (2) upper tertile fraction of exhaled nitric oxide (range 20–122 ppb, n = 64), and (3) individuals with GG genotype in IL4 receptor (IL4R) variant rs8832 (n = 134 non-Hispanic white people). Of these 3 subgroups, the greatest relative reduction in incidence of asthma exacerbation at the highest anti-IL4 receptor dose compared with placebo (88%) was observed for IL4R/rs8832 GG subjects. Participants with the IL4R/rs8832 GG genotype randomized to active anti-IL4 receptor therapy had decreased asthma exacerbations and decreased nocturnal awakenings and activities limited by asthma. There was also a dose-dependent reduction in exacerbations in these subjects because the frequency of exacerbations in the placebo, 1-mg, 3-mg, and 10-mg treatment groups was 25%, 16%, 12%, and 3% respectively.[101–103] This analysis represents one of the largest pharmacogenetic investigations of the TH2 pathway in patients with uncontrolled, moderate to severe asthma, identifying an asthma subgroup with improved response to this therapy.

Issues such as statistical power, ability to generalize, and functional characterization, which are critical for all genetic studies, are especially important in pharmacogenetic studies. Identifying appropriate replication populations also remains a challenge, because of the highly specific treatment regimens specified in clinical trials. However, these studies may represent an important step in personalized medicine, because clinical decisions regarding appropriate therapy for patients with asthma may rely on these types of studies in the future.

GENE/ENVIRONMENT INTERACTIONS AND ASTHMA

Despite the importance of environmental factors to the development of asthma (see **Fig. 1**), few gene/environment interactions have been consistently identified and replicated for asthma severity. Challenges in genetic association studies such as adequate sample size, population stratification, gene coverage, and adjustment for false-positives can be compounded in gene/environment interaction studies and accurately measuring environmental factors presents additional obstacles.

Several gene/environment studies have evaluated the interaction between genes and smoke exposure, including a genetic linkage analysis in 200 Dutch families. Linkage signals for asthma and BHR were observed on chromosomes 3p and 5q, although passive smoke exposure accounted for BHR linkage to 5q.[15] Similar results were observed in US populations.[104] Additional studies in candidate genes such as A disintegrin and metalloproteinase 33 (ADAM33) have also shown the effect of smoke exposure on increased risk of asthma. The ADAM33 gene was identified through positional cloning[6] and replicated as an asthma susceptibility gene in several candidate gene studies. ADAM33 variants have also been tested in 200 Dutch asthma cases with more than 25 years of longitudinal data and the S_2 polymorphism was a significant predictor of increased decline in FEV_1.[105] This gene has also been associated with risk of COPD in a Dutch cohort[106] and in a cross-sectional population of 880 long-term tobacco smokers,[107] suggesting that this gene may be related to disease progression in asthma and other respiratory diseases.

Investigators in the GABRIELA (GABRIEL Advanced) Study Group conducted a genome-wide interaction analysis for asthma and atopy testing 500,000 SNPs and rural farm-related exposures in 1708 European children. Overall, no significant interactions were identified and the investigators concluded that common genetic polymorphisms were unlikely to moderate the influence of the farming environment on childhood asthma, although rare variants may play a role.[108] This analysis emphasizes that new statistical and measurement tools are needed to address these issues genome-wide.[109,110]

There have been other studies in families to investigate gene/environment interaction on a genome-wide basis or in candidate gene analysis. The Childhood Asthma Management Program conducted a genome-wide study of genes and modulation of vitamin D levels related to asthma exacerbations using population-based and family-based approaches in 403 individuals and trios. Three common variants in the class I MHC-restricted T-cell–associated molecule (CRTAM) gene were associated with an increased rate of asthma exacerbations based on low vitamin D levels; these results were replicated in 584 children from a Costa Rican cohort. Functional studies then explored the interaction of vitamin D and the non-synonymous coding polymorphism rs2272094 on CRTAM expression. The results suggest that maintaining adequate vitamin D levels may be especially important in subsets of patients with asthma based on genotype.[111] In another candidate gene analysis, variants in the purinergic receptor P2Y (P2Y12) gene, which is necessary for leukotriene E4–induced inflammation, were tested for interaction with house dust mite exposure and association with lung function. Five P2RY12 SNPs were predictors of multiple lung function measures ($P = .006$–0.025) in 422 children with asthma and their parents. Individuals homozygous for minor alleles in P2RY12 exposed to house dust mite had lower lung function than those who were unexposed (P interaction $= 0.0028$–0.040).[112]

Despite the obvious challenges involved in gene/environment interaction studies, these types of analyses may account for some of the missing heritability that GWAS variants do not explain in common diseases such as asthma.[113] Perhaps even more challenging than systematic and comprehensive evaluation of gene/environment interactions is defining how environmental exposures lead to disease. It is likely that epigenetic mechanisms are an important component for understanding the development of asthma. Several studies are now focusing on understanding how epigenetic modifications such as methylation regulate gene expression and may ultimately affect disease susceptibility and severity.[114] Interaction studies can also provide insight into which environmental exposures contribute to asthma severity and risk of exacerbations and may guide interventions in the future.[110,115]

SUMMARY AND FUTURE STUDIES

More than 10 years have passed since the first human genome was sequenced in 2001,[116,117] and GWAS is currently the most effective approach to studying the genetics of human diseases. Several genes/regions have been consistently associated with asthma susceptibility through this method: ORMDL3/GSDMB, IL33, IL1RL1, RAD50/IL13, HLA-DR/DQ, TSLP, and SMAD3 (see **Table 1**).[2,3,11] In many cases, the effect of each individual genetic variant is small,[113] suggesting that the additive effect of multiple risk

variants should be taken into account. An important goal of the genetic approach in complex disease is to identify a group of variants that will reliably predict risk of the development (susceptibility) or progression (severity) of disease. Improved phenotyping approaches will also improve the ability to link genotype and phenotype. There is a need to understand asthma disease heterogeneity because different phenotypes may reflect several pathogenic pathways that have different underlying genetic architecture.[40]

Genes that contribute to phenotypes such as lung function and biomarker levels provide insight into mechanisms of asthma progression (see **Table 2**). However, additional studies evaluating genes and environmental factors leading to disease severity are needed. This will lead to greater understanding of the biologic pathways that contribute to disease progression. Future genetic studies in asthma severity will also incorporate whole-genome or exome-specific sequencing to identify more common and rare genetic variants. Exome and complete genome sequencing will provide better genomic coverage than existing genotyping platforms and will discover biologically relevant causal variants. For example, resequencing the IL4 gene in African Americans identified an excess of private noncoding SNPs in asthma cases compared with unaffected individuals ($P = .031$).[118] New genotyping technologies and comprehensive phenotyping should elucidate the genetics of asthma severity in the future. Understanding the functional biology of these novel variants discovered through genome-wide sequencing will also become increasing important. Using these variants identified in comprehensively phenotyped studies, personalized therapy for all individuals with asthma may more effectively be developed.

REFERENCES

1. Slager RE, Li X, Meyers DA, et al. Recent developments in the genetics of asthma susceptibility and severity. In: Chung KF, Bel EH, Wenzel SE, editors. Difficult-to-treat severe asthma. Sheffield (United Kingdom): European Respiratory Society Journals; 2011. p. 82–96.
2. Li X, Howard TD, Zheng SL, et al. Genome-wide association study of asthma identifies RAD50-IL13 and HLA-DR/DQ regions. J Allergy Clin Immunol 2010;125:328–35.
3. Moffatt MF, Gut IG, Demenais F, et al. A large-scale, consortium-based genomewide association study of asthma. N Engl J Med 2010;363:1211–21.
4. Ober C, Hoffjan S. Asthma genetics 2006: the long and winding road to gene discovery. Genes Immun 2006;7:95–100.

5. Ober C, Tan Z, Sun Y, et al. Effect of variation in CHI3L1 on serum YKL-40 level, risk of asthma, and lung function. N Engl J Med 2008;358:1682–91.

6. Van Eerdewegh P, Little RD, Dupuis J, et al. Association of the ADAM33 gene with asthma and bronchial hyperresponsiveness. Nature 2002;418: 426–30.

7. Vercelli D. Discovering susceptibility genes for asthma and allergy. Nat Rev Immunol 2008;8: 169–82.

8. Moffatt MF, Kabesch M, Liang L, et al. Genetic variants regulating ORMDL3 expression contribute to the risk of childhood asthma. Nature 2007;448:470–3.

9. Himes BE, Hunninghake GM, Baurley JW, et al. Genome-wide association analysis identifies PDE4D as an asthma-susceptibility gene. Am J Hum Genet 2009;84:581–93.

10. Reijmerink NE, Postma DS, Bruinenberg M, et al. Association of IL1RL1, IL18R1, and IL18RAP gene cluster polymorphisms with asthma and atopy. J Allergy Clin Immunol 2008;122:651–654.e8.

11. Torgerson DG, Ampleford EJ, Chiu GY, et al. Meta-analysis of genome-wide association studies of asthma in ethnically diverse North American populations. Nat Genet 2011;43:887–92.

12. Moffatt MF, Schou C, Faux JA, et al. Association between quantitative traits underlying asthma and the HLA-DRB1 locus in a family-based population sample. Eur J Hum Genet 2001;9:341–6.

13. Meyers DA. Genetics of asthma and allergy: what have we learned? J Allergy Clin Immunol 2010; 126:439–46.

14. Allen M, Heinzmann A, Noguchi E, et al. Positional cloning of a novel gene influencing asthma from chromosome 2q14. Nat Genet 2003;35:258–63.

15. Meyers DA, Postma DS, Stine OC, et al. Genome screen for asthma and bronchial hyperresponsiveness: interactions with passive smoke exposure. J Allergy Clin Immunol 2005;115:1169–75.

16. Xu J, Meyers DA, Ober C, et al. Genomewide screen and identification of gene-gene interactions for asthma-susceptibility loci in three U.S. populations: collaborative Study on the Genetics of Asthma. Am J Hum Genet 2001;68:1437–46.

17. Koppelman GH, Meyers DA, Howard TD, et al. Identification of PCDH1 as a novel susceptibility gene for bronchial hyperresponsiveness. Am J Respir Crit Care Med 2009;180:929–35.

18. Hershey GK, Friedrich MF, Esswein LA, et al. The association of atopy with a gain-of-function mutation in the alpha subunit of the interleukin-4 receptor. N Engl J Med 1997;337:1720–5.

19. Ober C, Leavitt SA, Tsalenko A, et al. Variation in the interleukin 4-receptor alpha gene confers susceptibility to asthma and atopy in ethnically diverse populations. Am J Hum Genet 2000;66: 517–26.

20. Howard TD, Koppelman GH, Xu J, et al. Gene-gene interaction in asthma: IL4RA and IL13 in a Dutch population with asthma. Am J Hum Genet 2002;70:230–6.

21. Kabesch M, Schedel M, Carr D, et al. IL-4/IL13 pathway genetics strongly influence serum IgE levels and childhood asthma. J Allergy Clin Immunol 2006;117:269–74.

22. Chen W, Ericksen MB, Levin LS, et al. Functional effect of the R110Q IL13 genetic variant alone and in combination with IL4RA genetic variants. J Allergy Clin Immunol 2004;114:553–60.

23. Fang Q, Zhao H, Wang A, et al. Association of genetic variants in chromosome 17q21 and adult-onset asthma in a Chinese Han population. BMC Med Genet 2011;12:133.

24. Hancock DB, Romieu I, Shi M, et al. Genome-wide association study implicates chromosome 9q21.31 as a susceptibility locus for asthma in Mexican children. PLoS Genet 2009;5:e1000623.

25. Wjst M. ORMDL3–guilt by association? Clin Exp Allergy 2008;38:1579–81.

26. Durbin RM, Abecasis GR, Altshuler DL, et al. A map of human genome variation from population-scale sequencing. Nature 2010;467:1061–73.

27. Wenzel SE, Busse WW. Severe asthma: lessons from the Severe Asthma Research Program. J Allergy Clin Immunol 2007;119:14–21.

28. Gupta RS, Carrion-Carire V, Weiss KB. The widening black/white gap in asthma hospitalizations and mortality. J Allergy Clin Immunol 2006; 117:351–8.

29. Mathias RA, Grant AV, Rafaels N, et al. A genome-wide association study on African-ancestry populations for asthma. J Allergy Clin Immunol 2010;125: 336–46. e4.

30. Hirota T, Takahashi A, Kubo M, et al. Genome-wide association study identifies three new susceptibility loci for adult asthma in the Japanese population. Nat Genet 2011;43:893–6.

31. Noguchi E, Sakamoto H, Hirota T, et al. Genome-wide association study identifies HLA-DP as a susceptibility gene for pediatric asthma in Asian populations. PLoS Genet 2011;7:e1002170.

32. Dolan CM, Fraher KE, Bleecker ER, et al. Design and baseline characteristics of The Epidemiology and Natural History of Asthma: Outcomes and Treatment Regimens (TENOR) study: a large cohort of patients with severe or difficult-to-treat asthma. Ann Allergy Asthma Immunol 2004;92: 32–9.

33. Haselkorn T, Fish JE, Zeiger RS, et al. Consistently very poorly controlled asthma, as defined by the impairment domain of the Expert Panel Report 3 guidelines, increases risk for future severe asthma exacerbations in The Epidemiology and Natural History of Asthma: Outcomes and Treatment

Regimens (TENOR) study. J Allergy Clin Immunol 2009;124:895–902, e1–4.

34. Howard TD, Whittaker PA, Zaiman AL, et al. Identification and association of polymorphisms in the interleukin-13 gene with asthma and atopy in a Dutch population. Am J Respir Cell Mol Biol 2001;25:377–84.

35. Grunig G, Warnock M, Wakil AE, et al. Requirement for IL13 independently of IL-4 in experimental asthma. Science 1998;282:2261–3.

36. Wills-Karp M, Luyimbazi J, Xu X, et al. Interleukin-13: central mediator of allergic asthma. Science 1998;282:2258–61.

37. Booth M, Shaw MA, Carpenter D, et al. Carriage of DRB1*13 is associated with increased posttreatment IgE levels against Schistosoma mansoni antigens and lower long-term reinfection levels. J Immunol 2006;176:7112–8.

38. Munthe-Kaas MC, Carlsen KL, Carlsen KH, et al. HLA Dr-Dq haplotypes and the TNFA-308 polymorphism: associations with asthma and allergy. Allergy 2007;62:991–8.

39. Moore WC, Bleecker ER, Curran-Everett D, et al. Characterization of the severe asthma phenotype by the National Heart, Lung, and Blood Institute's Severe Asthma Research Program. J Allergy Clin Immunol 2007;119:405–13.

40. Moore WC, Meyers DA, Wenzel SE, et al. Identification of asthma phenotypes using cluster analysis in the Severe Asthma Research Program. Am J Respir Crit Care Med 2010;181:315–23.

41. Hancock DB, Eijgelsheim M, Wilk JB, et al. Meta-analyses of genome-wide association studies identify multiple loci associated with pulmonary function. Nat Genet 2010;42:45–52.

42. Repapi E, Sayers I, Wain LV, et al. Genome-wide association study identifies five loci associated with lung function. Nat Genet 2010;42:36–44.

43. Li X, Howard TD, Moore WC, et al. Importance of hedgehog interacting protein and other lung function genes in asthma. J Allergy Clin Immunol 2011;127:1457–65.

44. Meyers DA, Wjst M, Ober C. Description of three data sets: Collaborative Study on the Genetics of Asthma (CSGA), the German Affected-Sib-Pair Study, and the Hutterites of South Dakota. Genet Epidemiol 2001;21(Suppl 1):S4–8.

45. Xu J, Zheng SL, Isaacs SD, et al. Inherited genetic variant predisposes to aggressive but not indolent prostate cancer. Proc Natl Acad Sci U S A 2010; 107:2136–40.

46. Zheng SL, Sun J, Wiklund F, et al. Cumulative association of five genetic variants with prostate cancer. N Engl J Med 2008;358:910–9.

47. Soler Artigas M, Loth DW, Wain LV, et al. Genome-wide association and large-scale follow up identifies 16 new loci influencing lung function. Nat Genet 2011;43:1082–90.

48. Ruse CE, Hill MC, Tobin M, et al. Tumour necrosis factor gene complex polymorphisms in chronic obstructive pulmonary disease. Respir Med 2007; 101:340–4.

49. Wu H, Romieu I, Sienra-Monge JJ, et al. Parental smoking modifies the relation between genetic variation in tumor necrosis factor-alpha (TNF) and childhood asthma. Environ Health Perspect 2007; 115:616–22.

50. Chu HW, Balzar S, Seedorf GJ, et al. Transforming growth factor-beta2 induces bronchial epithelial mucin expression in asthma. Am J Pathol 2004; 165:1097–106.

51. Febbraio MA, Rose-John S, Pedersen BK. Is interleukin-6 receptor blockade the Holy Grail for inflammatory diseases? Clin Pharmacol Ther 2010;87:396–8.

52. Ammit AJ, Moir LM, Oliver BG, et al. Effect of IL-6 trans-signaling on the pro-remodeling phenotype of airway smooth muscle. Am J Physiol Lung Cell Mol Physiol 2007;292:L199–206.

53. Yokoyama A, Kohno N, Fujino S, et al. Circulating interleukin 6 levels in patients with bronchial asthma. Am J Respir Crit Care Med 1995;151: 1354–8.

54. Garrod R, Marshall J, Barley E, et al. The relationship between inflammatory markers and disability in chronic obstructive pulmonary disease (COPD). Primary Care Resp J 2007;16:236–40.

55. Schols AM, Buurman WA, Staal van den Brekel AJ, et al. Evidence for a relation between metabolic derangements and increased levels of inflammatory mediators in a subgroup of patients with chronic obstructive pulmonary disease. Thorax 1996;51:819–24.

56. Karadag F, Karul AB, Cildag O, et al. Biomarkers of systemic inflammation in stable and exacerbation phases of COPD. Lung 2008;186:403–9.

57. Broekhuizen R, Wouters EF, Creutzberg EC, et al. Raised CRP levels mark metabolic and functional impairment in advanced COPD. Thorax 2006;61: 17–22.

58. Lee TM, Lin MS, Chang NC. Usefulness of C-reactive protein and interleukin-6 as predictors of outcomes in patients with chronic obstructive pulmonary disease receiving pravastatin. Am J Cardiol 2008;101:530–5.

59. Morjaria JB, Babu KS, Vijayanand P, et al. Sputum IL-6 concentrations in severe asthma and its relationship with FEV1. Thorax 2011;66:537.

60. Ferreira MA, Matheson MC, Duffy DL, et al. Identification of IL6R and chromosome 11q13.5 as risk loci for asthma. Lancet 2011;378:1006–14.

61. Hawkins GA, Robinson MB, Hastie AT, et al. IL6R variation Asp358Ala is a potential modifier of lung

function in asthma. J Allergy Clin Immunol 2012. [Epub ahead of print].

62. Simeone-Penney MC, Severgnini M, Tu P, et al. Airway epithelial STAT3 is required for allergic inflammation in a murine model of asthma. J Immunol 2007;178:6191–9.

63. Litonjua AA, Tantisira KG, Lake S, et al. Polymorphisms in signal transducer and activator of transcription 3 and lung function in asthma. Respir Res 2005;6:52.

64. Gao H, Guo RF, Speyer CL, et al. Stat3 activation in acute lung injury. J Immunol 2004;172: 7703–12.

65. Gao H, Ward PA. STAT3 and suppressor of cytokine signaling 3: potential targets in lung inflammatory responses. Expert Opin Ther Targets 2007;11: 869–80.

66. Rose-John S, Waetzig GH, Scheller J, et al. The IL-6/sIL-6R complex as a novel target for therapeutic approaches. Expert Opin Ther Targets 2007;11: 613–24.

67. Plushner SL. Tocilizumab: an interleukin-6 receptor inhibitor for the treatment of rheumatoid arthritis. Ann Pharmacother 2008;42:1660–8.

68. Brulhart L, Nissen MJ, Chevallier P, et al. Tocilizumab in a patient with ankylosing spondylitis and Crohn's disease refractory to TNF antagonists. Joint Bone Spine 2010;77:625–6.

69. Rose-John S, Mitsuyama K, Matsumoto S, et al. Interleukin-6 trans-signaling and colonic cancer associated with inflammatory bowel disease. Curr Pharm Des 2009;15:2095–103.

70. De Bandt M, Saint-Marcoux B. Tocilizumab for multirefractory adult-onset Still's disease. Ann Rheum Dis 2009;68:153–4.

71. Hagihara K, Kawase I, Tanaka T, et al. Tocilizumab ameliorates clinical symptoms in polymyalgia rheumatica. J Rheumatol 2010;37:1075–6.

72. Kawabata H, Tomosugi N, Kanda J, et al. Anti-interleukin 6 receptor antibody tocilizumab reduces the level of serum hepcidin in patients with multicentric Castleman's disease. Haematologica 2007;92: 857–8.

73. Kluger N, Bessis D, Guillot B. Tocilizumab as a potential treatment in Schnitzler syndrome. Med Hypotheses 2009;72:479–80.

74. Tanaka T, Ogata A, Narazaki M. Tocilizumab for the treatment of rheumatoid arthritis. Expert Rev Clin Immunol 2010;6:843–54.

75. Weidinger S, Gieger C, Rodriguez E, et al. Genome-wide scan on total serum IgE levels identifies FCER1A as novel susceptibility locus. PLoS Genet 2008;4:e1000166.

76. Granada M, Wilk JB, Tuzova M, et al. A genome-wide association study of plasma total IgE concentrations in the Framingham Heart Study. J Allergy Clin Immunol 2012;129:840–5.

77. Esparza-Gordillo J, Weidinger S, Folster-Holst R, et al. A common variant on chromosome 11q13 is associated with atopic dermatitis. Nat Genet 2009;41:596–601.

78. O'Regan GM, Campbell LE, Cordell HJ, et al. Chromosome 11q13.5 variant associated with childhood eczema: an effect supplementary to filaggrin mutations. J Allergy Cin Immunol 2010;125:170–4, e1–2.

79. Barrett JC, Hansoul S, Nicolae DL, et al. Genome-wide association defines more than 30 distinct susceptibility loci for Crohn's disease. Nat Genet 2008;40:955–62.

80. Li X, Ampleford EJ, Howard TD, et al. The C11orf30-LRRC32 region is associated with total serum IgE levels in asthmatic patients. J Allergy Clin Immunol 2012;129:575–8.

81. Gudbjartsson DF, Bjornsdottir US, Halapi E, et al. Sequence variants affecting eosinophil numbers associate with asthma and myocardial infarction. Nat Genet 2009;41:342–7.

82. Rothenberg ME, Spergel JM, Sherrill JD, et al. Common variants at 5q22 associate with pediatric eosinophilic esophagitis. Nat Genet 2010;42: 289–91.

83. Pascual RM, Bleecker ER. Pharmacogenetics of asthma. Curr Opin Pharmacol 2010;10:226–35.

84. Adcock IM, Barnes PJ. Molecular mechanisms of corticosteroid resistance. Chest 2008;134:394–401.

85. Barnes PJ, Adcock IM. Glucocorticoid resistance in inflammatory diseases. Lancet 2009;373:1905–17.

86. Tantisira KG, Lake S, Silverman ES, et al. Corticosteroid pharmacogenetics: association of sequence variants in CRHR1 with improved lung function in asthmatics treated with inhaled corticosteroids. Hum Mol Genet 2004;13:1353–9.

87. Hawkins GA, Lazarus R, Smith RS, et al. The glucocorticoid receptor heterocomplex gene STIP1 is associated with improved lung function in asthmatic subjects treated with inhaled corticosteroids. J Allergy Clin Immunol 2009;123:1376–83. e7.

88. Tantisira KG, Lasky-Su J, Harada M, et al. Genome-wide association between GLCCI1 and response to glucocorticoid therapy in asthma. N Engl J Med 2011;365:1173–83.

89. Lima JJ, Blake KV, Tantisira KG, et al. Pharmacogenetics of asthma. Curr Opin Pulm Med 2009;15: 57–62.

90. Green SA, Turki J, Innis M, et al. Amino-terminal polymorphisms of the human beta 2-adrenergic receptor impart distinct agonist-promoted regulatory properties. Biochemistry 1994;33:9414–9.

91. Green SA, Turki J, Bejarano P, et al. Influence of beta 2-adrenergic receptor genotypes on signal transduction in human airway smooth muscle cells. Am J Respir Crit Care Med 1995;13:25–33.

92. Bleecker ER, Nelson HS, Kraft M, et al. Beta2-receptor polymorphisms in patients receiving

salmeterol with or without fluticasone propionate. Am J Respir Crit Care Med 2010;181:676–87.

93. Bleecker ER, Postma DS, Lawrance RM, et al. Effect of ADRB2 polymorphisms on response to longacting beta2-agonist therapy: a pharmacogenetic analysis of two randomised studies. Lancet 2007;370:2118–25.

94. Israel E, Chinchilli VM, Ford JG, et al. Use of regularly scheduled albuterol treatment in asthma: genotype-stratified, randomised, placebo-controlled cross-over trial. Lancet 2004;364:1505–12.

95. Israel E, Drazen JM, Liggett SB, et al. The effect of polymorphisms of the beta(2)-adrenergic receptor on the response to regular use of albuterol in asthma. Am J Respir Crit Care Med 2000;162:75–80.

96. Wechsler ME, Kunselman SJ, Chinchilli VM, et al. Effect of beta2-adrenergic receptor polymorphism on response to longacting beta2 agonist in asthma (LARGE trial): a genotype-stratified, randomised, placebo-controlled, crossover trial. Lancet 2009; 374:1754–64.

97. Liggett SB, Wagoner LE, Craft LL, et al. The Ile164 beta2-adrenergic receptor polymorphism adversely affects the outcome of congestive heart failure. J Clin Invest 1998;102:1534–9.

98. Hawkins GA, Tantisira K, Meyers DA, et al. Sequence, haplotype, and association analysis of ADRbeta2 in a multiethnic asthma case-control study. Am J Respir Crit Care Med 2006;174:1101–9.

99. Ortega VE, Hastie A, Sadeghnejad A, et al. Rare beta2-adrenergic receptor gene polymorphisms in asthma cases and controls from the Severe Asthma Research Program. Am J Respir Crit Care Med 2011;183:A1357.

100. Corren J, Lemanske RF, Hanania NA, et al. Lebrikizumab treatment in adults with asthma. N Engl J Med 2011;365:1088–98.

101. Wenzel SE, Ind PW, Otulana BA, et al. A phase 2b study of inhaled pitrakinra, an IL-4/IL13 antagonist, successfully identified responder subpopulations of patients with uncontrolled asthma. Am J Respir Crit Care Med 2011;183:A6179.

102. Slager RE, Hawkins GA, Otulana BA, et al. Interleukin 4 receptor polymorphisms predict therapeutic pitrakinra treatment response in moderate to severe asthma. Am J Respir Crit Care Med 2011;183:A6178.

103. Slager RE, Otulana BA, Hawkins GA, et al. Interleukin 4 receptor polymorphisms predict reduction in asthma exacerbations during response to an anti-interleukin 4 alpha receptor antagonist. J Allergy Clin Immunol 2012. [Epub ahead of print].

104. Colilla S, Nicolae D, Pluzhnikov A, et al. Evidence for gene-environment interactions in a linkage study of asthma and smoking exposure. J Allergy Clin Immunol 2003;111:840–6.

105. Jongepier H, Boezen HM, Dijkstra A, et al. Polymorphisms of the ADAM33 gene are associated with accelerated lung function decline in asthma. Clin Exp Allergy 2004;34:757–60.

106. van Diemen CC, Postma DS, Vonk JM, et al. A disintegrin and metalloprotease 33 polymorphisms and lung function decline in the general population. Am J Respir Crit Care Med 2005;172: 329–33.

107. Sadeghnejad A, Ohar JA, Zheng SL, et al. Adam33 polymorphisms are associated with COPD and lung function in long-term tobacco smokers. Respir Res 2009;10:21, e1–9.

108. Ege MJ, Strachan DP, Cookson WO, et al. Gene-environment interaction for childhood asthma and exposure to farming in Central Europe. J Allergy Clin Immunol 2011;127:138–44, 144.e1–4.

109. Khoury MJ, Wacholder S. Invited commentary: from genome-wide association studies to gene-environment-wide interaction studies–challenges and opportunities. Am J Epidemiol 2009;169: 227–30.

110. Ober C, Vercelli D. Gene-environment interactions in human disease: nuisance or opportunity? Trends Genet 2011;27:107–15.

111. Du R, Litonjua AA, Tantisira KG, et al. Genome-wide association study reveals class I MHC-restricted T cell-associated molecule gene (CRTAM) variants interact with vitamin D levels to affect asthma exacerbations. J Allergy Clin Immunol 2012;129:368–73.

112. Bunyavanich S, Boyce JA, Raby BA, et al. Gene-by-environment effect of house dust mite on purinergic receptor P2Y12 (P2RY12) and lung function in children with asthma. Clin Exp Allergy 2012;42: 229–37.

113. Eichler EE, Flint J, Gibson G, et al. Missing heritability and strategies for finding the underlying causes of complex disease. Nat Rev Genet 2010; 11:446–50.

114. Ho SM. Environmental epigenetics of asthma: an update. J Allergy Clin Immunol 2010;126:453–65.

115. Vercelli D. Gene-environment interactions: the road less traveled by in asthma genetics. J Allergy Clin Immunol 2009;123:26–7.

116. Venter JC, Adams MD, Myers EW, et al. The sequence of the human genome. Science 2001; 291:1304–51.

117. Lander ES, Linton LM, Birren B, et al. Initial sequencing and analysis of the human genome. Nature 2001;409:860–921.

118. Haller G, Torgerson DG, Ober C, et al. Sequencing the IL4 locus in African Americans implicates rare noncoding variants in asthma susceptibility. J Allergy Clin Immunol 2009;124: 1204–9, e9.

How to Diagnose and Phenotype Asthma

Parameswaran Nair, MD, PhD, FRCP, FRCPC[a,*], Angira Dasgupta, MD, MRCP (UK)[a], Christopher E. Brightling, MB, PhD, FRCP[b], Kian Fan Chung, MD, DSc, FRCP[c]

KEYWORDS

• Asthma • Phenotyping • Inflammation

KEY POINTS

• The diagnosis of asthma depends on objective measurements of variable airflow obstruction, airway hyperresponsiveness, and airway inflammation.
• Phenotyping of asthma is complex because of the overlap of the various phenotypes, which makes it difficult to recognize a particular phenotype and direct treatment strategies accordingly.
• The authors recommend using clinical and physiologic characteristics combined with the knowledge of biomarkers to guide the treatment of asthma, especially when it is severe, persistent, or refractory.

INTRODUCTION

Asthma is characterized by variable airflow obstruction over short periods of time.[1] It has been defined in current guidelines according to the functional consequences of airway inflammation.[2] Asthma has been described as a chronic disease of the airways characterized by variable airflow obstruction, airway hyperresponsiveness (AHR), and airway inflammation.[2,3] The diagnosis of asthma, therefore, depends on the presence of one or more of these 3 fundamental components of airway diseases[1] and not on the identification of specific causative agents as is true for most other diseases.

The cause of asthma remains unknown. It has been recognized as a heterogeneous disease with complex interactions between genes and the environment. A large number of clinical variants have been described based on causal or exacerbating factors,[4–7] pattern of airflow obstruction,[8–10] clinical presentation,[9,11] severity of disease,[12] pattern of cellular inflammation,[3] and structural changes among patients with asthma of both genders and in all ethnic groups. However, there seems to be considerable overlap among these clinical variants, making accurate and comprehensive phenotyping difficult in asthma.

This review discusses the diagnosis and phenotyping of asthma, with a special emphasis on phenotyping based on the nature of cellular inflammation and radiological imaging and how this could be used to direct the treatment of asthma and, in the future, to apply specifically directed therapies to specifically diagnosed phenotypes.

THE DIAGNOSIS OF ASTHMA

Asthma is often suspected clinically by symptoms, such as chest tightness, cough, wheezes, or episodic breathlessness, which are all nonspecific for the disease. Therefore, a diagnosis of asthma necessitates objective measurements of each of the 3 fundamental components of asthma (**Fig. 1**).[3] However, the relationship between these

Dr Nair is supported by a Canada Research Chair in Airway Inflammometry.
[a] Department of Medicine, St Joseph's Healthcare, McMaster University, 50 Charlton Avenue East, Hamilton, Ontario L8N4A6, Canada; [b] Infection and Inflammation Institute, Glenfield Hospital, University of Leicester, Groby Road, Leicester, LE39QP, UK; [c] National Heart & Lung Institute, Imperial College & NIHR Biomedical Research Unit, Royal Brompton Hospital, Sydney Street, London, SW3 6NP, UK
* Corresponding author. Firestone Institute for Respiratory Health, St Joseph's Healthcare, 50 Charlton Avenue East, Hamilton, Ontario L8N4A6, Canada.
E-mail address: parames@mcmaster.ca

Clin Chest Med 33 (2012) 445–457
http://dx.doi.org/10.1016/j.ccm.2012.05.003
0272-5231/12/$ – see front matter © 2012 Elsevier Inc. All rights reserved

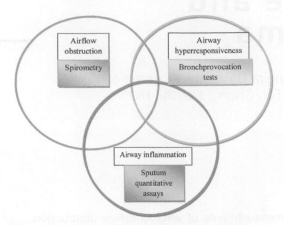

Fig. 1. Diagnosis of the components of asthma.

components is complex and each can occur disso-ciated from the other. Therefore, in asthma, airflow obstruction may occur alone or together with AHR and airway inflammation or bronchitis. In fact, airflow obstruction may even be absent in stable disease.

Variable Airflow Obstruction

The presence of airflow obstruction that is variable over short periods of time and often reversible either spontaneously or with treatment distin-guishes asthma from chronic obstructive pulmo-nary disease (COPD). Airflow obstruction is said to be present when the forced expiratory volume in the first second of expiration (FEV_1)/forced vital capacity ratio is greater than 0.7, whereas revers-ible airflow obstruction is defined as a change of 12% and 200 mL in FEV_1 or peak expiratory flow (PEF) from the prebronchodilator value after the inhalation of a bronchodilator (usually 200–400 mcg of salbutamol).[13,14] The variability of airflow obstruction is usually measured as the variability of the peak flow. Peak flows are measured in the morning prebronchodilator (expected to be lowest) and at night (expected to be higher). The difference between these 2 measurements expressed as a percentage of the mean daily peak flow for the individual is the variability. Often the average over 1 to 2 weeks is used for clinical purposes. Another method of measuring variability of peak flow is by expressing the minimum morning pre-bronchodilator peak flow over a week as a percentage of the recent best value. This method is easier than the former and has been held to be the best index of assessing variability of airflow obstruction in asthma.[15] A diurnal variation in PEF of more than 20% suggests a diagnosis of asthma.[16] Measuring peak flows over periods at work and away from work also help in diagnosing occupational asthma.

AHR

AHR is the limitation of airflow in response to stimuli that would not affect airflow in healthy indi-viduals. The measurement of AHR is more sensi-tive to identify variable airflow limitation than the beta-agonist reversibility of FEV_1 and is needed to validate the diagnosis of asthma when symp-toms raise the possibility of asthma and spirometry is normal.[13,17] It is objectively measured by bron-choprovocation tests, such as the methacholine or histamine challenge test, whereby these bron-choconstrictor agents directly cause airway smooth muscle constriction. Other available methods for bronchoprovocation tests are mannitol, 4.5% hypertonic saline or adenosine monophosphate challenge tests, eucapnic volun-tary hyperpnea (or isocapnic voluntary hyperventi-lation), or exercise challenge tests that provoke bronchoconstriction indirectly by inducing the release of bronchoconstrictor mediators from inflammatory cells or by neural mechanisms. In general, airway responsiveness to methacholine or histamine by the tidal breathing method is more sensitive in demonstrating AHR than the indi-rect methods, and patients with very mild asthma who are well controlled on inhaled corticosteroids may not respond to the indirect test.[18] However, hyperresponsiveness to an appropriate indirect stimulus might be needed to validate asthma when histamine or methacholine responsiveness is normal. An example is when current exercise symptoms are associated with current normal methacholine airway responsiveness.[18] Some-times bronchoprovocation with specific agents is used to diagnose occupational asthma. The prin-ciple of these tests is to expose patients to a graded increase in the concentration of the chal-lenge medication or stimulus and measure the concentration at which a given amount of airflow limitation occurs. In the case of methacholine or the histamine challenge test, the result is usually expressed as the PC20, that is, the provocative concentration that causes a 20% decrease in FEV_1. If the PC20 is less than 2 mg/mL, it indicates severe current airway hyperresponsiveness, whereas values more than 16 mg/mL indicate the absence of current asthma. These tests are, however, only sensitive for a diagnosis of current asthma but lack specificity.[19] Hence, the results of these tests need to be interpreted with caution.[20] When interpreting results that are normal, it is important to appreciate that these only reflect the current status of patients. They do not exclude past asthma, which might have been reversed completely by allergen or occupational sensitizer avoidance, the clearing of infection, or by corticosteroid treatment. If patients with a normal PC20 are symptomatic, it may be from causes other than asthma.[3]

Recently, indirect methods have received a lot of interest because they are more specific to the diagnosis of asthma. The mannitol challenge test is often preferred because of its operational ease.[21] The test has also been reported to be safe and well tolerated.[22] The mannitol dry powder is delivered in progressively increasing doses (0, 5, 10, 20, 40, 80, 160, 160, 160 mg), with FEV_1 measured 1 minute after each dose. A positive response is a 15% decrease in FEV_1 at a total cumulative dose of less than or equal to 635 mg or a 10% decrease in FEV_1 from the baseline between doses.[23] A positive test result to mannitol is consistent with the presence of inflammatory cells (eg, eosinophils or mast cells) and their mediators (eg, prostaglandins, leukotrienes, and histamine) in the airways. Indeed, most patients with mannitol hyperresponsiveness have abnormal fractional exhaled nitric oxide (FeNO), sputum eosinophilia, atopy, and AHR to methacholine. Therefore, this test can confirm a diagnosis of current asthma in treated or untreated patients. A negative test could mean that there is a low number of inflammatory cells or that the bronchial smooth muscles are unresponsive to the mediators as occurs in eosinophilic bronchitic with asthma.[22]

Airway Inflammation

Airway inflammation or bronchitis is thought to be the central component because it is responsible for all the physiologic consequences of asthma.[24] It can be assessed objectively and noninvasively by sputum quantitative assays[3] or by estimating the FeNO. Other measurements in exhaled breath, such as fraction of exhaled carbon monoxide, exhaled breath temperature, and pH, have not been studied as widely as the other tests in clinical trials.[25]

Airway inflammation cannot be estimated by measuring airflow by spirometry and it cannot be surmised clinically. In fact, only a weak association has been observed between airway inflammation and spirometry,[26] and the clinical assessment of the presence or type of cellular bronchitis has been shown to be inaccurate in almost 50% of the times because uncontrolled bronchitis may be present even in the absence of clinical symptoms.[27] Sputum quantitative assays can reflect airway inflammation reliably, specifically, comprehensively, and discriminatively.[28–30] The normal values are also well established.[31] The test entails the selection of a small quantity of sputum from either a spontaneous or induced sample, treatment with dithiothreitol and buffered saline, and the subsequent filtering to obtain a homogenous

suspension of cells. Total cell counts and viability are then determined in a hemocytometer, whereas differential counts are obtained from Wright stained cytospins.[29,32]

The estimation of FeNO has several advantages when used in clinical practice.[33] It is easier, the results are available immediately, and there seems to be a high degree of acceptance by patients. Unlike sputum assays, it does not require a wet laboratory and the expertise of a trained laboratory technician. However, it has been criticized as being not as valid or discriminative as sputum quantitative assays and of having a wide range in healthy individuals.[34] It also does not directly measure bronchitis or correlate with airway eosinophilia in patients with severe prednisone-dependent asthma.[35] FeNO is influenced by many factors[36] other than airway eosinophilia, such as spirometry, smoking, and ingestion of nitrate-containing food or viral infections. Furthermore, FeNO is not able to discriminate between bacterial versus nonbacterial causes of neutrophilic bronchitis. Most importantly, the treatment of asthma guided by algorithms to normalize FeNO has not generally been shown to decrease asthma exacerbations compared with standard guideline-based treatment.[37] Its utility is perhaps limited to situations when patients are unable to produce sufficient sputum for the analysis of cell counts.

PHENOTYPING OF ASTHMA

A phenotype is the outward manifestation of a gene or genes, may involve more than one organ system, and is dynamic, changing over time or in response to the environment.[38] In contrast, genotypes are stable over the lifespan of an individual. The accurate classification of disease phenotypes is important because the information may be used to predict prognosis, select patients for enrollment into clinical trials, personalize treatment, and provide the foundation for studies exploring the pathobiology of disease.

Over the years, many different clinical phenotypes of asthma have been described in the literature. These phenotypes may be classified into broad categories (**Box 1**), such as phenotyping according to causation, differing pattern of airflow obstruction, disease severity, radiologic pattern, and type of airway inflammation. However, there is considerable overlap between the various phenotypes, which often makes it difficult to recognize a particular phenotype and direct treatment strategies accordingly.

Phenotypes According to Causation and Trigger Factors

The earliest attempt to phenotype asthma was probably made by Rackemann[4] who proposed

---

Box 1
Phenotypes of asthma

1. According to causal or trigger factor
- Atopy
- Aspirin
- Infection
- Occupation
- Exercise
- Obesity

2. According to type of airflow obstruction
- Brittle asthma: type1 and 2
- Irreversible/fixed airflow obstruction

3. According to severity and response to treatments
- Mild-moderate asthma
- Severe refractory asthma
- Corticosteroid-insensitive asthma

4. According to radiological findings
- Airway dilatation
- Bronchial wall thickening
- Air trapping

5. According to nature of airway inflammation
- Eosinophilic
- Neutrophilic
- Combined/mixed inflammatory
- Paucigranulocytic

---

classifying asthma into extrinsic and intrinsic based on the presence or absence of allergic sensitization.[4] Later, these phenotypes came to be known as atopic and nonatopic asthma based on the presence or absence of atopy as diagnosed by a positive skin prick test or specific immunoglobulin E (IgE) antibodies against common allergens. However, it is now well known that the mere presence of atopy cannot be used to divide patients with asthma into the allergic and nonallergic phenotypes because of a high prevalence of atopy among nonasthmatics too. The prevalence of atopy in patients with asthma is mainly determined by the prevalence of atopy in the general population.[39] The association between atopy and asthma is weak and both IgE and non-IgE mechanisms have been suggested.

Extrinsic or allergic or atopic asthma are likely to account for slightly more than 50% of the patients with asthma. These patients have early onset disease, are more likely to be men with a positive

family history, have a history of allergies, have a better response to steroids, and a greater FEV_1.[40,41] Paroxysmal sneezing and seasonal rhinorrhea are also more common in atopic asthma. The Third National Health and Nutrition Examination Survey suggested that 4 allergens are associated with most patients with atopic asthma: *Alternaria* spp, cat, and white oak, with an inverse association with perennial rye.[42] When allergic asthma is severe, persistent, and associated with high IgE levels, treatment with omalizumab (anti-IgE) has been shown to be beneficial in reducing exacerbation rates and steroid requirement.[43–45]

Patients with intrinsic or nonatopic asthma, on the other hand, have a late onset of their airway disease, are more likely to be women, do not have a family history of asthma or allergic disease, and have a greater incidence of sinusitis, nasal polyps, and aspirin sensitivity.[40] They tend to have more severe disease and are more commonly triggered by infection, irritants, gastroesophageal reflux disease, and stress.[41]

Other phenotypes of asthma based on causation are aspirin sensitive asthma, occupational asthma, and exercise-induced asthma. The estimated prevalence of aspirin-sensitive asthma varies and is likely to be approximately between 10% and 20% of adult asthma.[46] Aspirin-sensitive asthma, which is characterized by late-onset asthma, nonatopy, and rhinosinusitis, is a severe form of asthma that can be provoked by ingestion of aspirin or nonsteroidal antiinflammatory agents.[5] These patients respond particularly well to leukotriene inhibitors, aspirin desensitization, nasal polypectomy, and topical steroids.

The prevalence of exercise-induced asthma (EIA) varies from 5% to 20%.[47] Various mechanisms have been postulated, including hyperventilation leading to increased irritant and cold, dry air exposure and the subsequent desiccation of the airways.[7,48] These mechanisms may lead to the activation of neutrophils, mast cells, and proinflammatory cytokines, causing significant airway inflammation. Elite athletes seem to have a higher prevalence of symptoms of EIA. Some of these cases may be simply misdiagnosed vocal cord dysfunction presenting soon after exercise with the feeling of obstruction in the throat or inspiratory stridor.[48] There is evidence to suggest the usefulness of the prophylactic β-agonist inhaler, or cromolyn administered 10 to 15 minutes before exercise can also decrease symptoms.[7]

Obesity has also been associated with asthma.[49] However, the relationship between these 2 diseases seems to be complex and may be simply caused by lower lung volumes and their consequent effect on AHR. Larger and longitudinal studies looking at airway inflammation studies and lung volume assessments are required to better address the association of obesity and asthma.

Phenotypes According to Differing Patterns of Airflow Obstruction

Asthma may be phenotyped according to the nature of airflow obstruction as being brittle or associated with irreversible airflow obstruction. Brittle asthma has been described to be of 2 different types.[8,9] Type 1 brittle asthma is asthma that is characterized by a maintained wide PEF variability (>40% diurnal variation for >50% of the time over a period of at least 150 days) despite considerable medical therapy, including a dose of inhaled steroids of at least 1500 µg of beclomethasone (or equivalent), whereas type 2 brittle asthma is characterized by sudden acute attacks occurring in less than 3 hours without an obvious trigger on a background of apparent normal airway function or well-controlled asthma. This finding needs validation.

Fixed or irreversible airflow obstruction in asthma is likely to be caused by airway remodeling and has been observed to be associated with the ADAM33 gene.[50,51] The clinical importance of recognizing this phenotype lies in limiting the overuse of bronchodilators during the treatment of these patients. This characteristic can be most difficult to ascertain because the airflow obstruction may respond minimally to bronchodilators or to corticosteroid therapy. Unless there has been a clear-cut documented history of asthma in the past, these patients may be classified as COPD.

Phenotypes According to Severity of Disease

The phenotype of severe asthma constitutes only about 5% to 10% of the asthma population.[52] However, its impact on the economic burden of asthma is much larger and the reasons for which are obvious. Much work has gone into the definition of patients with severe asthma[12,53]; recently, the phenotypic characterization of severe asthma subgroups has been focused on patients particularly at the severe end of the disease spectrum. It is of interest that these patients are usually characterized as asthma with either 1 of 3 pathophysiological features: the demonstration of variable airflow obstruction, such as daily PEF measurements, reversibility tests with a bronchodilator drug, challenge tests with a bronchoconstrictor agent, or a steroid-sparing trial.[54]

The definitions of severe asthma imply that these patients are less responsive to the therapeutic benefits of corticosteroid therapy and corticosteroid insensitivity or dependence is a feature of many of these patients. This finding has been related to neutrophilic or nonresponsive persistent eosinophilic airway inflammation. The underlying mechanism has been thought to be caused by a relative inefficacy of steroids to inhibit the release of stimulated proinflammatory cytokine release from alveolar macrophages and blood mononuclear cells.[55,56] However, a convenient biomarker for corticosteroid insensitivity is not available. Various other conditions have been associated with corticosteroid insensitivity in asthma, namely obesity, cigarette smoking, and vitamin D deficiency; there is evidence that increased activity of the mitogen-activated protein kinase (MAPK) of the p38 pathway may underlie the pathogenesis of corticosteroid insensitivity in severe asthma, although other mechanisms may also be operative. Transcriptomic studies of peripheral blood mononuclear cells from patients with glucocorticoid-sensitive and glucocorticoid-resistant asthma showed a differential expression pattern of 11 genes, including MAPK phosphatase, nuclear factor kappaB DNA-binding subunit, interleukin 4 (IL-4) receptor, and the signal transducer and activator of transcription 4, that could predict corticosteroid response in patients with asthma with 84% accuracy.[57]

The largest severe-asthma cohort that has been reported is from the Severe Asthma Research Program (SARP), which observed patients with severe asthma as defined by the American Thoracic Society.[12,52] The general characteristics of the patients with severe asthma in this program were older age, longer duration of disease, lower lung function that was responsive to bronchodilators, a history of sinopulmonary infections, persistent symptoms, and increased health care utilization. However, unlike other studies, an association with gender or body mass index was not found.[58,59] Further analyses of this cohort has provided insight into risk factors, including genetic factors and oxidative stress for developing severe asthma, airway inflammation and remodeling and lung-structure function relationships, together with inflammatory biomarker profiles.[57,60–64] One particular aspect that has been studied is the partitioning of chronic airflow obstruction into components of air trapping and airflow limitation.[60] Thus, patients with severe asthma have been observed to have prominent air trapping with increases in total lung capacity and functional reserve capacity.

Radiological Phenotypes

Recent advances in imaging using multidetector-row computed tomography (CT) scanners and postprocessing software for CT images now permits multiplanar reconstructions, 3-dimensional surface and volume images of the airway tree and lung parenchyma, detailed quantitative analysis, and virtual bronchoscopy. Quantitative imaging techniques have given us the ability to obtain direct measurements by 3-dimensional assessment of the large airways and indirect assessment of the small airways by densitometric measures of paired inspiratory and expiratory scans. In addition, CT can now also provide the functional assessment of ventilation and perfusion.

CT assessments of asthma have identified 3 main radiologic phenotypes: bronchiectasis, bronchial wall thickening, and air trapping in asthma. Although a high prevalence of bronchiectasis, bronchial wall thickening, and air trapping have been observed in patients with asthma compared with healthy controls, its clinical significance is not yet completely understood. Both bronchial wall thickening and bronchiectasis in patients with asthma have been associated with longer disease duration[65–68] and poorer lung function.[65,69] However, the association with disease severity was not consistent across all studies.[66,70,71] Whether or not these simply represent a comorbidity in severe asthma resulting in difficult-to-manage asthma or represent structural change or remodeling with natural progression of the disease[72] is not yet known and longitudinal studies are required to ascertain this differentiation. Airway wall thickening has been correlated with airflow limitation,[63,72] airway hyperresponsiveness,[63,73] and air trapping on expiratory CT.

There have also been attempts trying to correlate specific types of airway inflammation to bronchial wall remodeling as assessed by CT scans in a small number of studies. A single study demonstrated an association between bronchoalveolar lavage eosinophil cationic protein levels and airway wall thickening in a childhood severe asthma cohort.[74] The other studies have not shown any association between sputum neutrophils or eosinophils and airway wall geometry.[73,75] It has, however, been observed that although severe asthma and eosinophilic bronchitis both have a similar degree of airway eosinophilic inflammation, patients with eosinophilic bronchitis lacked airway wall thickening with maintained patency of the RB1 lumen area as compared with patients with severe asthma.[73]

Air trapping in asthma is an indirect evidence of small airway disease and has been shown to correlate with asthma severity. Various indices to quantify air trapping in asthma on CT have been developed, including -850 HU attenuation threshold at functional residual capacity,[76] percentage of pixels less than -900 HU in expiratory scans,[77] mean lung density expiratory to inspiratory ratio,[78] difference between inspiratory and expiratory lung attenuation,[79] and median lung attenuation or

lowest 10th percentile lung attenuation frequency distribution.[80] It has been reported[76] that patients with air trapping are significantly more likely to have a history of asthma-related hospitalization and intensive care visits compared with those without air trapping, which suggests that CT-assessed air trapping could potentially be used to identify the at-risk asthma phenotype. CT-assessed air trapping has also been associated with AHR,[78,81] disease duration,[76] airflow limitation,[76–78] and used for the evaluation of the response to inhaled corticosteroid therapy.[79] There is a wide variation of scanning protocols and indices of air trapping used by researchers. Yet, quantitative CT assessment of small airways in asthma will undoubtedly further our understanding of the disease pathogenesis in asthma. Functional magnetic resonance imaging holds promise but its role in phenotyping in asthma has yet to be fully realized. It may provide better insight into the contribution of the small airways and air trapping.

Phenotyping by Nature of Underlying Airway Inflammation

Phenotyping asthma based on the predominant cellular nature of airway infiltrate as assessed by sputum quantitative assays seems to be the most scientific method because it also provides an insight to the underlying pathobiology of the disease. This insight further helps to guide the management of asthma, especially when the disease is severe. According to the predominant type of cell in sputum quantitative assay, asthma may be eosinophilic, neutrophilic, combined (eosinophilic and neutrophilic), and paucigranulocytic. However, it is not necessary that a single patient will belong to one specific phenotype only at all times. It has been observed that the nature of airway inflammation or bronchitis may vary over time in the same patient during successive periods of exacerbations.[82]

Eosinophilic asthma or asthma with eosinophilic bronchitis is the predominant and the most clearly described phenotype. An analysis of a large sputum database has reported the prevalence of eosinophilic bronchitis in stable and exacerbated asthma to be 36% and 35% respectively.[83] Eosinophilic asthma is diagnosed by a raised eosinophil differential count (particularly >3%) and is usually a T-helper 2 (Th2)-driven process. In most cases, the total cell count remains normal unless associated with infection. Sputum eosinophil or the presence of moderate to many eosinophil-free granules predicts steroid responsiveness in asthma.[84,85] This information helps to guide treatment strategies aimed at maintaining the sputum eosinophil count within the normal range. In fact, it has been shown in clinical trials that this strategy is superior to that using the clinical strategy for guiding treatments.[86]

Neutrophilic asthma and its pathobiology is not completely understood. Its prevalence has been estimated to be between 20% and 30% in adults with persistent asthma.[87,88] An increased number of neutrophils has been reported in the airways of patients with severe asthma,[89–91] asthma exacerbations,[92] life-threatening severe asthma exacerbations,[93] and fatal asthma.[94] When asthma is associated with neutrophilic bronchitis (>65% or more neutrophils) with a raised total cell count (>9.7 million cells per gram of sputum), it is likely caused by airway infection (viral or bacterial). An intense neutrophilic bronchitis characterized by more than 50 million cells per gram of sputum and greater than 80% neutrophils points toward a possible bacterial cause because current evidence suggests that infective bronchitis of viral origin is generally milder (neutrophils <80% with a lower total cell count).[95,96] However, this requires further validation in studies designed to identify bacterial or viral organisms by both standard and molecular methods. There seems to be a subset of patients with asthma with neutrophilic bronchitis without identifiable airway infections, and the exact role of neutrophils in this subset of patients has not been established. There is some thought that patients with neutrophilic asthma have been sensitized by irritants, endotoxins, or infection, thus activating innate immunity initially.[97] These patients show an increased expression of toll-like receptor 2, toll-like receptor 4, CD 14, and increased levels of IL-8 (CXCL8), myeloperoxidase, and leukotriene B4 in bronchoalveolar lavage, or induced sputum that is consistent with inflammation from irritants and infection or possibly from high-dose steroids.[97,98] Indeed, eosinophilic bronchitis may sometimes be masked by neutrophilia and it may be helpful in such situations to repeat cell counts after the neutrophilia has resolved.[99] Persistent or recurrent intense neutrophilia might indicate an underlying bronchiectasis.[100] Because possible mechanisms for activation of innate immunity include biofilm formation, endotoxin exposure, or infection with Chlamydia or Mycoplasma spp, it may be reasonable to treat such patients with macrolides.[6]

Asthma with a combination of eosinophilic and neutrophilic airway inflammation may suggest allergic sensitization to fungi, such as Aspergillus associated with bronchiectasis. However, this phenotype has not been extensively looked at. When asthma is associated with a paucigranulocytic or normal sputum, it indicates an absence or controlled airway inflammation. Such patients generally have milder disease.

Phenotyping by Cluster Analysis

Statistical approaches, such as the unsupervised hierarchical cluster analysis, have been used increasingly to identify phenotypes in an unbiased approach. Using 34 qualitative and quantitative clinical and physiologic variables of the SARP cohort that also included nonsevere asthma, 5 clusters were revealed that were differentiated through the age of onset of asthma, baseline lung function, bronchodilator response, and the use of β-agonist medication.[52] Patients with early onset asthma and an allergic background with mild to severe disease constituted 40% of these patients, whereas patients with late-onset asthma, usually nonatopic female patients with reduced FEV_1 and frequent use of oral corticosteroids, formed the rest of the clusters with severe asthma. However, this analysis did not consider the airway inflammatory characteristics of the patients. A cluster analysis that did include sputum quantitative assays reported 3 phenotypes for milder disease: early onset atopic, obese noneosinophilic, and benign. The refractory group had 2 specific clusters: a group showing concordance between eosinophils and symptom expression and a group that did not.[58]

Although these initial analyses have yielded certain specific phenotypes of a clinical nature, this cannot be the final answer because better discriminatory analyses may ensue from the inclusion of other biomarkers of not only inflammation but also those from imaging, transcriptomics, and proteomics. This information should eventually provide a framework for a more comprehensive approach to subject characterization in severe asthma and potentially to better stratified management.

TREATMENT OF ASTHMA ACCORDING TO INFLAMMATORY PHENOTYPES

Treating asthma based on the nature of airway inflammation has been evaluated in clinical trials (**Box 2**). The first step is to identify the presence and the predominant cellular pattern of the airway inflammation.

If the predominant type of cells are eosinophils and the numbers are elevated to more than 3%, treatment is initiated with inhaled corticosteroids if patients are steroid naïve or additional doses of inhaled or ingested steroids are considered if patients are already on treatment. There is a gray area when the counts are between 1% and 3% because a clinical benefit can occur in some patients.[24] It is advisable not to reduce the dose of antiinflammatory therapy if the sputum eosinophils are in this range, even if the patients are

---

Box 2
Treatment titration based on cell counts

Eosinophilic bronchitis

    Less than 1%: consider decreasing dose of inhaled/ingested steroid

    1% to 2%: leave current dose of inhaled/ingested steroid unchanged

    2% to 3%: increase inhaled/ingested steroids if symptomatic

    More than 3%: increase inhaled/ingested steroids even if asthma is clinically controlled

    Persistent eosinophilia less than 3%: exclude other causes and ongoing allergen exposure; consider biologics (anti-IL5)

Neutrophilic bronchitis

    Total cell count (TCC) less than 10×10^6 cells per gram, neutrophils = 65% to 80%: antibiotics not necessary

    TCC 10 to 25×10^6 cells per gram, neutrophils greater than 80%: consider antibiotics

    TCC greater than 25×10^6 cells per gram, neutrophils greater than 80%: antibiotics

    Persistent or recurrent neutrophilia: exclude ongoing environmental exposures, long-term macrolides

Recheck sputum cell counts 4 to 6 weeks after a treatment change

Add long-acting β-agonist after controlling bronchitis if the patient continues to have symptomatic variable airflow obstruction

---

asymptomatic.[101] If sputum eosinophilia is in this grey area and is associated with symptomatic variable airflow obstruction, additional bronchodilators may be considered.

In patients with persistent eosinophilia despite high doses of prednisone, corticosteroid insensitivity should be considered. However, other causes of persistent eosinophilia, such as chronic rhinosinusitis, ongoing allergen exposure, eosinophilic vasculitis, hypereosinophilic syndrome, and chronic eosinophilic pneumonias, should also be looked for. This subset of patients is likely to benefit from novel biologic therapies, like anti-IL-5 (mepolizumab or reslizumab). Indeed, both reslizumab and mepolizumab have been observed to be beneficial in eosinophilic asthma.[102–104] Reslizumab reduced Asthma control questionnaire scores, whereas mepolizumab was successful in reducing the exacerbation rates and the steroid dosage in patients with prednisone-dependent severe asthma. Ramatroban, a chemoattractant receptor-homologous molecule expressed on TH2 cells (CHTR2) antagonist that acts via thromboxane A2–mediated pathways, may inhibit eosinophil trafficking to the lungs and has been observed to reduce AHR in patients with asthma in a single clinical trial.[105] Other novel therapies that are still under investigation for use in eosinophilic asthma are mostly agents targeted at cytokines and chemokines known to mediate airway eosinophilia, such as lebrikizumab (anti-IL-13), anti–receptor for C-C chemokine, and

anti–thymic stromal lymphopoietin. The biomarker periostin has been shown to be predictive of a clinical benefit from lebrikizumab.[106]

In patients treated with inhaled steroid or with prednisone, absent eosinophils suggest that the steroid treatment might be excessive and can be reduced. When the dose is adjusted to keep sputum eosinophils to less than 2% or 3%, eosinophilic exacerbations are reduced without the need for increased steroid treatment.[86] Such monitoring has not been shown to reduce noneosinophilic exacerbations.

Neutrophilic asthma is treated with appropriate antibiotics when there is evidence of bacterial infection as indicated by intense bronchitis with a higher degree of neutrophilia.[96] The clinical implication for isolated neutrophilia is not yet known. When neutrophilia persists or recurs in asthma despite all efforts at identifying and treating infection and patients continue to be symptomatic, long-term macrolide antibiotics may be helpful.[107,108] This latter observation may be related to the altered microbiome of severe asthma or to the antineutrophilic potential of macrolide antibiotics. Antineutrophil agents, like anti-IL-8, have not met with much success in the past. Recently, however, a small molecule antagonist of receptor for cxc chemokine (CXCR2) has been successful in reducing sputum neutrophil numbers in severe asthma with suggestions toward improvement in clinical outcomes.[109] Other ongoing environmental exposures known to cause airway

Table 1
Treatment of asthma according to clinical phenotypes and biomarkers

Clinical Phenotype	Biomarker	Drug
Atopy, reversible airflow obstruction	Serum IgE	Omalizumab
Atopy, mucus hypersecretion, AHR	Serum periostin	Lebrikizumab
Severe asthma, frequent exacerbations	Sputum eosinophils	Mepolizumab, reslizumab
Atopy, rhinosinusitis, aspirin sensitivity, AHR	Sputum eosinophils	Leukotriene receptor antagonist, CRTH2 antagonist (ramatroban)
Severe asthma, AHR	Increased expression of TNFα and TNFαR1 on peripheral blood monocyte	Anti-TNFα (etanercept)
Severe asthma without infections	Sputum neutrophils	Anti-CXCR2

neutrophilia, such as occupational asthma; smoking; and environmental pollution, such as ozone or diesel exhaust particle exposure, should also be considered.

If airway inflammation is absent, there is unlikely to be any benefit from additional steroids or antibiotics. Treatment in such situations should be aimed at improving variable airflow limitation by additional bronchodilators if patients are bronchoconstricted or have AHR. This treatment may not be helpful if the airflow obstruction is irreversible. But this approach requires further validation. Antagonists to tumor necrosis factor (TNF)-α, such as etanercept, may also be beneficial in such situations because it has improved PC20, FEV1, and asthma-related quality of life in severe asthma clinical trials without any effect on sputum eosinophils or neutrophils.[110,111] The clinical response in these studies correlated closely with the expression of TNFα and TNFαR1 on monocytes.[111] However, safety concerns have precluded its further evaluation in asthma clinical trials. The role of bronchial thermoplasty in this specific phenotype of patients with asthma remains to be determined.

It may be seen that treatment of asthma based on a specific type of phenotyping is difficult because the disease is extremely heterogeneous. Personalizing treatment based on the patients' clinical and physiologic characteristics and combining this with the knowledge of biomarkers predictive of clinical response to a particular drug may be the best way to manage patients with severe asthma (**Table 1**).

SUMMARY

The diagnosis of asthma depends on objective measurements of variable airflow obstruction,

AHR and airway inflammation. Phenotyping of asthma is complex because of the overlap of the various phenotypes, which makes it difficult to recognize a particular phenotype and direct treatment strategies accordingly. The authors recommend using clinical and physiologic characteristics combined with the knowledge of biomarkers to guide the treatment of asthma, especially when it is severe, persistent, or refractory.

REFERENCES

1. Hargreave FE, Nair P. The definition and diagnosis of asthma. Clin Exp Allergy 2009;39:1652–8.
2. Global Initiative for Asthma. GINA report, global strategy for asthma management and prevention. Updated December 2011. Available at: http://www.ginasthma.org. Accessed April 4, 2012.
3. Scadding JG. Principles of definition in medicine with special reference to chronic bronchitis and emphysema. Lancet 1959;1:323–5.
4. Rackemann FM. A clinical classification of asthma. Am J Med Sci 1921;12:802–3.
5. Szczeklik A, Stevenson DD. Aspirin-induced asthma: advances in pathogenesis, diagnosis, and management. J Allergy Clin Immunol 2003; 111:913–21 [quiz: 922].
6. MacDowell AL, Bacharier LB. Infectious triggers of asthma. Immunol Allergy Clin North Am 2005;25: 45–66.
7. Weiler JM, Bonini S, Coifman R, et al. American Academy of Allergy, Asthma & Immunology Work Group report: exercise-induced asthma. J Allergy Clin Immunol 2007;119:1349–58.
8. Turner-Warwick M. On observing patterns of airflow obstruction in chronic asthma. Br J Dis Chest 1977; 71:73–86.

9. Ayres JG, Miles JF, Barnes PJ. Brittle asthma. Thorax 1998;53:315–21.

10. Covar RA, Spahn JD, Murphy JR, et al. Progression of asthma measured by lung function in the childhood asthma management program. Am J Respir Crit Care Med 2004;170:234–41.

11. Wenzel SE. Asthma: defining of the persistent adult phenotypes. Lancet 2006;368:804–13.

12. American Thoracic Society. Proceedings of the ATS workshop on refractory asthma: current understanding, recommendations, and unanswered questions. Am J Respir Crit Care Med 2000;162:2341–51.

13. British Thoracic Society Scottish Intercollegiate Guidelines Network. British guideline on the management of asthma. Thorax 2008;63(Suppl 4): iv1–121.

14. Pellegrino R, Viegi G, Brusasco V, et al. Interpretative strategies for lung function tests. Eur Respir J 2005;26(5):948–68.

15. Reddel HK, Salome CM, Peat JK, et al. Which index of peak expiratory flow is most useful in the management of stable asthma? Am J Respir Crit Care Med 1995;151(5):1320–5.

16. Dekker FW, Schrier AC, Sterk PJ, et al. Validity of peak expiratory flow measurement in assessing reversibility of airflow obstruction. Thorax 1992; 47(3):162–6.

17. Ryan G, Latimer KM, Dolovich J, et al. Bronchial responsiveness to histamine: relationship to diurnal variation of peak flow rate, improvement after bronchodilator and airway caliber. Thorax 1982;37: 423–9.

18. Cockcroft DW, Davis BE. Diagnostic and therapeutic value of airway challenges in asthma. Curr Allergy Asthma Rep 2009;9:247–53.

19. Cockcroft DW, Murdock KY, Berscheid BA, et al. Sensitivity and specificity of histamine PC20 determination in a random selection of young college students. J Allergy Clin Immunol 1992;89(1 Pt 1): 23–30.

20. Boulet LP. Asymptomatic airway hyperresponsiveness: a curiosity or an opportunity to prevent asthma? Am J Respir Crit Care Med 2003;167(3): 371–8.

21. Anderson SD, Brannan J, Spring J, et al. A new method for bronchial-provocation testing in asthmatic subjects using a dry powder of mannitol. Am J Respir Crit Care Med 1997;156(3 Pt 1): 758–65.

22. Brannan JD, Anderson SD, Perry CP, et al. The safety and efficacy of inhaled dry powder mannitol as a bronchial provocation test for airway hyperresponsiveness: a phase 3 comparison study with hypertonic (4.5%) saline. Respir Res 2005;6:144.

23. Anderson SD. Indirect challenge tests: airway hyperresponsiveness in asthma: its measurement and clinical significance. Chest 2010;138(Suppl 2): 25S–30S.

24. Nair P, Hargreave FE. Measuring bronchitis in airway diseases: clinical implementation and application: airway hyperresponsiveness in asthma: its measurement and clinical significance. Chest 2010;138(Suppl 2):38S–43S.

25. Hunt J. Exhaled breath condensate: an evolving tool for noninvasive evaluation of lung disease. J Allergy Clin Immunol 2002;110(1):28–34.

26. Rosi E, Ronchi MC, Grazzini M, et al. Sputum analysis, bronchial hyperresponsiveness and airway function in asthma: results of a factor analysis. J Allergy Clin Immunol 1999;103:232–7.

27. Parameswaran K, Pizzichini E, Pizzichini MM, et al. Clinical judgment of airway inflammation versus sputum cell counts in patients with asthma. Eur Respir J 2000;15:486–90.

28. Nair PK, Hargreave FE. Airway diseases, inflammometry and individualized therapy. In: Holgate ST, Polosa R, editors. Therapeutic strategies in asthma: current treatments. Oxford (England): Clinical Publishing; 2007. p. 155–64.

29. Pizzichini E, Pizzichini MM, Efthimiadis A, et al. Indices of airway inflammation in induced sputum: reproducibility and validity of cell and fluid-phase measurements. Am J Respir Crit Care Med 1996; 154(2 Pt 1):308–17.

30. Lemière C, Ernst P, Olivenstein R, et al. Airway inflammation assessed by invasive and noninvasive means in severe asthma: eosinophilic and noneosinophilic phenotypes. J Allergy Clin Immunol 2006;118(5):1033–9.

31. Belda J, Leigh R, Nair P, et al. Induced sputum cell counts in healthy adults. Am J Respir Crit Care Med 2000;161:475–8.

32. Kelly MM, Efthimiadis A, Hargreave FE. Induced sputum: selection method. In: Rogers DF, Donnelly LE, editors. Methods in molecular medicine. Human airway inflammation: sampling techniques and analytical protocols. London: Humana Press; 2001. p. 77–92.

33. Pendharkar S, Mehta S. The clinical significance of exhaled nitric oxide in asthma. Can Respir J 2008; 15:99–106.

34. Taylor DR, Pijnenburg MW, Smith AD. Exhaled nitric oxide measurements: clinical application and interpretation. Thorax 2006;61(9):817–27.

35. Nair P, Kjarsgaard M, Armstrong S, et al. Fraction of exhaled nitric oxide does not correlate with eosinophils in sputum in prednisone-dependent asthma. J Allergy Clin Immunol 2010;126(2):404–6.

36. Spitale N, Popat N, McIvor A. Update on exhaled nitric oxide in pulmonary disease. Expert Rev Respir Med 2012;6(1):105–15.

37. Smith AD, Cowan JO, Brassell KP, et al. Use of exhaled nitric oxide measurements to guide

treatment in chronic asthma. N Engl J Med 2005; 352:2163–73.

38. Schulze TG, McMahon FJ. Defining the phenotype in human genetic studies: forward genetics and reverse phenotyping. Hum Hered 2004;58: 131–8.

39. Ronchetti R, Jesenak M, Rennerova Z, et al. Relationship between atopic asthma and the population prevalence rates for asthma or atopy in children: atopic and nonatopic asthma in epidemiology. Allergy Asthma Proc 2009;30(1):55–63.

40. Romanet-Manent S, Charpin D, Magnan A, et al. Allergic vs nonallergic asthma: what makes the difference? Allergy 2002;57:607–13.

41. Novak N, Bieber T. Allergic and nonallergic forms of atopic diseases. J Allergy Clin Immunol 2003; 112:252–62.

42. Arbes SJ Jr, Gergen PJ, Vaughn B, et al. Asthma cases attributable to atopy: results from the Third National Health and Nutrition Examination Survey. J Allergy Clin Immunol 2007;120:1139–45.

43. Busse W, Corren J, Lanier BQ, et al. Omalizumab, anti-IgE recombinant humanized monoclonal antibody, for the treatment of severe allergic asthma. J Allergy Clin Immunol 2001;108:184–90.

44. Solèr M, Matz J, Townley R, et al. The anti-IgE antibody omalizumab reduces exacerbations and steroid requirement in allergic asthmatics. Eur Respir J 2001;18:254–61.

45. Humbert M, Beasley R, Ayres J, et al. Benefits of omalizumab as add-on therapy in patients with severe persistent asthma who are inadequately controlled despite best available therapy (GINA 2002 step 4 treatment): INNOVATE. Allergy 2005; 60:309–16.

46. Szczeklik A, Sanak M. The broken balance in aspirin hypersensitivity. Eur J Pharmacol 2006; 533:145–55.

47. Handoyo S, Rosenwasser LJ. Asthma phenotypes. Curr Allergy Asthma Rep 2009;9(6):439–45.

48. Fitch KD, Sue-Chu M, Anderson SD, et al. Asthma and the elite athlete: summary of the International Olympic Committee's consensus conference, Lausanne, Switzerland, January 22–24, 2008. J Allergy Clin Immunol 2008;122:254–60, 260.e1–7.

49. Jensen ME, Wood LG, Gibson PG. Obesity and childhood asthma - mechanisms and manifestations. Curr Opin Allergy Clin Immunol 2012;12(2): 186–92.

50. Canonica GW. Treating asthma as an inflammatory disease. Chest 2006;130(Suppl 1):21S–8S.

51. Lee JY, Park SW, Chang HK, et al. A disintegrin and metalloproteinase 33 protein in patients with asthma: relevance to airflow limitation. Am J Respir Crit Care Med 2006;173:729–35.

52. Moore WC, Bleecker ER, Curran-Everett D, et al. Characterization of the severe asthma phenotype by the National Heart, Lung, and Blood Institute's Severe Asthma Research Program. J Allergy Clin Immunol 2007;119:405–13.

53. Chung KF, Godard P, Adelroth E, et al. Difficult/therapy-resistant asthma: the need for an integrated approach to define clinical phenotypes, evaluate risk factors, understand pathophysiology and find novel therapies. ERS Task Force on Difficult/Therapy-Resistant Asthma. European Respiratory Society. Eur Respir J 1999;13(5): 1198–208.

54. Bel EH, Sousa A, Fleming L, et al. Unbiased Biomarkers for the Prediction of Respiratory Disease Outcome (U-BIOPRED) Consortium, Consensus Generation. Diagnosis and definition of severe refractory asthma: an international consensus statement from the Innovative Medicine Initiative (IMI). Thorax 2011;66(10):910–7.

55. Bhavsar P, Hew M, Khorasani N, et al. Relative corticosteroid insensitivity of alveolar macrophages in severe asthma compared with non-severe asthma. Thorax 2008;63(9):784–90.

56. Hew M, Bhavsar P, Torrego A, et al. Relative corticosteroid insensitivity of peripheral blood mononuclear cells in severe asthma. Am J Respir Crit Care Med 2006;174(2):134–41.

57. Hakonarson H, Bjornsdottir US, Halapi E, et al. Profiling of genes expressed in peripheral blood mononuclear cells predicts glucocorticoid sensitivity in asthma patients. Proc Natl Acad Sci U S A 2005;102(41):14789–94.

58. Haldar P, Pavord ID, Shaw DE, et al. Cluster analysis and clinical asthma phenotypes. Am J Respir Crit Care Med 2008;178(3):218–24.

59. Lessard A, Turcotte H, Cormier Y, et al. Obesity and asthma: a specific phenotype? Chest 2008;134: 317–23.

60. Sorkness RL, Bleecker ER, Busse WW, et al. Lung function in adults with stable but severe asthma: air trapping and incomplete reversal of obstruction with bronchodilation. J Appl Physiol 2008;104(2): 394–403.

61. Wenzel SE, Balzar S, Ampleford E, et al. IL4R Alpha mutations are associated with asthma exacerbations and mast Cell/IgE expression. Am J Respir Crit Care Med 2007;175(6):570–6.

62. Li X, Howard TD, Moore WC, et al. Importance of hedgehog interacting protein and other lung function genes in asthma. J Allergy Clin Immunol 2011;127(6):1457–65.

63. Aysola RS, Hoffman EA, Gierada D, et al. Airway remodeling measured by multidetector CT is increased in severe asthma and correlates with pathology. Chest 2008;134(6):1183–91.

64. Hastie AT, Moore WC, Meyers DA, et al. Analyses of asthma severity phenotypes and inflammatory proteins in subjects stratified by

sputum granulocytes. J Allergy Clin Immunol 2010;125(5):1028–36.

65. British Thoracic Society. British guideline on the management of asthma - A national clinical guideline. Thorax 2008;63(Suppl 4):iv1–121.

66. Gupta S, Siddiqui S, Haldar P, et al. Qualitative analysis of high-resolution CT scans in severe asthma. Chest 2009;136(6):1521–8.

67. Grenier P, Mourey-Gerosa I, Benali K, et al. Abnormalities of the airways and lung parenchyma in asthmatics: CT observations in 50 patients and inter- and intraobserver variability. Eur Radiol 1996;6(2):199–206.

68. Lynch DA, Newell JD, Tschomper BA, et al. Uncomplicated asthma in adults: comparison of CT appearance of the lungs in asthmatic and healthy subjects. Radiology 1993;188(3):829–33.

69. Bumbacea D, Campbell D, Nguyen L, et al. Parameters associated with persistent airflow obstruction in chronic severe asthma. Eur Respir J 2004;24(1): 122–8.

70. Paganin F, Seneterre E, Chanez P, et al. Computed tomography of the lungs in asthma: influence of disease severity and etiology. Am J Respir Crit Care Med 1996;153(1):110–4.

71. Yilmaz S, Ekici A, Ekici M, et al. High-resolution computed tomography findings in elderly patients with asthma. Eur J Radiol 2006;59(2):238–43.

72. Niimi A, Matsumoto H, Amitani R, et al. Airway wall thickness in asthma assessed by computed tomography. Relation to clinical indices. Am J Respir Crit Care Med 2000;162(4 Pt 1):1518–23.

73. Siddiqui S, Gupta S, Cruse G, et al. Airway wall geometry in asthma and nonasthmatic eosinophilic bronchitis. Allergy 2009;64(6):951–8.

74. de Blic J, Tillie-Leblond I, Emond S, et al. High-resolution computed tomography scan and airway remodeling in children with severe asthma. J Allergy Clin Immunol 2005;116(4):750–4.

75. Little SA, Sproule MW, Cowan MD, et al. High resolution computed tomographic assessment of airway wall thickness in chronic asthma: reproducibility and relationship with lung function and severity. Thorax 2002;57(3):247–53.

76. Busacker A, Newell JD Jr, Keefe T, et al. A multivariate analysis of risk factors for the air-trapping asthmatic phenotype as measured by quantitative CT analysis. Chest 2009;135(1):48–56.

77. Newman KB, Lynch DA, Newman LS, et al. Quantitative computed tomography detects air trapping due to asthma. Chest 1994;106(1):105–9.

78. Gono H, Fujimoto K, Kawakami S, et al. Evaluation of airway wall thickness and air trapping by HRCT in asymptomatic asthma. Eur Respir J 2003;22(6): 965–71.

79. Tunon-de-Lara JM, Laurent F, Giraud V, et al. Air trapping in mild and moderate asthma: effect of

inhaled corticosteroids. J Allergy Clin Immunol 2007;119(3):583–90.

80. Goldin JG, McNitt-Gray MF, Sorenson SM, et al. Airway hyperreactivity: assessment with helical thin-section CT. Radiology 1998;208(2):321–9.

81. Ueda T, Niimi A, Matsumoto H, et al. Role of small airways in asthma: investigation using high-resolution computed tomography. J Allergy Clin Immunol 2006;118(5):1019–25.

82. D'silva L, Cook RJ, Allen CJ, et al. Changing types of bronchitis during successive exacerbations of airway disease. Respir Med 2007;101: 2217–20.

83. D'silva L, Hassan N, Wang HY, et al. Heterogeneity of bronchitis in airway diseases in tertiary care clinical practice. Can Respir J 2011;18(3):144–8.

84. Green RH, Brightling CE, McKenna S, et al. Asthma exacerbations and sputum eosinophil counts: a randomised controlled trial. Lancet 2002; 360(9347):1715–21.

85. Pizzichini MM, Pizzichini E, Clelland L, et al. Sputum in severe exacerbations of asthma: kinetics of inflammatory indices after prednisone treatment. Am J Respir Crit Care Med 1997; 155(5):1501–8.

86. Jayaram L, Pizzichini MM, Cook RJ, et al. Determining asthma treatment by monitoring sputum cell counts: effect on exacerbations. Eur Respir J 2006;27(3):483–94.

87. Simpson JL, Scott R, Boyle MJ, et al. Inflammatory subtypes in asthma: assessment and identification using induced sputum. Respirology 2006;11(1): 54–61.

88. Green RH, Brightling CE, Woltmann G, et al. Analysis of induced sputum in adults with asthma: identification of subgroup with isolated sputum neutrophilia and poor response to inhaled corticosteroids. Thorax 2002;57:875–9.

89. The ENFUMOSA cross-sectional European multicentre study of the clinical phenotype of chronic severe asthma. European Network for Understanding Mechanisms of Severe Asthma. Eur Respir J 2003;22:470–7.

90. Jatakanon A, Uasuf C, Maziak W, et al. Neutrophilic inflammation in severe persistent asthma. Am J Respir Crit Care Med 1999;160:1532–9.

91. Gibson PG, Simpson JL, Saltos N. Heterogeneity of airway inflammation in persistent asthma. Chest 2001;119:1329–36.

92. Fahy JV, Kim KW, Liu J, et al. Prominent neutrophilic inflammation in sputum from subjects with asthma exacerbation. J Allergy Clin Immunol 1995;95:843–52.

93. Lamblin C, Gosset P, Tillie-Leblond I, et al. Bronchial neutrophilia in patients with noninfectious status asthmaticus. Am J Respir Crit Care Med 1998;157:394–402.

94. Carroll N, Carello S, Cooke C, et al. Airway structure and inflammatory cells in fatal attacks of asthma. Eur Respir J 1996;9:709–15.

95. Wark PA, Johnston SL, Moric I, et al. Neutrophil degranulation and cell lysis is associated with clinical severity in virus-induced asthma. Eur Respir J 2002;19(1):68–75.

96. Pizzichini MM, Pizzichini E, Efthimiadis A, et al. Asthma and natural colds. Inflammatory indices in induced sputum: a feasibility study. Am J Respir Crit Care Med 1998;158(4):1178–84.

97. Simpson JL, Grissell TV, Douwes J, et al. Innate immune activation in neutrophilic asthma and bronchiectasis. Thorax 2007;62(3):211–8.

98. Borish L, Culp JA. Asthma: a syndrome composed of heterogeneous diseases. Ann Allergy Asthma Immunol 2008;101:1–8 [quiz: 8–11, 50].

99. D'silva L, Allen CJ, Hargreave FE, et al. Sputum neutrophilia can mask eosinophilic bronchitis during exacerbations. Can Respir J 2007;14(5):281–4.

100. Drost N, D'silva L, Rebello R, et al. Persistent sputum cellularity and neutrophils may predict bronchiectasis. Can Respir J 2011;18(4):221–4.

101. Belda J, Parameswaran K, Lemière C, et al. Predictors of loss of asthma control induced by corticosteroid withdrawal. Can Respir J 2006; 13(3):129–33.

102. Castro M, Mathur S, Hargreave F, et al, Res-5-0010 Study Group. Reslizumab for poorly controlled, eosinophilic asthma: a randomized, placebo-controlled study. Am J Respir Crit Care Med 2011;184(10):1125–32.

103. Nair P, Pizzichini MM, Kjarsgaard M, et al. Mepolizumab for prednisone-dependent asthma with sputum eosinophilia. N Engl J Med 2009;360(10):985–93.

104. Haldar P, Brightling CE, Hargadon B, et al. Mepolizumab and exacerbations of refractory eosinophilic asthma. N Engl J Med 2009;360:973–84.

105. Aizawa H, Shigyo M, Nogami H, et al. BAY u3405, a thromboxane A2 antagonist, reduces bronchial hyperresponsiveness in asthmatics. Chest 1996; 109:338–42.

106. Corren J, Lemanske RF, Hanania NA, et al. Lebrikizumab treatment in adults with asthma. N Engl J Med 2011;365(12):1088–98.

107. Hatipoglu U, Rubinstein I. Low-dose, long-term macrolide therapy in asthma: an overview. Clin Mol Allergy 2004;2(1):4.

108. Simpson JL, Powell H, Boyle MJ, et al. Clarithromycin targets neutrophilic airway inflammation in refractory asthma. Am J Respir Crit Care Med 2008;177(2):148–55.

109. Nair P, Gaga M, Zervas E, et al. Safety and efficacy of a CXCR2 antagonist in patients with severe asthma and sputum neutrophils: a randomized, placebo-controlled clinical trial. Clin Exp 2012;42:1097–103.

110. Howarth PH, Babu KS, Arshad HS, et al. Tumour necrosis factor (TNFalpha) as a novel therapeutic target in symptomatic corticosteroid dependent asthma. Thorax 2005;60(12):1012–8.

111. Berry MA, Hargadon B, Shelley M, et al. Evidence of a role of tumor necrosis factor alpha in refractory asthma. N Engl J Med 2006;354(7):697–708.

Biomarkers in Asthma
A Real Hope to Better Manage Asthma

Serpil C. Erzurum, MD[a],*, Benjamin M. Gaston, MD[b]

KEYWORDS

- Asthma • Biomarkers • Asthma management

KEY POINTS

- Diagnosis and treatment of asthma are currently based on assessment of patient symptoms and physiologic tests of airway reactivity.
- This article provides an overview of blood, urine and airway biomarkers that can provide information on airway inflammation and asthma severity.
- Mechanistic biomarkers that identify pathologic pathways also provide critical insight for new therapeutic approaches for asthma.

THE CLINICAL NEED FOR BIOMARKERS TO INFORM THE CARE OF PATIENTS WITH ASTHMA

Asthma is defined as reversible airflow obstruction in the setting of airway inflammation. Asthma prevalence increased dramatically between 1970 and 2000, with more than 22 million people, of whom over 4.8 million are children, now living with asthma in the United States.[1,2] The increase of asthma has been variously ascribed to improved hygiene worldwide, acetaminophen use, increased exposure to allergens and pollution, and/or increased transmission of respiratory viruses.[3] This epidemic has occurred against a backdrop of a variety of genetic, biochemical, and immunologic host characteristics that substantially affect asthma phenotype.

Currently, standard clinical practice relies on patient history of symptoms and the measure of bronchial obstruction and reactivity, which are surrogates of the inflammatory and biochemical processes that give rise to the inflammation underlying all asthma.[4] For example, the phenotype of severe asthma, which comprises up to 5% of patients with asthma, is based on a compilation of criteria, the most important of which is the documentation of the lack of clinical treatment response.[5,6] Asthma treatment is directed equally toward reversing bronchoconstriction and treating airway inflammation. Common, noninvasive measures of airflow are usually able to quantitate the efficacy of the treatment of bronchoconstriction in adults. However, commonly available methods do not precisely measure the biology of inflammation underlying the bronchoconstriction. Further, the care of children with asthma is often inadequate because of the lack of bronchial obstruction on lung function tests even when symptoms are severe, and the reluctance to prescribe corticosteroids because of actual or perceived associated morbidities in children.[7] Thus, quantifiable noninvasive biomarkers that are informative for asthma control and, optimally, for assessing

Funding sources: Dr Erzurum: National Heart Lung Blood Institute, American Asthma Foundation, Cardiovascular Medical Research Education Foundation, and Asthmatx Inc. Dr Gaston: National Heart Lung and Blood Institute: P01HL101871; U10HL109250; R01 HL59337.
Conflict of interests: Dr Erzurum: None. Dr Gaston: Intellectual property and minority shareholder in Respiratory Research, Inc, and In Airbase Pharmaceuticals. Intellectual property in N30 Pharma.
[a] Department of Pathobiology, Lerner Research Institute, and the Respiratory Institute, Cleveland Clinic Lerner College of Medicine-CWRU, 9500 Euclid Avenue, NC22, Cleveland, OH 44195-0001, USA; [b] Department of Pediatric Pulmonary Medicine, University of Virginia School of Medicine, Box 800386, UVA HSC, Charlottesville, VA 22908, USA
* Corresponding author.
E-mail address: erzurus@ccf.org

Clin Chest Med 33 (2012) 459–471
http://dx.doi.org/10.1016/j.ccm.2012.06.007
0272-5231/12/$ – see front matter © 2012 Elsevier Inc. All rights reserved.

the pathobiologic pathways leading to the chronic airway inflammation in a specific patient will be of clinical utility in designing successful personalized treatment plans.

Based on this rationale, the National Institutes of Health and the Agency for Health Care Quality Research have launched efforts to promote the use of biomarkers in clinical studies of new therapies of asthma and ultimately in the evaluation of routine clinical care. A recent National Heart, Lung, and Blood Institute (NHLBI) report identifies biomarkers, most of which assess atopic inflammation, such as the multiallergen screen, sputum and blood eosinophil numbers, serum IgE, exhaled nitric oxide, and urine leukotrienes.[8] Although asthma tends to be particularly problematic in patients with allergies, and more than 40% of some populations suffer from allergies, allergic diathesis genes do not seem to be uniquely associated with asthma.[2,6,9] Thus, whatever is driving the asthma epidemic, the asthma syndrome has affected a tremendous spectrum of individuals with diverse immunologic and biochemical responses.[9,10] This heterogeneity in the human population has resulted in a heterogeneity among asthma phenotypes.[10–12] Therefore, biomarker tests were recently developed and extended to identify and quantitate specific pathways of inflammation to identify specific asthma phenotypes, particularly those amenable to biologically based antiinflammatory therapy. The benefit of a noninvasive biomarker in assessing therapeutic strategies is clear; the alternative is inspection and biopsy of the airway using invasive bronchoscopy.[13]

The mechanism-based biomarker approach avoids the limitations that occur with unbiased genotyping and phenotyping approaches.[10] For example, unbiased genetic analyses did not reveal a unifying asthma gene. Rather, asthma susceptibility genes are manifest in populations depending on environmental exposures, such as secondhand cigarette smoke.[14] Similarly, unbiased asthma clinical phenotypes, although clearly revealing the heterogeneity of asthma,[15] require association with underlying pathobiologic mechanisms for clinically meaningful use. In a large asthma population of nonsevere and severe asthma, nonbiased hierarchical cluster analysis of clinical variables, such as age at asthma onset, duration of episodes, gender, race, lung functions, atopy, and questionnaire data, identified three phenotype clusters that contained patients with the most severe asthma.[15] Similar cluster analyses of children confirmed heterogeneity in childhood severe asthma.[16] This variety supports that asthma encompasses a range of underlying biochemical

and immunologic disorders. Thus, an informed biochemical and pathophysiologic approach is most likely to lead directly to clinical applications. This article describes biomarkers and their potential use to stratify patients into medically meaningful unique asthma phenotypes (**Table 1**).

THE EOSINOPHILIC OR T-HELPER TYPE 2 HIGH INFLAMMATION PHENOTYPE: SPUTUM EOSINOPHILS, URINARY 3-BROMOTYROSINE, AND PERIOSTIN

Asthma phenotyping was first performed based on atopic status (ie, classification of asthma as extrinsic allergic or intrinsic nonallergic).[9] Allergic asthma is common, and documentation of this phenotype has been helpful in avoiding allergen triggers and considering immunologic-based therapies. Classification as atopic asthma, which is typified by interleukin (IL)-4, IL-5, and IL-13 cytokines, has traditionally used standard clinical tests, including circulating numbers of eosinophils and total and allergen-specific IgE. These biomarkers are used in planning immunotherapy and anti-IgE therapy. In extension of these biomarkers, several groups describe that the number of eosinophils in sputum is closely related to airway obstruction and hyperresponsiveness.[17–19] Exciting early data suggested that sputum eosinophils predict asthma control and loss of control, particularly in children who predominantly experience atopic asthma.[20,21] The presence of more than 2% eosinophils in sputum has been used to define the eosinophilic or atopic asthma phenotype, which is also usually corticosteroid-responsive.[22] A recent study of severe asthma validates that sputum eosinophils can identify individuals with poor asthma control, and greater health care use[23]; however, the test requires sputum induction, specialized processing of the sputum sample, and an experienced cytotechnologist for accurate counting, all of which have limited the use of sputum eosinophils in general clinical care. More recently, Woodruff and colleagues[24] further identified a T-helper type 2 (Th2)–high inflammation phenotype based on a combination of biomarkers, which include the presence of high serum IgE (>100 ng/mL), blood eosinophilia (>0.14 x 10^9 eosinophils/L), and high sputum eosinophils.[25] The use of microarrays has also identified a Th2-high blood biomarker, periostin, which is an IL-13–inducible protein produced by the airway epithelium. The use of periostin as a biomarker of the Th2-high phenotype to select patients who benefitted the most from treatment with an inhibitor of IL-13[25] provided a proof of concept that biomarkers may be used to stratify patients for

Table 1
Biomarkers of asthma

Biomarker Phenotype	Pathogenetic Pathways	Implications for Mechanistic Management
In blood		
Eosinophils[a]	Atopic; excessive Th2 pathways activation	Immunotherapy depending on clinical signs and symptoms of asthma
IgE[a]	Atopic; excessive Th2 pathways activation	Immunotherapy depending on clinical signs and symptoms of asthma
Allergen specific IgE[a]	Atopic; excessive Th2 pathways activation	Avoidance of allergens, immunotherapy, anti-IgE therapies
Periostin	IL-13–driven asthma (Th2 pathway gene)	May benefit from biologic blockade of IL-4/IL-13 receptors
Superoxide dismutase (SOD)	Oxidative and nitrative inflammation and injury leading to reducing-oxidizing (redox) imbalance and loss of SOD activity	Associated with greater airflow obstruction and bronchial hyperreactivity; evaluate environmental oxidative exposures, such as secondhand smoke and air pollutants; may benefit from redox regulation in the future
$CD34^+CD133^+$ progenitor cells	Circulating myeloid progenitors are increased in asthma, and increase further with exacerbations; differentiate into proangiogenic monocytic cells and mast cells in the airway	Promote remodeling and inflammation in the airway; anti-cKIT–directed therapies to decrease bone marrow precursors
Airway-derived		
Sputum eosinophils	Atopic asthma; excessive Th2 pathways activation	Avoidance of allergens, Immunotherapy, anti-IgE therapies
Exhaled NO (FeNO)[a]	High: excessive iNOS; when used with GSNO challenge, may indicate greater GSNO reductase or low pH	Risk for exacerbation; may need to step up antiinflammatory therapies (eg, corticosteroids decrease iNOS)
	Low or normal: limited arginine bioavailability because of consumption by arginases (activated by Th2 cytokines) or competition by methylarginines (when dimethylarginine dimethylamino hydrolase [DDAH] activity is low)	Metabolic abnormalities in arginine metabolism
Exhaled breath condensate (EBC) pH and formate	Airway acidification because of infection, low airway glutaminase, or, when formate is high, greater activity of GSNO reductase	Buffered solutions and/or glutamine inhalation
Ethyl nitrite challenge and measure of FeNO	High GSNO reductase in the airway, low levels of GSNO (loss of bronchodilator response)	Therapies to block GSNO reductase or supplement beneficial S-nitrosothiols in the airways
In urine		
Bromotyrosine (BrY)	Activation of eosinophil peroxidase for specific bromination pathways	Unstable asthma, predicts exacerbations, particularly in children; step up of antiinflammatory therapy (ie, corticosteroids)
Leukotriene E_4 (LTE$_4$)	Cysteinyl leukotriene pathway overactivity	Aspirin avoidance and/or desensitization; leukotriene receptor or 5-lipoxygenase inhibition
F2 isoprostanes (F2IsoP)	Nonspecific peroxidation of membrane lipids to generate F2IsoP (8-epi-PGF$_{2\alpha}$ and 2,3-dinor-8-epi-PGF$_{2\alpha}$) through excessive generation of reactive oxygen species	Nonspecific inflammation by neutrophils or eosinophils; evaluate environmental oxidative exposures, such as secondhand smoke and air pollutants; may benefit from leukotriene receptor or 5-lipoxygenase inhibition

Abbreviations: GSNO, S-nitrosoglutathione; IL, interleukin; iNOS, inducible nitric oxide synthase; NO, nitric oxide; Th2, T-helper type 2.

[a] Currently readily available to general practitioners and approved for asthma evaluation, others are not generally available or are emerging or experimental.

biologic-based therapies. Conversely, the data also validate the important point that a substantial number of patients with asthma have non–Th2-predominant inflammation.

A high sputum eosinophil count correlates with a high fractional excretion of NO (FeNO) in the exhaled breath, which is often suggested as a biomarker of inflammation. However, low FeNO has been found to be a much better predictor of a noneosinophilic phenotype than a high FeNO is for an eosinophilic phenotype. Hence, FeNO should be considered as a unique metabolic biomarker of asthma, as discussed later. However, eosinophils generate high levels of reactive oxygen species,[26] and the eosinophil peroxidase is unique in its ability to convert hydrogen peroxide to hypobromous acid,[27,28] which oxidizes tyrosines to 3-bromotyrosine (BrY) (**Fig. 1**). BrY is highly stable and can be measured noninvasively in urine as a biomarker highly specific for eosinophil activation.[29,30] Because BrY is a biomarker

of eosinophil activation, its levels increase dramatically after experimental or clinical asthma exacerbations,[29] and early studies show that urinary BrY in children with asthma seems highly correlated with asthma control and predicts risk of asthma exacerbations.[31] Studies are needed to evaluate the relationship of BrY and periostin in the Th2-high phenotype, but given that BrY is unrelated to IgE or blood eosinophils, these biomarkers may be nonredundant and possibly complementary in predicting asthma phenotypes for clinical treatments.

A subpopulation of patients with asthma has increased activity of the enzyme S-nitrosoglutathione (GSNO) reductase (see **Fig. 1**).[32–34] GSNO is an endogenous nitric oxide synthase (NOS) product that causes cyclic guanosine monophosphate (cGMP)–independent relaxation of human airway smooth muscle.[35,36] It can directly prevent actin-myosin interaction[37] and can S-nitrosylate G protein–coupled kinase 2 (GRK2), tachyphylaxis

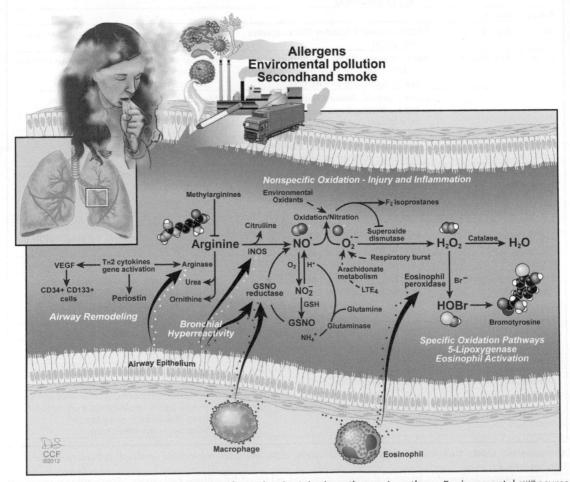

Fig. 1. Biomarkers of specific and nonspecific pathophysiologic pathways in asthma. Environmental exposures trigger and/or amplify underlying pathophysiology. *Abbreviations:* CD, cluster of differentiation; iNOS, inducible nitric oxide synthase; LTE4, leukotriene E4; TH2, T-helper 2; VEGF, vascular endothelial growth factor.

induced by β_2-adrenergic agonist stimulation.[38] GSNO is broken down in vivo by GSNO reductase.[32-34,39] Antigen-sensitized mice deficient in GSNO reductase are protected from methacholine-induced increased airway resistance. Further, mice deficient in GSNO reductase are prevented from having pulmonary tachyphylaxis to isoproterenol.[33] In children with asthmatic respiratory failure, GSNO reductase activity is upregulated and GSNO levels are profoundly low,[32] creating an endogenous airway smooth muscle relaxant that is deficient in the asthmatic airway. This deficiency also exacerbates refractoriness to β_2-agonist–based treatment.

Gain-of-function single nucleotide polymorphisms (SNPs) in GSNO reductase are associated with refractory asthma in certain subpopulations. Biopsies with increased GSNO reductase expression are anatomically associated with areas of poor airflow, as analyzed with hyperpolarized xenon or helium imaging. Thus, GSNO reductase is an important mechanism in the origins of a reactive asthma phenotype, but bronchoalveolar lavage studies show that GSNO reductase activity is not increased in all patients with asthma.[34] Further, essentially no differences are seen among stable, ambulatory severe, and nonsevere asthma with regard to GSNO reductase activity (Marozkina NV, unpublished observation, 2012). How can this important subpopulation with high GSNO reductase activity be identified in the clinic to target therapy with S-nitrosoglutathione replacement and/or S-nitrosoglutathione reductase inhibition? The importance of this question is highlighted by recent evidence showing that chronic excessive inhibition of S-nitrosoglutathione reductase has the potential to be associated with the development of cancer in patients exposed to chronic nitrosative stress.[40]

The authors envision the following clinical paradigm to approach this type of question. First, the clinical disease phenotype must be identified. The clinical characteristics of patients with increased airway GSNO reductase activity must be determined, which can be done through defining the phenotype of those who are identified through biochemical analysis of bronchoscopic samples. It can also be done through SNP-wide analysis of phenotype.

Next, biomarkers that validate the biochemical abnormality should be developed. In the example of GSNO reductase, there are at least two possible biomarkers. GSNO reductase also serves as an S-formylglutathione dehydrogenase.[41,42] The product of the latter enzymatic activity is formic acid, which can be measured in breath condensate. Levels are high in a subpopulation of patients with asthma, and these seem to be the same patients as those with high GSNO reductase activity. This hypothesis requires validation.

Another approach is challenge testing. In cystic fibrosis, GSNO replacement is associated with an increase of FeNO.[43] The faster the rate of GSNO breakdown, the faster the decline of FeNO after GSNO inhalation. This principle can likely also be applied to asthma. A challenge with GSNO or a GSNO precursor is associated with an increase in FeNO. The decay rate of FeNO after GSNO inhalation can be used as a surrogate for airway GSNO reductase activity. FeNO will likely be used as a readout in challenge testing for several subpopulations, including those with low pH,[36,44] high levels of eosinophils, or high levels of GSNO reductase activity. The authors believe that the challenge test may serve as a useful paradigm for identifying treatable subpopulations.

THE REDUCING-OXIDIZING IMBALANCE PHENOTYPE: LIPID OXIDATION AND LOSS OF ANTIOXIDANT SUPEROXIDE DISMUTASE

Recruitment and activation of inflammatory cells, both eosinophils and neutrophils, causes a respiratory burst in the airways that produces reactive oxygen species and reactive nitrogen species.[45-48] Certain of these species can damage proteins via specific enzyme-catalyzed oxidations or nonspecific oxidation of susceptible molecules. For example, eosinophil peroxidase and neutrophil myeloperoxidase cause halogenation, ie, bromination and chlorination respectively, of tyrosine residues; the halogenated products serve as molecular fingerprints of eosinophilic or neutrophilic inflammation. However, peroxidation of membrane lipids occurs spontaneously and results in the F_2-isoprostanes (F_2IsoPs), 8-epi-PGF$_{2\alpha}$ and its metabolite 2,3-dinor-8-epi-PGF$_{2\alpha}$. These structurally stable products are renally excreted, making them quantifiable noninvasive biomarkers of nonspecific reducing-oxidizing (redox) imbalance and inflammation.[49-51] In support of an increase of nonspecific oxidation, urine F_2IsoPs are higher in patients with asthma than healthy controls, and urine levels rise on an allergen-induced asthma exacerbation.[49,52,53] Biomarkers of enzyme-catalyzed oxidation pathways, such as urine BrY, and nonspecific oxidation pathways, such as F_2IsoPs, allow multiple opportunities to monitor asthma control and plan appropriate treatments. For example, stepping up corticosteroid therapy may be warranted in individuals with high urine BrY, but may be less helpful in those with low or normal BrY and high urine F_2IsoPs. In the latter case, neutrophilic inflammation or environmental oxidant-mediated inflammation might be suspect.

Nonspecific oxidation events also indicate a relative inadequacy of protective antioxidants. A wide array of antioxidants are present in the airways,[54] but oxidative and nitrosative stress can overwhelm these defenses, resulting in redox imbalance and oxidative injury.[10,48] The airway contains nonenzymatic antioxidants, such as glutathione, and enzymatic antioxidants, such as superoxide dismutases (SOD) and catalase (see **Fig. 1**). Asthmatic airways have increased total glutathione levels but loss of SOD and catalase enzymic activities.[48] The loss of SOD activity is found in the airways and serum of patients with asthma, allowing the serum SOD to be used as a biomarker of redox imbalance.[48,55–60] SOD activity is inversely related to airway reactivity and airflow obstruction, with higher levels of SOD related to lower airway reactivity and better airflow.[60] Murine models of asthma confirm that SOD plays a mechanistic role in airway hyperresponsiveness and inflammation (eg, SOD transgenic mice have less allergen-induced airway inflammation and reactivity than wild-type mice).[61]

In patients with asthma and in the murine model of asthma, SOD activity loss is partly related to the oxidation of the manganese SOD (MnSOD) protein and is linked to epithelial apoptosis and airway remodeling.[60,62] Low levels of serum SOD activity was an independent biomarker for airflow obstruction in patients with severe asthma nonresponsive to corticosteroids.[59] Furthermore, secondhand smoke exposure is associated with poorer lung functions and lower levels of serum SOD activity.[58] These findings suggest that strategies aimed at restoration of normal redox balance, perhaps through the use of SOD mimetics, may help patients with noneosinophilic inflammation in whom corticosteroids may have little impact on asthma control.

THE LOW pH PHENOTYPE

During acute exacerbations of asthma, breath condensate pH is decreased.[63] This reaction is associated with decreased serum and airway activity of glutaminase, activated downstream of Th1 cytokines associated with viral asthma exacerbations, preventing airway buffering.[63,64] Decreased airway pH promotes ciliary dysfunction, mucus hypersecretion, and cough.[63–65] Recent evidence suggests that this decreased airway pH might be successfully treated with inhaled buffer.[36,44] However, most patients with stable asthma seen in day-to-day practice do not have decreased pH.[66] In the NHLBI Severe Asthma Research Program (SARP) study of 572 subjects with stable asthma, only 7% had breath condensate pH less than 6.5 at baseline. This group was characterized by prominently low FeNO, low

forced expiratory volume in 1 second, high body mass index, low levels of airway eosinophils, and gastric esophageal reflux symptoms, along with other features. Because most nebulized treatments are in acidic solutions, this subpopulation of outpatients with asthma with decreased airway pH might benefit from less acidic therapy, and might even experience improvement with inhaled base.

To identify these patients, initial medical suspicion should be based on the phenotype described earlier. Patients who have a characteristic phenotype can then be diagnosed through biomarker analysis. Because nitrite has a acid dissociation constant (pKa) of 3.6 and, once protonated, dissociates to form NO, increasing airway pH decreases FeNO. Therefore, inhaled buffer followed by serial FeNO measures can be used to diagnose the low pH phenotype.[36,44] Patients with a decrease in FeNO after inhaled buffer should be those whose asthma will improve with inhaled base or glutamine supplement as a targeted therapy.

AIRWAY REMODELING PHENOTYPE: AIRWAY ANGIOGENIC BIOMARKERS

Increased number of blood vessels is universally found in asthmatic airway remodeling of children and adults.[67,68] The mouse model of asthma suggests that the switch to a proangiogenic airway and neovascularization occurs early and well in advance of eosinophilic inflammation.[69] This finding suggests that angiogenesis participates in the genesis of asthma. In fact, several lines of evidence indicate that angiogenesis and chronic inflammation are mutually supportive.[70] Inflammatory cells produce many proangiogenic factors in asthmatic lungs,[71] chief among which is vascular endothelial growth factor (VEGF). VEGF levels are increased in asthma bronchoalveolar lavage fluid, and related to blood vessel numbers in the mucosa.[69,71] High VEGF levels in sputum are associated with airflow obstruction, and levels of VEGF increase in sputum during an asthma attack.[67] Likewise in model systems, allergen- or virus-induced inflammation increases airway VEGF levels.[72,73] In support of a mechanistic role, VEGF overexpression in airways of transgenic mice leads to an asthma-like phenotype.[74] Mast cells and eosinophils can produce high levels of proangiogenic factors, including VEGF.[75,76] Proangiogenic factors such as VEGF cause neovascularization largely through effects on myeloid progenitor cell proliferation and mobilization from the bone marrow. Cell surface markers CD34 and CD133 define the subset of proangiogenic myeloid progenitors,[77,78] and can thus easily be enumerated through flow cytometric analysis. Studies identify high levels of

CD34+CD133+ cells in blood of patients with asthma and show that the levels correlate with airflow obstruction. Intriguingly, this same population of CD34+CD133+ cells also contains the mast cell progenitor. Further work is needed to determine if quantitation of circulating CD34+CD133+ cells can serve as a biomarker of airway remodeling and/or mast cell numbers and types in asthma.

THE ARGININE/NO PHENOTYPE: FENO, ARGINASE, METHYLARGININES

Measure of NO in the exhaled breath has been labeled as a sensitive and reliable biomarker of airway inflammation in adults and children.[79–84] Based on this finding, the U.S. Food and Drug Administration approved FeNO for evaluating antiinflammatory treatment responses of patients with asthma.[84] However, FeNO exhibits a broad range of values in these patients[85]; it is useful for identifying patients characterized by the greatest airflow obstruction and most frequent use of emergency care.

Inflammation, as characteristic in asthmatic airways, results in the expression of the inducible NO synthase (iNOS).[86–88] iNOS is expressed in many airway cells, but is prominent in the airway epithelial cells, where it catalyzes the conversion of L-arginine into NO and L-citrulline[86,87] (see **Fig. 1**). The synthesized gaseous NO may be measured noninvasively in the exhaled breath as a biomarker of chronic airway inflammation induction of the iNOS.[79,80,86] Eosinophils are not necessary for iNOS production of NO, and Th2 cytokines are not essential for iNOS expression. Hence, FeNO does not uniformly track with airway eosinophils, urine BrY, or periostin. Although studies suggest that monitoring antiinflammatory therapy through FeNO is useful, it does not necessarily diminish the rate of asthma exacerbations.[81,89,90] This limitation is likely because not all inflammatory processes are reflected by FeNO measurements.[8,91,92] This finding supports the concept that biomarkers of asthma may be more informative when used in combination with challenge testing (ie, FeNO measures with inhalation of base or in combination with other biomarkers such as urine BrY levels). In this context, although FeNO, urine BrY, and urine F2IsoP each are useful as a biomarker of asthma, pooled together they serve as a highly sensitive and specific biomarker panel for diagnosing asthma.[93]

Although a multitude of studies focus on the meaning of high FeNO in asthma,[29,62,86,94–97] asthma patients may often have values within the normal range (<25 parts per billion). Patients with low to normal FeNO values usually do not have eosinophilic inflammation but may still have signs of inflammation and remodeling. Low FeNO is helpful in that it suggests a phenotype that is less responsive to corticosteroids, preventing excessive medication use that may cause substantial morbidity. Patients with low FeNO may have non-Th2 inflammation and/or abnormalities in arginine metabolism and/or increased oxidative consumption of NO in the airway. Additionally, FeNO may be low because of low levels of GSNO in the airways caused by catabolism by higher than normal levels of GSNO reductase. Chronic loss of airway nitrite in the context of low airway pH leads to low baseline FeNO in the low pH phenotype.

Patients with asthma often have greater metabolism of arginine via iNOS and the arginase enzymes, which identifies a subpopulation of asthma as a disease of increased arginine catabolism[98] (see **Fig. 1**). High levels of arginase activity in asthma are often associated with increased levels of methylarginines, which are endogenous NOS inhibitors. This finding suggests that methylarginines may impact arginine availability as a substrate for iNOS.[97,99,100] Serum arginase increases during acute asthma exacerbations and decreases with improved asthma control, and is inversely related to airflow.[97,98] Studies indicate that arginase expression and activity is increased by allergen-induced gene activation in asthma, and Th2 cytokines.[86,99–105] However, oxidative stress can decrease the metabolism of methylarginines through effects on dimethylarginine dimethylaminohydrolase (DDAH).[106] This diminished metabolism of methylarginines may block iNOS and contribute to low FeNO in some patients with asthma, particularly those with severe corticosteroid-resistant asthma. Serum arginase also provides insight into mechanisms of airway remodeling.[107] Arginase regulates polyamine synthesis, which is required for DNA synthesis in cell proliferation.[108,109] Arginase also regulates precursors for the synthesis of proline, required for collagen production.[110,111] Thus, serum arginase and FeNO are unique biomarkers of inflammation in severe asthma and independent of the eosinophilic phenotype. Increased arginase is associated with low FeNO in adults with severe asthma.[98] Decreased SOD activity is also associated with low FeNO in adults with severe asthma, suggesting an oxidative consumption of NO that may lead to low normal values of FeNO (see **Fig. 1**).[98]

THE LEUKOTRIENE PHENOTYPE: LEUKOTRIENE E4, LIPOXINS AND PROTECTANTS

Endogenous lipid mediators can help maintain tissue homeostasis, yet they can also contribute to inflammation and bronchoconstriction.[112] Leukotrienes are examples of potent proinflammatory and bronchoconstricting agents. Inhibitors of the cysteinyl leukotriene receptor and the upstream cysteinyl leukotriene synthetic enzyme, 5-lipoxygenase (5-LO), are in clinical use for asthma treatment.[113] However, many patients with asthma are not effectively treated with leukotriene receptor antagonists. Further, 5-LO inhibition can cause hepatotoxicity. Therefore, identification of asthma subpopulations in whom these specific antileukotriene agents may be effective has for some time been a focus of genetic studies in asthma. Genetic testing for polymorphisms and 5-LO has also been proposed as a screening tool for identifying responsive subpopulations.[52,114] Additionally, biomarkers have been sought, including urinary leukotrienes and FeNO, to try to identify patients who would be most responsive.[115,116]

Urine leukotriene E_4 (LTE_4) has been validated as a biomarker of cysteinyl leukotriene overactivity. Levels of LTE_4 increase with acute asthma attacks and with aspirin-exacerbated respiratory disease, and decrease with cysteinyl leukotriene synthesis blockade but not with corticosteroids.[117–124] Although the use of therapies in the leukotriene pathway are valuable, lack of widespread availability of clinical testing for LTE_4 limit the use of this biomarker in optimizing asthma therapies. Specific lipid mediators can also prevent airway inflammation. For example, lipoxins have antiinflammatory properties affecting epithelial cells, airway leukocytes, and the pulmonary endothelium. They inhibit eosinophil and neutrophil migration into the airway and block the cytotoxicity of natural killer cells.[112,125]

The dysregulation and site of effect of lipoxins and other potentially beneficial lipid mediators (such as resolvins and protectins) in asthma is complex.[112,126] Lipoxin A4 levels are decreased in the bronchoalveolar lavage of patients with severe asthma, and lipoxin synthesis is inhibited in the circulation of many patients with severe asthma.[127,128] Decreased levels of lipoxin A4 in exhaled breath condensate have been proposed as a biomarker of lipoxin pathway abnormalities in severe asthma.

Levels of protectin D1 are similarly decreased in breath condensate during acute asthma exacerbations.[129] The identification of these biomarkers may permit targeted pharmacologic interventions for specific patients; they might ultimately be used to predict whether interventions can benefit, fail to benefit, or even harm patients based on their lipid-mediator phenotypes. It is increasingly apparent that the use of blood, sputum, and/or breath condensate biomarker analysis will be critically important in tailoring specific pharmacotherapy for specific patients with asthma.

ADDITIONAL CONSIDERATIONS FOR FUTURE STUDY

Biologic understanding is improving for several risk factors for severe asthma, including sex, race, obesity, and environmental tobacco exposure. Severe asthma is more prevalent in women after puberty.[130,131] Obesity is associated with asthma severity in adult-onset disease.[6] The greater prevalence of severe asthma among obese women may be related to menstrual cycle effects on circulating $CD34^+CD133^+$ cells[130] or adipose-related factors.[132,133] Additionally, circulating chitinase-like protein (YKL-40) levels are higher among patients with severe asthma in several cohorts, including SARP.[134] Asthma is characterized by air trapping.[6,15,135] Although in the early stages, CT studies may allow measurements of airways[136,137] and parenchyma,[137] which can serve as biomarkers of airway remodeling and air-trapping phenotypes. In studies of patients with severe asthma, CT determinations of air trapping were associated with disease severity.[138,139] New applications of molecular imaging promise the ability to track specific mechanistic biomarkers to specific structures using coregistered CT images, opening the door to imaging biomarkers in clinical practice. Biomarkers for severe asthma symptoms are likely to emerge from these studies.

SUMMARY

Asthma occurs in individuals with a broad range of different inflammatory and biochemical phenotypes. Most of these phenotypes have the potential to be targeted with specific treatments. Targeted treatment of the underlying disease process has the potential to be corticosteroid-sparing, particularly in patients with severe asthma. Many biomarkers are being developed to identify these specific phenotypes noninvasively. This development is grounded in a medically meaningful paradigm in which an underlying pathophysiology is suspected based on clinical presentation, a biomarker test is used to confirm the cause/diagnosis, and a targeted treatment is provided.

This article discusses several phenotypes of asthma, and more phenotypes associated with additional underlying processes almost certainly exist. The authors anticipate that each pathophysiology-based phenotype will ultimately be diagnosed by a defining biomarker, a panel of biomarkers, and/or a biomarker challenge test. Phenotypes may overlap in specific patients and may change over time. Hence, patients will likely profit from repetitive testing to define asthma pathophysiologic phenotypes and to tailor therapy. Providing targeted therapy, particularly for severe patients, based on interpretation of biomarker profiles may ultimately be the role of the asthma specialist. The authors believe that this approach will provide a clear path forward to improve treatment and minimize adverse effects.

REFERENCES

1. Yawn BP, Brenneman SK, Allen-Ramey FC, et al. Assessment of asthma severity and asthma control in children. Pediatrics 2006;118:322–9.

2. National Heart Lung and Blood Institute. Expert panel report 3: guidelines for the diagnosis and management of asthma full report. Available at: http://www.nhlbi.nih.gov/guidelines/asthma/asthgdln.pdf. Accessed July 2, 2012.

3. Wenzel S, Holgate ST. The mouse trap: it still yields few answers in asthma. Am J Respir Crit Care Med 2006;174:1173–6 [discussion: 6–8].

4. Masoli M, Fabian D, Holt S, et al. The global burden of asthma: executive summary of the GINA dissemination Committee report. Allergy 2004;59:469–78.

5. Busse WW, Banks-Schlegel S, Wenzel SE. Pathophysiology of severe asthma. J Allergy Clin Immunol 2000;106:1033–42.

6. Moore WC, Bleecker ER, Curran-Everett D, et al. Characterization of the severe asthma phenotype by the National Heart, Lung, and Blood Institute's Severe Asthma Research Program. J Allergy Clin Immunol 2007;119:405–13.

7. Paull K, Covar R, Jain N, et al. Do NHLBI lung function criteria apply to children? A cross-sectional evaluation of childhood asthma at National Jewish Medical and Research Center, 1999-2002. Pediatr Pulmonol 2005;39:311–7.

8. ATS Workshop Proceedings: exhaled nitric oxide and nitric oxide oxidative metabolism in exhaled breath condensate: executive summary. Am J Respir Crit Care Med 2006;173:811–3.

9. Wenzel SE. Asthma: defining of the persistent adult phenotypes. Lancet 2006;368:804–13.

10. Gaston B. The biochemistry of asthma. Biochim Biophys Acta 2011;1810:1017–24.

11. Anderson GP. Endotyping asthma: new insights into key pathogenic mechanisms in a complex, heterogeneous disease. Lancet 2008;372:1107–19.

12. Leckie MJ, ten Brinke A, Khan J, et al. Effects of an interleukin-5 blocking monoclonal antibody on eosinophils, airway hyper-responsiveness, and the late asthmatic response. Lancet 2000;356:2144–8.

13. Pavord ID, Shaw DE, Gibson PG, et al. Inflammometry to assess airway diseases. Lancet 2008;372:1017–9.

14. Meyers DA, Postma DS, Stine OC, et al. Genome screen for asthma and bronchial hyperresponsiveness: interactions with passive smoke exposure. J Allergy Clin Immunol 2005;115:1169–75.

15. Moore WC, Meyers DA, Wenzel SE, et al. Identification of asthma phenotypes using cluster analysis in the Severe Asthma Research Program. Am J Respir Crit Care Med 2010;181:315–23.

16. Fitzpatrick AM, Teague WG, Meyers DA, et al. Heterogeneity of severe asthma in childhood: confirmation by cluster analysis of children in the National Institutes of Health/National Heart, Lung, and Blood Institute Severe Asthma Research Program. J Allergy Clin Immunol 2010;127:382–9 e1–13.

17. Woodruff PG, Khashayar R, Lazarus SC, et al. Relationship between airway inflammation, hyperresponsiveness, and obstruction in asthma. J Allergy Clin Immunol 2001;108:753–8.

18. Polosa R, Renaud L, Cacciola R, et al. Sputum eosinophilia is more closely associated with airway responsiveness to bradykinin than methacholine in asthma. Eur Respir J 1998;12:551–6.

19. Louis R, Lau LC, Bron AO, et al. The relationship between airways inflammation and asthma severity. Am J Respir Crit Care Med 2000;161:9–16.

20. Covar RA, Spahn JD, Martin RJ, et al. Safety and application of induced sputum analysis in childhood asthma. J Allergy Clin Immunol 2004;114:575–82.

21. Gibson PG. Use of induced sputum to examine airway inflammation in childhood asthma. J Allergy Clin Immunol 1998;102:S100–101.

22. Berry M, Morgan A, Shaw DE, et al. Pathological features and inhaled corticosteroid response of eosinophilic and non-eosinophilic asthma. Thorax 2007;62:1043–9.

23. Hastie AT, Moore WC, Meyers DA, et al. Analyses of asthma severity phenotypes and inflammatory proteins in subjects stratified by sputum granulocytes. J Allergy Clin Immunol 2010;125:1028–36. e13.

24. Woodruff PG, Modrek B, Choy DF, et al. T-helper type 2-driven inflammation defines major subphenotypes of asthma. Am J Respir Crit Care Med 2009;180:388–95.

25. Corren J, Lemanske RF, Hanania NA, et al. Lebrikizumab treatment in adults with asthma. N Engl J Med 2011;365:1088–98.

26. MacPherson JC, Comhair SA, Erzurum SC, et al. Eosinophils are a major source of nitric oxide-derived oxidants in severe asthma: characterization of pathways available to eosinophils for generating reactive nitrogen species. J Immunol 2001;166:5763–72.

27. Aldridge RE, Chan T, van Dalen CJ, et al. Eosinophil peroxidase produces hypobromous acid in the airways of stable asthmatics. Free Radic Biol Med 2002;33:847–56.

28. Erpenbeck VJ, Hohlfeld JM, Petschallies J, et al. Local release of eosinophil peroxidase following segmental allergen provocation in asthma. Clin Exp Allergy 2003;33:331–6.

29. Wu W, Chen Y, d'Avignon A, et al. 3-Bromotyrosine and 3,5-dibromotyrosine are major products of protein oxidation by eosinophil peroxidase: potential markers for eosinophil-dependent tissue injury in vivo. Biochemistry 1999;38:3538–48.

30. Mita H, Higashi N, Taniguchi M, et al. Urinary 3-bromotyrosine and 3-chlorotyrosine concentrations in asthmatic patients: lack of increase in 3-bromotyrosine concentration in urine and plasma proteins in aspirin-induced asthma after intravenous aspirin challenge. Clin Exp Allergy 2004;34:931–8.

31. Wedes SH, Wu W, Comhair SA, et al. Urinary bromotyrosine measures asthma control and predicts asthma exacerbations in children. J Pediatr 2011; 159;248–255. e1.

32. Gaston B, Sears S, Woods J, et al. Bronchodilator S-nitrosothiol deficiency in asthmatic respiratory failure. Lancet 1998;351:1317–9.

33. Que LG, Liu L, Yan Y, et al. Protection from experimental asthma by an endogenous bronchodilator. Science 2005;308:1618–21.

34. Que LG, Yang Z, Stamler JS, et al. S-nitrosoglutathione reductase: an important regulator in human asthma. Am J Respir Crit Care Med 2009;180: 226–31.

35. Gaston B, Reilly J, Drazen JM, et al. Endogenous nitrogen oxides and bronchodilator S-nitrosothiols in human airways. Proc Natl Acad Sci U S A 1993;90:10957–61.

36. Gaston B, Kelly R, Urban P, et al. Buffering airway acid decreases exhaled nitric oxide in asthma. J Allergy Clin Immunol 2006;118:817–22.

37. Evangelista AM, Rao VS, Filo AR, et al. Direct regulation of striated muscle myosins by nitric oxide and endogenous nitrosothiols. PloS One 2010;5: e11209.

38. Whalen EJ, Foster MW, Matsumoto A, et al. Regulation of beta-adrenergic receptor signaling by S-nitrosylation of G-protein-coupled receptor kinase 2. Cell 2007;129:511–22.

39. Fang K, Johns R, Macdonald T, et al. S-nitrosoglutathione breakdown prevents airway smooth muscle relaxation in the guinea pig. Am J Physiol 2000;279:L716–21.

40. Marozkina NV, Wei C, Yemen S, et al. S-nitrosoglutathione reductase in human lung cancer. Am J Respir Cell Mol Biol 2011;46:63–70.

41. Jensen DE, Belka GK, Du Bois GC. S-nitrosoglutathione is a substrate for rat alcohol dehydrogenase

class III isoenzyme. Biochem J 1998;331(Pt 2): 659–68.

42. Greenwald R, Fitzpatrick AM, Gaston B, et al. Breath formate is a marker of airway S-nitrosothiol depletion in severe asthma. PloS One 2010;5: e11919.

43. Snyder AH, McPherson ME, Hunt JF, et al. Acute effects of aerosolized S-nitrosoglutathione in cystic fibrosis. Am J Respir Crit Care Med 2002;165:922–6.

44. Shin HW, Shelley DA, Henderson EM, et al. Airway nitric oxide release is reduced after PBS inhalation in asthma. J Appl Physiol 2007;102:1028–33.

45. Caramori G, Papi A. Oxidants and asthma. Thorax 2004;59:170–3.

46. Mak JC, Chan-Yeung MM. Reactive oxidant species in asthma. Curr Opin Pulm Med 2006;12: 7–11.

47. Andreadis AA, Hazen SL, Comhair SA, et al. Oxidative and nitrosative events in asthma. Free Radic Biol Med 2003;35:213–25.

48. Comhair SA, Erzurum SC. Redox control of asthma: molecular mechanisms and therapeutic opportunities. Antioxid Redox Signal 2010;12:93–124.

49. Dworski R, Murray JJ, Roberts LJ 2nd, et al. Allergen-induced synthesis of F(2)-isoprostanes in atopic asthmatics. Evidence for oxidant stress. Am J Respir Crit Care Med 1999;160:1947–51.

50. Morrow JD, Roberts LJ. The isoprostanes: their role as an index of oxidant stress status in human pulmonary disease. Am J Respir Crit Care Med 2002;166:S25–30.

51. Wood LG, Gibson PG, Garg ML. Biomarkers of lipid peroxidation, airway inflammation and asthma. Eur Respir J 2003;21:177–86.

52. Tse SM, Tantisira K, Weiss ST. The pharmacogenetics and pharmacogenomics of asthma therapy. Pharmacogen J 2011;11:383–92.

53. Dworski R, Sheller JR. Urinary mediators and asthma. Clin Exp Allergy 1998;28:1309–12.

54. Heffner JE, Repine JE. Pulmonary strategies of antioxidant defense. Am Rev Respir Dis 1989; 140:531–54.

55. De Raeve HR, Thunnissen FB, Kaneko FT, et al. Decreased Cu, Zn-SOD activity in asthmatic airway epithelium: correction by inhaled corticosteroid in vivo. Am J Physiol 1997;272:L148–54.

56. Comhair SA, Bhathena PR, Dweik RA, et al. Rapid loss of superoxide dismutase activity during antigen-induced asthmatic response. Lancet 2000;355:624.

57. Comhair SA, Erzurum SC. Antioxidant responses to oxidant-mediated lung diseases. Am J Physiol 2002;283:L246–55.

58. Comhair SA, Gaston BM, Ricci KS, et al. Detrimental effects of environmental tobacco smoke in relation to asthma severity. PloS One 2011;6: e18574.

59. Comhair SA, Ricci KS, Arroliga M, et al. Correlation of systemic superoxide dismutase deficiency to airflow obstruction in asthma. Am J Respir Crit Care Med 2005;172:306–13.

60. Comhair SA, Xu W, Ghosh S, et al. Superoxide dismutase inactivation in pathophysiology of asthmatic airway remodeling and reactivity. Am J Pathol 2005;166:663–74.

61. Larsen GL, White CW, Takeda K, et al. Mice that overexpress Cu/Zn superoxide dismutase are resistant to allergen-induced changes in airway control. Am J Physiol 2000;279:L350–9.

62. Ghosh S, Janocha AJ, Aronica MA, et al. Nitrotyrosine proteome survey in asthma identifies oxidative mechanism of catalase inactivation. J Immunol 2006;176:5587–97.

63. Hunt JF, Erwin E, Palmer L, et al. Expression and activity of pH-regulatory glutaminase in the human airway epithelium. Am J Respir Crit Care Med 2002;165:101–7.

64. Carraro S, Doherty J, Zaman K, et al. S-nitrosothiols regulate cell-surface pH buffering by airway epithelial cells during the human immune response to rhinovirus. Am J Physiol 2006;290:L827–32.

65. Hunt JF, Fang K, Malik R, et al. Endogenous airway acidification. Implications for asthma pathophysiology. Am J Respir Crit Care Med 2000;161:694–9.

66. Liu L, Teague WG, Erzurum S, et al. Determinants of exhaled breath condensate pH in a large population with asthma. Chest 2011;139:328–36.

67. Barbato A, Turato G, Baraldo S, et al. Epithelial damage and angiogenesis in the airways of children with asthma. Am J Respir Crit Care Med 2006;174:975–81.

68. Hashimoto M, Tanaka H, Abe S. Quantitative analysis of bronchial wall vascularity in the medium and small airways of patients with asthma and COPD. Chest 2005;127:965–72.

69. Asosingh K, Swaidani S, Aronica M, et al. Th1- and Th2-dependent endothelial progenitor cell recruitment and angiogenic switch in asthma. J Immunol 2007;178:6482–94.

70. Jackson JR, Seed MP, Kircher CH, et al. The codependence of angiogenesis and chronic inflammation. Faseb J 1997;11:457–65.

71. Chetta A, Zanini A, Foresi A, et al. Vascular endothelial growth factor up-regulation and bronchial wall remodelling in asthma. Clin Exp Allergy 2005;35:1437–42.

72. Psarras S, Volonaki E, Skevaki CL, et al. Vascular endothelial growth factor-mediated induction of angiogenesis by human rhinoviruses. J Allergy Clin Immunol 2006;117:291–7.

73. Avdalovic MV, Putney LF, Schelegle ES, et al. Vascular remodeling is airway generation-specific in a primate model of chronic asthma. Am J Respir Crit Care Med 2006;174:1069–76.

74. Lee CG, Link H, Baluk P, et al. Vascular endothelial growth factor (VEGF) induces remodeling and enhances TH2-mediated sensitization and inflammation in the lung. Nature Med 2004;10:1095–103.

75. Puxeddu I, Alian A, Piliponsky AM, et al. Human peripheral blood eosinophils induce angiogenesis. Int J Biochem Cell Biol 2005;37:628–36.

76. Ribatti D, Crivellato E, Roccaro AM, et al. Mast cell contribution to angiogenesis related to tumour progression. Clin Exp Allergy 2004;34:1660–4.

77. Prater DN, Case J, Ingram DA, et al. Working hypothesis to redefine endothelial progenitor cells. Leukemia 2007;21:1141–9.

78. Asahara T, Murohara T, Sullivan A, et al. Isolation of putative progenitor endothelial cells for angiogenesis. Science 1997;275:964–7.

79. Kharitonov SA, Yates D, Robbins RA, et al. Increased nitric oxide in exhaled air of asthmatic patients. Lancet 1994;343:133–5.

80. Ricciardolo FL, Gaston B, Hunt J. Acid stress in the pathology of asthma. J Allergy Clin Immunol 2004;113:610–9.

81. Smith AD, Cowan JO, Brassett KP, et al. Use of exhaled nitric oxide measurements to guide treatment in chronic asthma. N Engl J Med 2005;352:2163–73.

82. Dinakar C. Exhaled nitric oxide in pediatric asthma. Curr Allergy Asthma Rep 2009;9:30–7.

83. Nordvall SL, Janson C, Kalm-Stephens P, et al. Exhaled nitric oxide in a population-based study of asthma and allergy in schoolchildren. Allergy 2005;60:469–75.

84. Silkoff PE, Carlson M, Bourke T, et al. The Aerocrine exhaled nitric oxide monitoring system NIOX is cleared by the US Food and Drug Administration for monitoring therapy in asthma. J Allergy Clin Immunol 2004;114:1241–56.

85. Dweik RA, Sorkness RL, Wenzel S, et al. Use of exhaled nitric oxide measurement to identify a reactive, at-risk phenotype among patients with asthma. Am J Respir Crit Care Med 2010;181:1033–41.

86. Guo FH, Comhair SA, Zheng S, et al. Molecular mechanisms of increased nitric oxide (NO) in asthma: evidence for transcriptional and post-translational regulation of NO synthesis. J Immunol 2000;164:5970–80.

87. Guo FH, Erzurum SC. Characterization of inducible nitric oxide synthase expression in human airway epithelium. Environ Health Perspect 1998;106(Suppl 5):1119–24.

88. Guo FH, Uetani K, Haque SJ, et al. Interferon gamma and interleukin 4 stimulate prolonged expression of inducible nitric oxide synthase in human airway epithelium through synthesis of soluble mediators. J Clin Invest 1997;100:829–38.

89. Shaw DE, Berry MA, Thomas M, et al. The use of exhaled nitric oxide to guide asthma management: a randomized controlled trial. Am J Respir Crit Care Med 2007;176:231–7.

90. Szefler SJ, Mitchell H, Sorkness CA, et al. Management of asthma based on exhaled nitric oxide in addition to guideline-based treatment for inner-city adolescents and young adults: a randomised controlled trial. Lancet 2008;372: 1065–72.

91. Khatri SB, Hammel J, Kavuru MS, et al. Temporal association of nitric oxide levels and airflow in asthma after whole lung allergen challenge. J Appl Physiol 2003;95:436–40 [discussion: 5].

92. Proceedings of the ATS workshop on refractory asthma: current understanding, recommendations, and unanswered questions. American Thoracic Society. Am J Respir Crit Care Med 2000;162: 2341–51.

93. Wedes SH, Khatri SB, Zhang R, et al. Noninvasive markers of airway inflammation in asthma. Clin Transl Sci 2009;2:112–7.

94. Nelson BV, Sears S, Woods J, et al. Expired nitric oxide as a marker for childhood asthma. J Pediatr 1997;130:423–7.

95. Ceylan E, Aksoy N, Gencer M, et al. Evaluation of oxidative-antioxidative status and the L-arginine-nitric oxide pathway in asthmatic patients. Respir Med 2005;99:871–6.

96. Li H, Romieu I, Sienra-Monge JJ, et al. Genetic polymorphisms in arginase I and II and childhood asthma and atopy. J Allergy Clin Immunol 2006; 117:119–26.

97. Morris CR, Poljakovic M, Lavrisha L, et al. Decreased arginine bioavailability and increased serum arginase activity in asthma. Am J Respir Crit Care Med 2004;170:148–53.

98. Lara A, Khatri SB, Wang Z, et al. Alterations of the arginine metabolome in asthma. Am J Respir Crit Care Med 2008;178:673–81.

99. Zimmermann N, King NE, Laporte J, et al. Dissection of experimental asthma with DNA microarray analysis identifies arginase in asthma pathogenesis. J Clin Invest 2003;111:1863–74.

100. Zimmermann N, Rothenberg ME. The arginine-arginase balance in asthma and lung inflammation. Eur J Pharmacol 2006;533:253–62.

101. Maarsingh H, Leusink J, Bos IS, et al. Arginase strongly impairs neuronal nitric oxide-mediated airway smooth muscle relaxation in allergic asthma. Respir Res 2006;7:6.

102. King NE, Rothenberg ME, Zimmermann N. Arginine in asthma and lung inflammation. J Nutr 2004;134:2830S–6S [discussion: 53S].

103. Corraliza IM, Soler G, Eichmann K, et al. Arginase induction by suppressors of nitric oxide synthesis (IL-4, IL-10 and PGE2) in murine bone-marrow

104. Modolell M, Corraliza IM, Link F, et al. Reciprocal regulation of the nitric oxide synthase/arginase balance in mouse bone marrow-derived macrophages by TH1 and TH2 cytokines. Eur J Immunol 1995;25:1101–4.

105. Mistry SK, Zheng M, Rouse BT, et al. Induction of arginases I and II in cornea during herpes simplex virus infection. Virus Res 2001;73:177–82.

106. Ito A, Tsao PS, Adimoolam S, et al. Novel mechanism for endothelial dysfunction: dysregulation of dimethylarginine dimethylaminohydrolase. Circulation 1999;99:3092–5.

107. Cohen L, E X, Tarsi J, et al. Epithelial cell proliferation contributes to airway remodeling in severe asthma. Am J Respir Crit Care Med 2007;176:138–45.

108. Li H, Meininger CJ, Hawker JR Jr, et al. Regulatory role of arginase I and II in nitric oxide, polyamine, and proline syntheses in endothelial cells. Am J Physiol Endocrinol Metab 2001;280:E75–82.

109. Janne J, Alhonen L, Leinonen P. Polyamines: from molecular biology to clinical applications. Ann Med 1991;23:241–59.

110. Albina JE, Abate JA, Mastrofrancesco B. Role of ornithine as a proline precursor in healing wounds. J Surg Res 1993;55:97–102.

111. Kershenobich D, Fierro FJ, Rojkind M. The relationship between the free pool of proline and collagen content in human liver cirrhosis. J Clin Invest 1970; 49:2246–9.

112. Haworth O, Levy BD. Endogenous lipid mediators in the resolution of airway inflammation. Eur Respir J 2007;30:980–92.

113. O'Byrne PM, Israel E, Drazen JM. Antileukotrienes in the treatment of asthma. Ann Intern Med 1997; 127:472–80.

114. Kalayci O, Birben E, Sackesen C, et al. ALOX5 promoter genotype, asthma severity and LTC production by eosinophils. Allergy 2006;61:97–103.

115. Montuschi P, Mondino C, Koch P, et al. Effects of montelukast treatment and withdrawal on fractional exhaled nitric oxide and lung function in children with asthma. Chest 2007;132:1876–81.

116. Rabinovitch N, Graber NJ, Chinchilli VM, et al. Urinary leukotriene E4/exhaled nitric oxide ratio and montelukast response in childhood asthma. J Allergy Clin Immunol 2010;126. 545–551. e1–4.

117. Daffern PJ, Muilenburg D, Hugli TE, et al. Association of urinary leukotriene E4 excretion during aspirin challenges with severity of respiratory responses. J Allergy Clin Immunol 1999;104:559–64.

118. O'Shaughnessy KM, Wellings R, Gillies B, et al. Differential effects of fluticasone propionate on allergen-evoked bronchoconstriction and increased urinary leukotriene E4 excretion. Am Rev Respir Dis 1993; 147:1472–6.

119. O'Sullivan S, Roquet A, Dahlen B, et al. Urinary excretion of inflammatory mediators during allergen-induced early and late phase asthmatic reactions. Clin Exp Allergy 1998;28:1332–9.

120. Green SA, Malice MP, Tanaka W, et al. Increase in urinary leukotriene LTE4 levels in acute asthma: correlation with airflow limitation. Thorax 2004;59:100–4.

121. Liu MC, Dube LM, Lancaster J. Acute and chronic effects of a 5-lipoxygenase inhibitor in asthma: a 6-month randomized multicenter trial. Zileuton Study Group. J Allergy Clin Immunol 1996;98:859–71.

122. Wenzel SE, Trudeau JB, Kaminsky DA, et al. Effect of 5-lipoxygenase inhibition on bronchoconstriction and airway inflammation in nocturnal asthma. Am J Respir Crit Care Med 1995;152:897–905.

123. Pavord ID, Ward R, Woltmann G, et al. Induced sputum eicosanoid concentrations in asthma. Am J Respir Crit Care Med 1999;160:1905–9.

124. Miranda C, Busacker A, Balzar S, et al. Distinguishing severe asthma phenotypes: role of age at onset and eosinophilic inflammation. J Allergy Clin Immunol 2004;113:101–8.

125. Levy BD. Lipoxins and lipoxin analogs in asthma. Prostaglandins Leukot Essent Fatty Acids 2005; 73:231–7.

126. Haworth O, Cernadas M, Yang R, et al. Resolvin E1 regulates interleukin 23, interferon-gamma and lipoxin A4 to promote the resolution of allergic airway inflammation. Nat Immunol 2008;9:873–9.

127. Planaguma A, Kazani S, Marigowda G, et al. Airway lipoxin A4 generation and lipoxin A4 receptor expression are decreased in severe asthma. Am J Respir Crit Care Med 2008;178:574–82.

128. Levy BD, Bonnans C, Silverman ES, et al. Diminished lipoxin biosynthesis in severe asthma. Am J Respir Crit Care Med 2005;172:824–30.

129. Levy BD, Kohli P, Gotlinger K, et al. Protectin D1 is generated in asthma and dampens airway inflammation and hyperresponsiveness. J Immunol 2007;178:496–502.

130. Farha S, Asosingh K, Laskowski D, et al. Effects of the menstrual cycle on lung function variables in women with asthma. Am J Respir Crit Care Med 2009;180:304–10.

131. Tantisira KG, Colvin R, Tonascia J, et al. Airway responsiveness in mild to moderate childhood asthma: sex influences on the natural history. Am J Respir Crit Care Med 2008;178:325–31.

132. Holguin F, Bleecker ER, Busse WW, et al. Obesity and asthma: an association modified by age of asthma onset. J Allergy Clin Immunol 2011;127: 1486–93. e2.

133. Holguin F, Fitzpatrick A. Obesity, asthma, and oxidative stress. J Appl Physiol 2010;108:754–9.

134. Chupp GL, Lee CG, Jarjour N, et al. A chitinase-like protein in the lung and circulation of patients with severe asthma. N Engl J Med 2007;357: 2016–27.

135. Sorkness RL, Bleecker ER, Busse WW, et al. Lung function in adults with stable but severe asthma: air trapping and incomplete reversal of obstruction with bronchodilation. J Appl Physiol 2008;104: 394–403.

136. Little SA, Sproule MW, Cowan MD, et al. High resolution computed tomographic assessment of airway wall thickness in chronic asthma: reproducibility and relationship with lung function and severity. Thorax 2002;57:247–53.

137. Mitsunobu F, Ashida K, Hosaki Y, et al. Decreased computed tomographic lung density during exacerbation of asthma. Eur Respir J 2003;22:106–12.

138. Busacker A, Newell JD Jr, Keefe T, et al. A multivariate analysis of risk factors for the air-trapping asthmatic phenotype as measured by quantitative CT analysis. Chest 2009;135:48–56.

139. de Lange EE, Altes TA, Patrie JT, et al. Evaluation of asthma with hyperpolarized helium-3 MRI: correlation with clinical severity and spirometry. Chest 2006;130:1055–62.

Asthma: A Chronic Infectious Disease?

Gaetano Caramori, MD, PhD[a],
Nikos Papadopoulos, MD, PhD[b], Marco Contoli, MD, PhD[a],
Brunilda Marku, MD, PhD[a], Giacomo Forini, MD[a],
Alessia Pauletti, MD[a], Sebastian L. Johnston, MD, PhD[c],
Alberto Papi, MD[a],*

KEYWORDS

• Asthma • Respiratory infection • Bacterial infection • Rhinovirus

KEY POINTS

• There are increasing data to support the "hygiene" and "microbiota" hypotheses of a protective role of infections in modulating the risk of subsequent development of asthma.

• There is some evidence that rhinovirus respiratory infections are associated with the development of asthma, particularly in childhood, whereas these infections in later life seem to have a weaker association with the development of asthma.

• The role of bacterial infections in chronic asthma remains unclear, but there are emerging data for a potential role of Mycoplasma pneumoniae and Chlamydia pneumoniae and gut microbiota in increasing the risk of the development of asthma and in modulating the degree of asthma control.

INTRODUCTION

The "Global Strategy for Asthma Management," prepared by a panel convened by the National Institutes of Health and the World Health Organization, defines asthma as "a chronic inflammatory disorder of the airways, in which many cells and cellular elements play a role. The chronic inflammation is associated with airway hyperresponsiveness that leads to recurrent episodes of wheezing, breathlessness, chest tightness, and coughing, particularly at night or in the early morning. These episodes are usually associated with widespread, but variable, airflow limitation within the lung that is often reversible, either spontaneously or with treatment."[1]

The chronic airway inflammation seen in asthma is present even in those with very mild disease and is unique in that the airway wall is infiltrated by T lymphocytes of the T-helper (Th) type 2 phenotype, eosinophils, macrophages and monocytes, and mast cells.[1,2] In addition, an "acute-on-chronic" inflammation may be observed during exacerbations, with an increase in eosinophils and sometimes neutrophils.[1,2] Lower airway structural cells also produce inflammatory mediators. Thus, bronchial and bronchiolar epithelial cells, lung endothelial cells, lung fibroblasts, and bronchial and bronchiolar smooth muscle cells show an altered phenotype in asthma and express multiple inflammatory mediators, including cytokines, chemokines, and peptides.[2] Chronic inflammation in asthma may lead to structural changes in the lower airways, including reticular basement membrane fibrosis under the bronchial epithelium; increased thickness (mainly through hyperplasia) of lower airway smooth muscle cells; increased numbers of bronchial blood vessels (neoangiogenesis); and increased number or volume of

[a] Section of Respiratory Diseases, Department of Medical Sciences, Centro per lo Studio delle Malattie Infiammatorie Croniche delle Vie Aeree e Patologie Fumo Correlate dell'Apparato Respiratorio (CEMICEF), University of Ferrara, via Savonarola 9, 44121, Ferrara, Italy; [b] Allergy Department, 2nd Paediatric Clinic, University of Athens, 13 Levadias Street, 11527 Goudi, Athens, Greece; [c] MRC and Asthma UK Centre in Allergic Mechanisms of Asthma, Centre for Respiratory Infection, National Heart and Lung Institute, Imperial College London, Norfolk Place, London W2 1PG, UK
* Corresponding author. Sezione di Malattie dell'Apparato Respiratorio, University of Ferrara, Via Savonarola 9, 44121 Ferrara, Italy.
E-mail address: ppa@unife.it

Clin Chest Med 33 (2012) 473–484
http://dx.doi.org/10.1016/j.ccm.2012.06.009
0272-5231/12/$ – see front matter © 2012 Elsevier Inc. All rights reserved

mucus-secreting cells in the bronchial mucosa (surface epithelium and glands). These changes, often referred to as "airway remodeling," may not be fully reversible with current treatments.[3] The most objective method to confirm the diagnosis of asthma in a subject with symptoms of asthma remains the assessment of the presence of reversible airflow obstruction. The reversibility of airflow obstruction (spontaneous or induced by pharmacologic treatment) may be assessed either by measuring peak expiratory flow or FEV_1 before and after a single dose of a bronchodilator, or before and after a 3-month course of full antiasthma treatment including inhaled glucocorticoids.[4]

The cause of asthma is still unknown, and is probably multifactorial, involving complex interactions between many genetic and environmental factors. According to its presumed etiology asthma may still be defined as extrinsic (or atopic or allergic) or intrinsic. Although the term extrinsic refers to a well-recognized environmental agent, extrinsic asthma is usually defined as asthma that occurs in atopic individuals (ie, subjects with an increased amount of serum immunoglobulin E [IgE] antibodies against common environmental aeroallergens). Sometimes it is possible to identify the allergens responsible for the development and maintenance of asthma in an individual with atopy, but often it is possible to establish only the association of asthma and atopy and not the precise cause of asthma, because people with asthma and atopy can develop symptoms of asthma and airflow obstruction after exposure to a variety of provoking agents other than allergens. In addition, in some patients it is possible to identify the agents that trigger asthma exacerbations in individuals who are nonatopic. This is the case in occupational asthma induced by low-molecular-weight chemicals and in subjects with asthma induced by some drugs (eg, aspirin-induced asthma). In these cases asthma may be considered extrinsic (ie, caused by a well-defined agent), but occurring in individuals without atopy.[4]

The existence of a group of patients in whom no environmental causal agent can be identified has strongly limited the classification of asthma according to its etiology. Asthma induced by unknown causes in a subject without atopy is still defined as intrinsic. Apart from some differences in onset, severity, and natural history, and some aspects of pathology, extrinsic and intrinsic asthma are very similar, particularly from pathologic, pathophysiologic, and pharmacologic points of view.[4]

Although a genetic basis for asthma is undeniable, elucidation of polymorphisms that are "causal" is greatly hampered by variability in the clinical phenotype, which is likely caused by the multiple molecular mechanisms underlying the complex pathologic processes involved in disease development and progression.[5] However, very expensive genome-wide association studies of asthma have recently discovered many novel susceptibility genes and this may further increase the understanding of asthma.[6]

An association between respiratory infections, mainly viral, and asthma exacerbations is well documented and accepted,[7] but less conclusive, mainly epidemiologic studies also suggest a possible role of many different infections in the cause of asthma. This article reviews the available evidence indicating that asthma may be considered as a chronic infectious disease.

DUAL ROLE OF INFECTIONS IN THE ETIOLOGY OF ASTHMA

The role of infections in the cause of asthma is complex. There is mounting evidence suggesting a protective role of a greater overall exposure to infectious agents or components thereof in reducing the risk of development of asthma and less convincing data suggesting instead a role of some infections in causing the development of asthma.

INFECTIONS PROTECT FROM THE DEVELOPMENT OF ASTHMA

Many epidemiologic studies suggest that the exposure to infections in early childhood may play a protective role in the later development of asthma, the so-called "hygiene hypothesis," first proposed by Strachan[8] in 1989 demonstrating that infections and contact with older siblings or through other exposures confer protection from the development of allergy and asthma. This hypothesis has evolved in various ways exploring the role of overt viral and bacterial infections, the significance of environmental exposure to microbial compounds, and their effect on underlying responses of innate and adaptive immunity.[9]

The hygiene hypothesis proposes that a greater load of infections in early life is protective toward the eventual development of asthma.[8] These associations are supported by observations showing an inverse relationship between the age of entering day care and the incidence of asthma later in life.[10] This inverse relationship is also present between the number of siblings or family size and asthma. However, these studies have used surrogate markers for increased exposure to infections; there is a need to investigate directly the real impact of respiratory infections. Whether infections have protective effect or not may have to do also with their location, frequency, intensity, and timing.[11]

It has been proposed that the protective effect related to more frequent infections may depend on their capacity to stimulate protective Th1 immunity.[12] Indeed, neonates are born with an immune response predominantly type 2.[13] Early infections skew the immune system toward a type 1 phenotype, inducing the production of interleukin (IL)-12 by dendritic cells.[14]

Because asthma is characterized by increased Th2 immune responses, by this mechanism a reduction in childhood infectious illnesses could lead to an increase in the prevalence of asthma, especially if there is also a genetic background of impaired type 1 immunity (infants with a family history of atopic diseases).

More recent studies suggest an alternative interpretation of the evidence supporting the "hygiene hypothesis," namely the "microbiota hypothesis." Particularly, it seems that exposure to nonpathogenic microbes may be more important in directing healthy immune development and reducing the risk of asthma.

There is increasing evidence that commensal bacterial flora (human microbiome or microbiota) in various sites, including gut, skin, and lungs, is an important modulator of immune function and development and a critical contributor to the maintenance of mucosal homeostasis. However, the mechanisms by which the human microbiome influences lung immunity and inflammation and its role in the development of asthma are still not well characterized.[15]

Microbes residing in the environment might shape an exposed subject's immune responses and thereby his or her risk of asthma. There is substantial evidence that a diversity of microbial exposure can exert a protective effect, particularly in childhood, against the development of asthma.[15]

Endotoxins from gram-negative bacteria have been the first agents associated with a reduced risk for asthma. In later studies, $\beta(1 \rightarrow 3)$glucans, extracellular polysaccharides, and muramic acid from, respectively, molds and gram-positive bacteria were associated with a reduced risk of asthma separately in rural and urban populations. These results already suggested that not just one but several independent microbial signals from gram-negative and -positive bacteria, and molds, might play a role in explaining the protective effects.[16] Surprisingly, the diversity of fungal and bacterial exposure seems to have protective effects. Such a concept of diversity is challenging when aiming at refining methods of exposure assessment for future studies. In turn, it might better grasp the nature of microbial exposures, which always relate to microbial communities and the shift in such communities rather than to single microorganisms.[15]

In animal models of asthma the presence of the microbiota is essential to protect from an exaggerated Th2 response, increased airway hyperresponsiveness, and airway inflammation after sensitization and challenge with ovalbumin.[17] Furthermore, in animals, antibiotic use during infancy may indeed quantitatively or qualitatively change the intestinal microflora and thereby prevent postnatal Th1 cell maturation, thus resulting in a Th2-polarized immune deviation.[18]

Epigenetic regulation is an important mechanism by which indigenous microbiota might interact with genes involved in asthma development. For example, in pregnant maternal mice prenatal administration of the farm-derived gram-negative bacterium *Acinetobacter lwoffii* F78 prevents the development of an asthmatic phenotype in the progeny, and this effect is interferon (IFN)-γ dependent. Furthermore, the IFN-γ promoter of CD4$^+$ T cells in the offspring has a significant protection against loss of histone 4 acetylation, which is closely associated with IFN-γ expression.[19]

Although epidemiologic data support a protective effect of parasitic infection on asthma development, this may be caused by other exposures. To date, there is no conclusive evidence that parasitic infection protects against asthma development.[20]

The strongest epidemiologic evidence suggests that helminthic intestinal hookworm infections may protect subjects from developing asthma.[20] In an animal model of asthma the application of excreted and secreted products (NES) of the helminth *Nippostrongylus brasiliensis* together with ovalbumin and alum during the sensitization period totally inhibited the development of eosinophilia and goblet-cell metaplasia in the airways and also strongly reduced the development of airway hyperresponsiveness.[21] Allergen-specific IgG1 and IgE serum levels are also strongly reduced. These findings correlated with decreased levels of IL-4 and IL-5 in the airways in NES-treated animals.[21] The suppressive effects on the development of allergic responses were independent of the presence of Toll-like receptors (TLR) 2 and 4, IFN-γ, and IL-10. Paradoxically, strong helminth NES-specific Th2 responses are induced in parallel with the inhibition of asthma-like responses.[21]

Th2 responses induced by allergens or helminths share many common features. However, allergen-specific IgE can almost always be detected in patients with atopy, whereas helminth-specific IgE is often not detectable and anaphylaxis often occurs in atopy but not with helminth infections.

This may be caused by T regulatory responses induced by the helminths or the lack of helminth-specific IgE. Alternatively nonspecific IgE induced by the helminths may protect from mast cell or basophil degranulation by saturating IgE binding sites. Both of these mechanisms have been implicated to be involved in helminth-induced protection from allergic responses.[22] However, a study has shown that N brasiliensis antigen (Nb-Ag1) specific IgE could only be detected for a short period of time during infection, and that these levels are sufficient to prime mast cells thereby leading to active cutaneous anaphylaxis after the application of Nb-Ag1. Taken together, at least for the model helminth N brasiliensis, the IgE blocking hypothesis can be discarded.[23] However, novel antigens binding helminth-specific IgE may be identified for other pathogenic helminths infecting humans. Identifying these antigens may aid in IgE/mast cell–dependent vaccine development for asthma.[22]

Epidemiologic studies suggest that a hookworm infection producing 50 eggs per gram of feces may protect against asthma.[24] A pilot dose-ranging study of experimental human infection with Necator americanus larvae has been performed to identify the dose of hookworm larvae necessary to achieve 50 eggs per gram of feces for therapeutic trials in asthma.[25] Experimental infection with 10 hookworm larvae in patients with asthma did not result in significant improvement in bronchial responsiveness or other measures of asthma control. However, infection was well tolerated and resulted in a nonsignificant improvement in airway responsiveness, indicating that further studies that mimic more closely natural infection are feasible and should be undertaken.[26] More controlled studies are ongoing in this area and will provide useful new data in the coming years.

RESPIRATORY INFECTIONS AND INCREASED RISK OF DEVELOPMENT OF ASTHMA

Some epidemiologic studies suggest that certain early life respiratory tract infections can favor the development of asthma later in life. However, it is unknown whether early childhood viral infections cause asthma or simply identify those who are predisposed to asthma development. Furthermore, if respiratory infections are a causal factor, it is not known which specific microorganisms are most likely to cause asthma development. Finally, the immunopathologic link between respiratory infections and asthma development is not known.

Studies that have directly analyzed infectious episodes during infancy (ie, by parental reports or doctor diagnosis) suggest that respiratory infections in early life favor the later development of asthma. Nystad and colleagues[27] have found a positive association between full-time day care and early respiratory tract infections and asthma. The association between early infections and asthma was stronger than that between day care and asthma. In this Oslo Birth Cohort, established in 1992 to 1993, early respiratory infections did not protect against the development of asthma during the first 10 years of life but increased the risk for asthma symptoms at age 10.[28] In another epidemiologic study (the Tucson study) a higher prevalence of asthma was found in children who had doctor-diagnosed pneumonia or lower respiratory tract infection, reported by parents, in early life.[29]

These studies report a positive association between asthma and infections but not the direction of this association. It is not clear whether this association is "causal" or "circumstantial." Indeed, children predisposed to asthma may simply be more likely to develop respiratory tract infections. Another hypothesis is that individuals at high risk of developing asthma are more likely to develop symptoms with respiratory tract infections, and therefore the seemingly higher incidence of infections is influenced by reporting bias. Another confounding factor to consider is the site and type of infection (ie, gastrointestinal rather than respiratory, or bacterial rather than viral) or the possibility that in the future a specific pathogenic strain associated with the subsequent onset of asthma can be identified.

RESPIRATORY VIRAL INFECTIONS AND INCREASED RISK OF DEVELOPMENT OF ASTHMA

Several epidemiologic studies suggest that infants who develop severe viral respiratory infections are more likely to have asthma later in childhood.[30] This evidence is strongest for respiratory infections caused by respiratory syncytial virus (RSV) and rhinoviruses (RVs). However, the link between respiratory viral infections and asthma development remains unclear. The four main causative mechanisms hypothesized in the association between viral respiratory infections and the subsequent development of asthma in children are (1) alterations in airway function and size; (2) dysregulation (congenital and acquired) of airway tone, (3) alterations in the immune response to infections; and (4) the genetic variants involved in immune response.[30] There is a need to better understand whether host factors, such as epithelial cell function or immune response or virulence of virus strain, are important in modulating the subsequent risk to develop asthma after a respiratory viral infection.[31]

In humans there is scarce evidence that respiratory viral infections in early life compromising the airway epithelial barrier lead to enhanced absorption of allergens across this barrier and enhance lung sensitization to aeroallergens, whereas there is more evidence that the airway epithelium of subjects with atopy and asthma is more prone to respiratory viral infections.[32–34] For example, allergens can damage antiviral responses of the airway epithelium and this can promote greater viral replication.[32]

RSV INFECTIONS AND INCREASED RISK OF DEVELOPMENT OF ASTHMA

RSV is the major cause of severe bronchiolitis in children less than 1 year of age; consequently, it is considered the most important respiratory tract pathogen of early childhood.[35] In animal studies neonatal RSV infection sensitizes the newborn to develop an asthma-like phenotype on reinfection.[30,36,37] Sigurs and colleagues[38] found that severe RSV bronchiolitis, linked to hospitalization, was associated with a significantly increased risk of asthma to 18 years of age, especially in children with a family history of atopy. These results are supported by another study conducted in Tennessee. Wu and colleagues[39] reported that children born 120 days before the peak of RSV season have the highest rate of hospitalization for wheezing illnesses and also the greatest risk of asthma between 4 and 5 years of age. Future reports from this cohort (The Tennessee Children's Respiratory Initiative) will help to clarify the complex relationship between infant respiratory viral infection severity, etiology, atopic predisposition, and the subsequent development of early childhood asthma.

However, not all the investigations have seen this positive relationship between RSV infections and a subsequent increased risk of development of asthma.[40] For example, the Tucson Children's Respiratory Study reported an association between RSV lower respiratory tract infections before 3 years of age and development of asthma in early childhood, but this association was not observed beyond age 11 years.[41] Thus, severe RSV infections did not cause asthma, but instead, interacted with other genetic, environmental, and developmental factors, changing the expression of the asthma phenotype over time. For example, in one study the infants who subsequently developed RSV bronchiolitis have lower cord blood levels of IL-12 at birth[42] suggesting that RSV does not induce a Th2 response but that in the subjects susceptible to RSV infections there is already a preexisting impaired Th1 immunity. A possible cause of this deficiency of IL-12 is a polymorphism in the CD14 gene, with lower levels of soluble CD14 (a coreceptor along with the TLR-4 for the detection of bacterial lipopolysaccharide) and consequently higher serum IgE levels and diminished Th1 function.[43] In addition, a recent study found that impaired cord-blood immune responses to RSV predict the susceptibility to acute respiratory tract illness during the first year of life.[44]

RV INFECTIONS OF THE RESPIRATORY TRACT AND INCREASED RISK OF DEVELOPMENT OF ASTHMA

RSV is not the only cause of bronchiolitis in infants; in 2% to 40% of cases the causative agent is RV infection.[45] Bronchiolitis associated with RV infections, occurring mainly during spring and fall, are associated with a 25% increased likelihood of early childhood asthma compared with those occurring during winter and associated mainly with RSV infections.[46] Furthermore, hospitalization for RV-associated wheezing Illnesses during the first 2 years of life increases fourfold the risk of childhood asthma compared with hospitalization for wheezing associated with other viruses.[46]

These findings suggest that RV infection is more strongly associated with the risk of asthma development than is RSV infection. Thus, the increased risk of development of asthma associated with respiratory viral infections seems to be related not only to the type of infection but also timing of this and the recurrence or not of wheezing over time.

The COAST study has demonstrated that the age at which RV wheezing illnesses occur is very important to define subsequent asthma risk at age 6 years.[47] Particularly, children who wheezed with RV during the third year of life have about a 32-fold increase in asthma risk at age 6 years, compared with those who wheezed during the first year of life.[47]

Moreover, children who began wheezing before age 3 and continued to wheeze at school-age had impairment in lung function that persisted at least to the teenage years.[48] In summary, children with persistent rather than transient wheezing are more likely to develop asthma. Transient wheezing may depend on mechanical factors, such as small airway size, and when these children grow older and their airway caliber increases their wheezing may resolve.

There is evidence suggesting that the immune response between these groups is different. In one study the group of children with persistent wheeze has increased eosinophils and mast cell number and eosinophilic cationic protein levels in bronchoalveolar lavage.[49] Other studies have found higher levels of serum IgE and eosinophilic cationic protein during viral infections in persistent wheezers than in transient wheezers,[50,51] and eosinophil activity in early life predicts the development of childhood asthma after hospitalization for wheezing in infancy.[51,52] These findings are suggestive of an underlying Th2-predominant immune response in children with persistent wheeze. Instead, transient wheezers may have an immune response less skewed toward a Th2 differentiation and other mechanisms are important to explain their wheezing. Furthermore, in persistent wheezing, inflammatory changes and remodeling typical of asthma develop between 1 and 3 years of age and not before, emphasizing the potential importance of virus infections and probably other environmental exposures during this period.[53]

Despite RV infections being the main respiratory viral infections associated with an increased risk of subsequent development of asthma, it is likely that RV infection does not cause asthma by itself, because RV infections are very common in the general population and not all children infected by RV develop later asthma. This suggests that, in addition to early respiratory viral infections, there are other factors that contribute to asthma development, such as the viral strain that could be more "asthmagenic"; environmental factors (ie, tobacco smoke exposure and allergic sensitization during early childhood); and host factors (ie, genetic predisposition to atopy with probably impaired Th1 immunity leading to defective antiviral responses).[54,55]

For example, the barrier function of the airway epithelium is an important component of the innate immune response to respiratory viral infection. Disruption of the airway epithelium could alter host antiviral responses and increase replication of RV. This is a potential mechanism by which various environmental exposures, such as tobacco smoke and allergens, may increase viral replication and determine more severe lower respiratory illnesses.

IFN deficiencies are another potential mechanism behind the susceptibility of people with asthma to more severe RV illnesses. Bronchial epithelial cells and alveolar macrophages from subjects with atopic asthma infected in vitro with RV produce less IFN-β and IFN-λ compared with control subjects and this is associated with increased RV replication,[33,34] and peripheral blood cells from patients with atopic asthma, when exposed to respiratory viruses, produce lower levels of IFN-α.[56] Studies have linked reduced peripheral blood IFN-γ responses at first months of life to an increased risk of wheezing in school-age children.[57]

BACTERIAL INFECTIONS AND INCREASED RISK OF DEVELOPMENT OF ASTHMA

There is some evidence to support a role for chronic bacterial infection or colonization of the lower airways with an increased risk of development of asthma, but it is also possible that a subject with altered immune function, biased toward atopy, may have altered host defenses that increase susceptibility to bacterial infections and an increased risk of developing asthma.[58,59] Indeed, there is evidence of impaired IFN responses in patients with atopic asthma to bacterial polysaccharides[34] and of an approximately threefold increased risk of severe respiratory bacterial infections in people with asthma.[59]

The potential role of atypical bacterial infection in the pathogenesis of asthma is a subject of continuing debate. There is an increasing body of literature concerning the association between the atypical intracellular bacteria Chlamydophila (formerly Chlamydia) pneumoniae and Mycoplasma pneumoniae and asthma pathogenesis; however, many studies investigating such a link have been uncontrolled and have provided conflicting evidence, in part because of the difficulty in accurately diagnosing infection with these atypical pathogens.[60]

Using highly sensitive molecular techniques the genome of M pneumoniae and C pneumoniae are frequently detected in samples from the lower airways of patients with asthma, although their exact contribution to asthma development or persistence remains to be determined and a definitive diagnosis of infection is often difficult to obtain because of limitations with sampling and detection.[61] It has been previously reported that approximately 40% of adult subjects with acute asthma exacerbations had evidence of reactivation of C pneumoniae infection, and that those with evidence of reactivation had four times greater neutrophilic and eosinophilic airway inflammation.[62]

Small uncontrolled serologic studies suggest also that in a subgroup of adults with severe persistent asthma a chronic infection with C pneumoniae may amplify the inflammation that occurs in asthma and improves with antibiotic therapy effective against C pneumonia.[61] However, other studies have shown that seropositivity to C pneumoniae is common in older adults and does not correlate with asthma.[63,64] Another study performed with methods (eg, culture, polymerase chain reaction [PCR]) that are more specific for persistent *C pneumoniae* infection than serology could not find any evidence of *C pneumoniae* infection in the airways of adults with stable persistent asthma.[65]

Numerous animal studies have outlined mechanisms by which these infections may promote allergic lung inflammation and airway remodeling.[61] *C pneumoniae* infection can induce allergic airway sensitization in animals modulating the action of T regulatory and dendritic cells.[66] There is evidence in animal models that chronic asymptomatic chlamydial infections may cause persistent airway inflammatory responses through innate and adaptive immune responses. Indeed, this chronic infection, through chronic antigenic stimulation, seems to promote continued specific IgE production, which causes bronchoconstriction, airway inflammation, and hyperreactivity.[66] Furthermore, the major *C pneumoniae* antigen, heat-shock protein 60, seems to be a powerful inducer of macrophage inflammatory response through the innate immune receptor complex TLR-4/MD-2.[67]

Case reports suggest the onset of persistent asthma after *M pneumoniae* infection[61] and a few studies suggest a chronic reduction of small airways function after childhood *M pneumoniae* infection.[61] A report has demonstrated that *M pneumoniae* is present by PCR (but not culture) in the lower airways (bronchoalveolar lavage or bronchial biopsies) of 9 of 18 adults with persistent asthma and only 1 of 11 control subjects.[65] In animals and human subjects during respiratory tract infections *M pneumoniae* is mainly localized to the cilia of bronchial epithelial cells.[61]

In animal studies *M pneumoniae* infection of the lungs is associated with an elevated IL-4/INF-γ ratio and development of airway hyperresponsiveness.[68] Studies in mice have shown that allergic airway inflammation impairs antibacterial host defenses: it particularly reduces the expression of TLR-2 and the production of IL-6, which play an important role in *M pneumoniae* response,[39] and markedly reduces short palate, lung, and nasal epithelium clone 1 protein expression, contributing to persistent *Mycoplasma* infection in allergic airway disease.[58]

Animal studies have also suggested that mycoplasmic infections may contribute to neurogenic inflammation in the airways.[69] Neurogenic inflammation is induced in a murine model of respiratory infection with *Mycoplasma pulmonis* and sensory nerve stimulation with capsaicin. The infected rat airway demonstrates an increased neurokinin 1 expression on blood vessels and enhanced mucus production in the trachea epithelial layer.[69]

Treatment with a tetracycline antibiotic in this animal model significantly reduced the airway neurogenic inflammation and the number of infecting organisms.[69] Increased expression of substance P or neurokinin 1 receptor has been shown in the lower airway tissue, especially in the bronchial epithelium, of subjects with asthma and *M pneumoniae* infection compared with normal control subjects and subjects with asthma without *M pneumoniae* infection.[69] Subjects with asthma treated with a macrolide antibiotic active against *M pneumoniae* show reduction of substance P, neurokinin 1, and mucus in the epithelium. Reduction of epithelial neurokinin 1 expression is more prominent in subjects with asthma and *M pneumoniae* than in those without *M pneumoniae* infection.[69] However, because macrolide antibiotics have been suggested to have some direct anti-inflammatory effects, it is not possible to exclude the possibility that these results may be caused by their anti-inflammatory effect. For example, clarithromycin treatment in patients with asthma could reduce the edematous area as identified by α_2-macroglobulin staining, which may lead to airway tissue shrinkage and cause an artificial increase in the number of blood vessels.[70]

It is possible that chronic airway infection by atypical bacteria promotes persistent airway inflammation that favors progression of asthma and action of viruses or allergens. The role of antimicrobials, particularly macrolide-ketolide antibiotics, directed against atypical bacteria in asthma is still under investigation.[61,71] Animal studies, case reports, and a few small, mainly uncontrolled, pilot studies suggested initially a potential benefit of these drugs in the chronic treatment of stable persistent asthma.[61,71] In a small controlled clinical trial 6 weeks of clarithromycin therapy improves lung function in adults with asthma, but only in those subjects with positive PCR findings for *M pneumoniae* or *C pneumonia*.[72]

However, more recently in a large controlled clinical trial, adding clarithromycin to fluticasone in adults with mild-to-moderate persistent asthma that was suboptimally controlled by low-dose inhaled glucocorticoids alone did not further improve asthma control. Although there is an improvement in airway hyperresponsiveness with clarithromycin, this benefit is not accompanied by improvements in other secondary outcomes.[73] In another controlled clinical trial performed in a subgroup subjects with asthma with serologic evidence of *C pneumoniae* infection, 6 weeks of treatment with roxithromycin led to an initial improvement in asthma control but this benefit is not sustained at 3 and 6 months after the end of treatment, where differences between the two groups are not significant.[74] Furthermore, in another controlled clinical trial azithromycin has not been an effective inhaled corticosteroid-sparing agent in children with moderate-to-severe persistent asthma.[75]

In analyzing the results of the controlled clinical trials using antibacterial agents for the treatment of chronic asthma it should also be noted that macrolide-ketolide antibiotics have been suggested to have in vitro and in vivo some direct anti-inflammatory, immunomodulatory, and antiviral effects independent from their antibacterial action.[76] Furthermore, telithromycin, like macrolides, is also a strong inhibitor of cytochrome P-450 (CYP) isoenzyme 3A4. Two inhaled glucocorticoids commonly used in clinical practice (budesonide and fluticasone) are metabolized to inactive catabolites predominantly by CYP3A enzymes in the liver. The CYP3A4 is also responsible for aliphatic oxidation of the long-acting inhaled β_2-agonist bronchodilator salmeterol, which is extensively metabolized by hydroxylation. Drug interactions may reduce CYP3A activity through inhibition or may increase metabolic activity through induction. Such interactions can expand the range of variability of its activity to about 400-fold.[77] Further controlled clinical trials are required to assess the role of these antimicrobals in the treatment of severe stable asthma.

A study has found that neonates colonized in the hypopharyngeal region with Streptococcus pneumoniae, Haemophilus influenzae, or Moraxella catarrhalis, or with a combination of these organisms, are at increased risk for recurrent wheeze and asthma early in life,[78] suggesting a potential role for neonatal extracellular bacteria colonization of the upper airways in modulating the risk of developing asthma. This interesting new area of research clearly requires more data.

Several experimental, epidemiologic, and clinical observations support the hypothesis that changes in human indigenous microbiota can be a predisposing risk factor for asthma.[79] The microbiota resides as a stable climax community. However, it is dynamic and has the ability to maintain its structure after a perturbation (resistance) and to return to its baseline structure after resistance is broken (resilience).[80] Although the adults' microbiota remains relatively stable over time, the microbiota's structure in the first months of life is strongly influenced by many environmental factors, such as antibiotic use, dietary changes, and other lifestyle differences.[81]

Chronic airway colonization by pathogenic bacteria (airway microbiota) may directly play a role in the pathogenesis of chronic asthma. Recent studies using molecular analysis of the polymorphic bacterial 16S-rRNA gene to characterize the composition of bacterial communities from the lower airways have demonstrated that the bronchial tree is not sterile, containing a mean of 2000 bacterial genomes per square centimeter surface sampled.[82] Pathogenic Proteobacteria, particularly Haemophilus spp., are more frequent in bronchi of adults with asthma than control subjects and there is a significant increase in Proteobacteria in children with asthma. Conversely, Bacteroidetes, particularly Prevotella spp., are more frequent in control subjects than people with asthma.[82] Compared with control subjects, 16S ribosomal RNA amplicon concentrations (an index of bacterial burden) and bacterial diversity are significantly higher among patients with asthma. Furthermore, the relative abundance of particular phylotypes, including members of the Comamonadaceae, Sphingomonadaceae, Oxalobacteraceae, and other bacterial families, are highly correlated with the degree of bronchial hyperresponsiveness of the patient with asthma.[83]

The highest concentration of microbes on the mucosal surface in the human body is in the gastrointestinal tract, and this "gut microbiota" is also thought to modulate the risk of developing asthma. In epidemiologic and clinical studies there is a correlation between an alteration in the fecal microbiota and the risk of developing asthma,[79,81] and early childhood antibiotic use slightly increases the risk of later development of asthma.[84]

There is evidence for the perinatal programing of asthma by the gastrointestinal microbiome.[85] Physiologic gastrointestinal microflora dominated by lactic acid bacteria is crucial for the maturation and proper functioning of the human immune system. Gut microbiota play a central role in the maintenance of oral and airway tolerance, because they seem tightly linked.[85] The colonization of the intestine begins during the birthing process and these commensal bacteria play an important role in shaping the immune system during infancy.[85] Gut microbes induce regulatory T cells that help guide the host's Th1/Th2 balance, keeping resident dendritic cells in an immature or noninflammatory state.[85] Infants who develop asthma probably harbor a distinct gut microbiota. In particular, the pathogen Clostridium difficile has been associated with increased future risk of asthma.[86]

Caesarean delivery, breastfeeding, probiotics, and antibiotics are the main modifiers of infant gut microbiota in the development of asthma. The association between caesarean delivery and increased risk of developing asthma in children is controversial.[87] Caesarean delivery may prevent exposure to maternal fecal microbes, resulting in less intestinal colonization by Bifidobacterium and *Bacteroides* and increased colonization by *C difficile*, and this effect persist for years.[88]

Breastfeeding protects against recurrent wheeze and asthma in later childhood; however, these benefits may not apply when the nursing mother has atopy.[85] Interestingly, the milk of mothers with atopy contains significantly lower amounts of *Bifidobacterium* compared with nonallergic mothers and this may increase the risk of asthma later in childhood.[89]

Direct and indirect (infants born to mothers who received antibiotics during pregnancy or while breastfeeding) early exposure to antibiotics may suppress commensal gut bacteria and permit the emergence of asthma-associated pathogens, such as *C. difficile*,[90] and these perturbations could last for years.[91] Two recent studies have found that this association is limited to nonatopic predisposed children,[92] probably because infants of mothers with atopy inherit low levels of commensal bacteria[89] and then antibiotic exposure would be less disruptive on commensal gut bacteria. However, in childhood, the antibiotic treatment is often prescribed in response to respiratory infections,[84] suggesting that respiratory infections and not antibiotic usage may increase the risk of asthma development.

Finally, studies have shown that administration of probiotics to pregnant women, nursing mothers, or newborns can influence the composition of gut microbiota.[93] In animal studies direct and indirect supplementation of probiotics is able to attenuate allergic airway responses.[94] However, the results of the controlled clinical trials in humans have been highly variable.[95] Probiotic supplementation may have clinical benefits for school-age children with asthma. Many more good-quality studies are needed to resolve this issue.

SUMMARY

There are increasing fascinating data to support the "hygiene" and "microbiota" hypotheses of a protective role of infections (mainly viral and bacterial, but also helminthic) in modulating the risk of subsequent development of asthma. However, there is less evidence that respiratory infections can actually cause the development of asthma. There is some evidence that RV respiratory infections are associated with the development of asthma, particularly in childhood, whereas these infections in later life seem to have a weaker association with the development of asthma. The role of bacterial infections in chronic asthma remains unclear, but there are emerging data for a potential role of *M pneumoniae* and *C pneumoniae* and gut microbiota in increasing the risk of the development of asthma and in modulating the degree of asthma control.

ACKNOWLEDGMENTS

The Section of Respiratory Diseases of the University of Ferrara - Italy - received unrestricted grants for research from the Chiesi Foundation, Parma, Italy.

REFERENCES

1. Global Initiative for Asthma. Global strategy for Asthma Management and Prevention. NHLBI/WHO Workshop report 2002. NHI Publication 02-3659. Last update 2011. Available at: http://www.ginasthma.com. Accessed July 10, 2012.
2. Barnes PJ, Chung KF, Page CP. Inflammatory mediators of asthma: an update. Pharmacol Rev 1998;50: 515–96.
3. Contoli M, Baraldo S, Marku B, et al. Fixed airflow obstruction due to asthma or chronic obstructive pulmonary disease: 5-year follow-up. J Allergy Clin Immunol 2010;125:830–7.
4. Maestrelli P, Caramori G, Franco F, et al. Definition, clinical features, investigations and differential diagnosis in asthma. In: Kay AB, Bousquet J, Holt P, et al, editors. Allergy and allergic disease, vol. 2, 2nd edition. London: Blackwell; 2008. p. 1597–620.
5. Barnes KC. Genetic studies of the etiology of asthma. Proc Am Thorac Soc 2011;8:143–8.
6. Torgerson DG, Ampleford EJ, Chiu GY, et al. Meta-analysis of genome-wide association studies of asthma in ethnically diverse North American populations. Nat Genet 2011;43:887–92.
7. Mallia P, Contoli M, Caramori G, et al. Exacerbations of asthma and chronic obstructive pulmonary disease (COPD): focus on virus induced exacerbations. Curr Pharm Des 2007;13:73–97.
8. Strachan DP. Family size, infection and atopy: the first decade of the "hygiene hypothesis." Thorax 2000;55(Suppl 1):S2–10.
9. von Mutius E. Allergies, infections and the hygiene hypothesis: the epidemiological evidence. Immunobiology 2007;212:433–9.
10. Ball TM, Castro-Rodriguez JA, Griffith KA, et al. Siblings, day-care attendance, and the risk of asthma and wheezing during childhood. N Engl J Med 2000;343:538–43.
11. Oddy WH, de Klerk NH, Sly PD, et al. The effects of respiratory infections, atopy, and breastfeeding on childhood asthma. Eur Respir J 2002;19:899–905.
12. Holt PG. Postnatal maturation of immune competence during infancy and childhood. Pediatr Allergy Immunol 1995;6:59–70.
13. Prescott SL, Macaubas C, Smallacombe T, et al. Development of allergen-specific T-cell memory

in atopic and normal children. Lancet 1999;353: 196–200.

14. Tschernig T, Debertin AS, Paulsen F, et al. Dendritic cells in the mucosa of the human trachea are not regularly found in the first year of life. Thorax 2001; 56:427–31.

15. von Mutius E. A fascinating look at the world with a new microscope. J Allergy Clin Immunol 2012; 129:1202–3.

16. Heederik D, von Mutius E. Does diversity of environmental microbial exposure matter for the occurrence of allergy and asthma? J Allergy Clin Immunol 2012; 130:44–50.

17. Herbst T, Sichelstiel A, Schar C, et al. Dysregulation of allergic airway inflammation in the absence of microbial colonization. Am J Respir Crit Care Med 2011;184:198–205.

18. Oyama N, Sudo N, Sogawa H, et al. Antibiotic use during infancy promotes a shift in the T(h)1/T(h)2 balance toward T(h)2-dominant immunity in mice. J Allergy Clin Immunol 2001;107:153–9.

19. Brand S, Teich R, Dicke T, et al. Epigenetic regulation in murine offspring as a novel mechanism for transmaternal asthma protection induced by microbes. J Allergy Clin Immunol 2011;128:618–25.

20. Cooper PJ, Barreto ML, Rodrigues LC. Human allergy and geohelminth infections: a review of the literature and a proposed conceptual model to guide the investigation of possible causal associations. Br Med Bull 2006;79–80:203–18.

21. Trujillo-Vargas CM, Werner-Klein M, Wohlleben G, et al. Helminth-derived products inhibit the development of allergic responses in mice. Am J Respir Crit Care Med 2007;175:336–44.

22. Erb KJ. Helminths, allergic disorders and IgE-mediated immune responses: where do we stand? Eur J Immunol 2007;37:1170–3.

23. Pochanke V, Koller S, Dayer R, et al. Identification and characterization of a novel antigen from the nematode Nippostrongylus brasiliensis recognized by specific IgE. Eur J Immunol 2007;37:1275–84.

24. Scrivener S, Yemaneberhan H, Zebenigus M, et al. Independent effects of intestinal parasite infection and domestic allergen exposure on risk of wheeze in Ethiopia: a nested case-control study. Lancet 2001;358:1493–9.

25. Mortimer K, Brown A, Feary J, et al. Dose-ranging study for trials of therapeutic infection with Necator americanus in humans. Am J Trop Med Hyg 2006; 75:914–20.

26. Feary JR, Venn AJ, Mortimer K, et al. Experimental hookworm infection: a randomized placebo-controlled trial in asthma. Clin Exp Allergy 2010;40: 299–306.

27. Nystad W, Skrondal A, Magnus P. Day care attendance, recurrent respiratory tract infections and asthma. Int J Epidemiol 1999;28:882–7.

28. Nafstad P, Brunekreef B, Skrondal A, et al. Early respiratory infections, asthma, and allergy: 10-year follow-up of the Oslo Birth Cohort. Pediatrics 2005; 116:e255–62.

29. Castro-Rodriguez JA, Holberg CJ, Wright AL, et al. Association of radiologically ascertained pneumonia before age 3 year with asthmalike symptoms and pulmonary function during childhood: a prospective study. Am J Respir Crit Care Med 1999; 159:1891–7.

30. Dakhama A, Lee YM, Gelfand EW. Virus-induced airway dysfunction: pathogenesis and biomechanisms. Pediatr Infect Dis J 2005;24:S159–69.

31. Papadopoulos NG, Gourgiotis D, Javadyan A, et al. Does respiratory syncytial virus subtype influences the severity of acute bronchiolitis in hospitalized infants? Respir Med 2004;98:879–82.

32. Rosenthal LA, Avila PC, Heymann PW, et al. Viral respiratory tract infections and asthma: the course ahead. J Allergy Clin Immunol 2010;125:1212–7.

33. Wark PA, Johnston SL, Bucchieri F, et al. Asthmatic bronchial epithelial cells have a deficient innate immune response to infection with rhinovirus. J Exp Med 2005;201:937–47.

34. Contoli M, Message SD, Laza-Stanca V, et al. Role of deficient type III interferon-lambda production in asthma exacerbations. Nat Med 2006;12:1023–6.

35. Psarras S, Papadopoulos NG, Johnston SL. Pathogenesis of respiratory syncytial virus bronchiolitis-related wheezing. Paediatr Respir Rev 2004; 5(Suppl A):S179–84.

36. Dakhama A, Lee YM, Ohnishi H, et al. Virus-specific IgE enhances airway responsiveness on reinfection with respiratory syncytial virus in newborn mice. J Allergy Clin Immunol 2009;123:138–45.

37. Culley FJ, Pollott J, Openshaw PJ. Age at first viral infection determines the pattern of T cell-mediated disease during reinfection in adulthood. J Exp Med 2002;196:1381–6.

38. Sigurs N, Aljassim F, Kjellman B, et al. Asthma and allergy patterns over 18 years after severe RSV bronchiolitis in the first year of life. Thorax 2010;65: 1045–52.

39. Wu P, Dupont WD, Griffin MR, et al. Evidence of a causal role of winter virus infection during infancy in early childhood asthma. Am J Respir Crit Care Med 2008;178:1123–9.

40. Stein RT, Sherrill D, Morgan WJ, et al. Respiratory syncytial virus in early life and risk of wheeze and allergy by age 13 years. Lancet 1999;354:541–5.

41. Taussig LM, Wright AL, Holberg CJ, et al. Tucson Children's Respiratory Study: 1980 to present. J Allergy Clin Immunol 2003;111:661–75.

42. Blanco-Quiros A, Gonzalez H, Arranz E, et al. Decreased interleukin-12 levels in umbilical cord blood in children who developed acute bronchiolitis. Pediatr Pulmonol 1999;28:175–80.

43. Baldini M, Lohman IC, Halonen M, et al. A polymorphism* in the 5' flanking region of the CD14 gene is associated with circulating soluble CD14 levels and with total serum immunoglobulin E. Am J Respir Cell Mol Biol 1999;20:976–83.

44. Sumino K, Tucker J, Shahab M, et al. Antiviral IFN-gamma responses of monocytes at birth predict respiratory tract illness in the first year of life. J Allergy Clin Immunol 2012;129:1267–73.

45. Papadopoulos NG, Moustaki M, Tsolia M, et al. Association of rhinovirus infection with increased disease severity in acute bronchiolitis. Am J Respir Crit Care Med 2002;165:1285–9.

46. Miller EK, Williams JV, Gebretsadik T, et al. Host and viral factors associated with severity of human rhinovirus-associated infant respiratory tract illness. J Allergy Clin Immunol 2011;127:883–91.

47. Jackson DJ, Gangnon RE, Evans MD, et al. Wheezing rhinovirus illnesses in early life predict asthma development in high-risk children. Am J Respir Crit Care Med 2008;178:667–72.

48. Morgan WJ, Stern DA, Sherrill DL, et al. Outcome of asthma and wheezing in the first 6 years of life: follow-up through adolescence. Am J Respir Crit Care Med 2005;172:1253–8.

49. Ennis M, Turner G, Schock BC, et al. Inflammatory mediators in bronchoalveolar lavage samples from children with and without asthma. Clin Exp Allergy 1999;29:362–6.

50. Martinez FD, Stern DA, Wright AL, et al. Differential immune responses to acute lower respiratory illness in early life and subsequent development of persistent wheezing and asthma. J Allergy Clin Immunol 1998;102:915–20.

51. Koller DY, Wojnarowski C, Herkner KR, et al. High levels of eosinophil cationic protein in wheezing infants predict the development of asthma. J Allergy Clin Immunol 1997;99:752–6.

52. Hyvarinen MK, Kotaniemi-Syrjanen A, Reijonen TM, et al. Eosinophil activity in infants hospitalized for wheezing and risk of persistent childhood asthma. Pediatr Allergy Immunol 2010;21:96–103.

53. Saglani S, Malmstrom K, Pelkonen AS, et al. Airway remodeling and inflammation in symptomatic infants with reversible airflow obstruction. Am J Respir Crit Care Med 2005;171:722–7.

54. Miller EK, Edwards KM, Weinberg GA, et al. A novel group of rhinoviruses is associated with asthma hospitalizations. J Allergy Clin Immunol 2009;123:98–104.

55. Message SD, Laza-Stanca V, Mallia P, et al. Rhinovirus-induced lower respiratory illness is increased in asthma and related to virus load and Th1/2 cytokine and IL-10 production. Proc Natl Acad Sci U S A 2008;105:13562–7.

56. Bufe A, Gehlhar K, Grage-Griebenow E, et al. Atopic phenotype in children is associated with decreased virus-induced interferon-alpha release. Int Arch Allergy Immunol 2002;127:82–8.

57. Stern DA, Guerra S, Halonen M, et al. Low IFN-gamma production in the first year of life as a predictor of wheeze during childhood. J Allergy Clin Immunol 2007;120:835–41.

58. Chu HW, Thaikoottathil J, Rino JG, et al. Function and regulation of SPLUNC1 protein in Mycoplasma infection and allergic inflammation. J Immunol 2007; 179:3995–4002.

59. Talbot TR, Hartert TV, Mitchel E, et al. Asthma as a risk factor for invasive pneumococcal disease. N Engl J Med 2005;352:2082–90.

60. Johnston SL, Martin RJ. Chlamydophila pneumoniae and Mycoplasma pneumoniae: a role in asthma pathogenesis? Am J Respir Crit Care Med 2005; 172:1078–89.

61. Metz G, Kraft M. Effects of atypical infections with Mycoplasma and Chlamydia on asthma. Immunol Allergy Clin North Am 2010;30:575–85.

62. Wark PA, Johnston SL, Simpson JL, et al. Chlamydia pneumoniae immunoglobulin A reactivation and airway inflammation in acute asthma. Eur Respir J 2002;20:834–40.

63. Mills GD, Lindeman JA, Fawcett JP, et al. Chlamydia pneumoniae serological status is not associated with asthma in children or young adults. Int J Epidemiol 2000;29:280–4.

64. Routes JM, Nelson HS, Noda JA, et al. Lack of correlation between Chlamydia pneumoniae antibody titers and adult-onset asthma. J Allergy Clin Immunol 2000;105:391–2.

65. Kraft M, Cassell GH, Henson JE, et al. Detection of Mycoplasma pneumoniae in the airways of adults with chronic asthma. Am J Respir Crit Care Med 1998;158:998–1001.

66. Crother TR, Schroder NW, Karlin J, et al. Chlamydia pneumoniae infection induced allergic airway sensitization is controlled by regulatory T-cells and plasmacytoid dendritic cells. PLoS One 2011; 6:e20784.

67. Bulut Y, Faure E, Thomas L, et al. Chlamydial heat shock protein 60 activates macrophages and endothelial cells through Toll-like receptor 4 and MD2 in a MyD88-dependent pathway. J Immunol 2002; 168:1435–40.

68. Koh YY, Park Y, Lee HJ, et al. Levels of interleukin-2, interferon-gamma, and interleukin-4 in bronchoalveolar lavage fluid from patients with Mycoplasma pneumoniae: implication of tendency toward increased immunoglobulin E production. Pediatrics 2001;107:E39.

69. Chu HW, Kraft M, Krause JE, et al. Substance P and its receptor neurokinin 1 expression in asthmatic airways. J Allergy Clin Immunol 2000;106:713–22.

70. Chu HW, Kraft M, Rex MD, et al. Evaluation of blood vessels and edema in the airways of asthma

patients: regulation with clarithromycin treatment. Chest 2001;120:416–22.

71. Good JT Jr, Rollins DR, Martin RJ. Macrolides in the treatment of asthma. Curr Opin Pulm Med 2012;18: 76–84.

72. Kraft M, Cassell GH, Pak J, et al. *Mycoplasma pneumoniae* and *Chlamydia pneumoniae* in asthma: effect of clarithromycin. Chest 2002;121:1782–8.

73. Sutherland ER, King TS, Icitovic N, et al. A trial of clarithromycin for the treatment of suboptimally controlled asthma. J Allergy Clin Immunol 2010; 126:747–53.

74. Black PN, Blasi F, Jenkins CR, et al. Trial of roxithromycin in subjects with asthma and serological evidence of infection with *Chlamydia pneumoniae*. Am J Respir Crit Care Med 2001;164:536–41.

75. Strunk RC, Bacharier LB, Phillips BR, et al. Azithromycin or montelukast as inhaled corticosteroid-sparing agents in moderate-to-severe childhood asthma study. J Allergy Clin Immunol 2008;122:1138–44.

76. Zarogoulidis P, Papanas N, Kioumis I, et al. Macrolides: from in vitro anti-inflammatory and immunomodulatory properties to clinical practice in respiratory diseases. Eur J Clin Pharmacol 2012;68:479–503.

77. Caramori G, Papi A. Telithromycin in acute exacerbations of asthma. N Engl J Med 2006;355:96.

78. Bisgaard H, Hermansen MN, Buchvald F, et al. Childhood asthma after bacterial colonization of the airway in neonates. N Engl J Med 2007;357:1487–95.

79. Noverr MC, Huffnagle GB. The 'microflora hypothesis' of allergic diseases. Clin Exp Allergy 2005;35: 1511–20.

80. Allison SD, Martiny JB. Colloquium paper: resistance, resilience, and redundancy in microbial communities. Proc Natl Acad Sci U S A 2008; 105(Suppl 1):11512–9.

81. Murgas Torrazza R, Neu J. The developing intestinal microbiome and its relationship to health and disease in the neonate. J Perinatol 2011;31(Suppl 1):S29–34.

82. Hilty M, Burke C, Pedro H, et al. Disordered microbial communities in asthmatic airways. PLoS One 2010;5:e8578.

83. Huang YJ, Nelson CE, Brodie EL, et al. Airway microbiota and bronchial hyperresponsiveness in patients with suboptimally controlled asthma. J Allergy Clin Immunol 2011;127:372–81.

84. Penders J, Kummeling I, Thijs C. Infant antibiotic use and wheeze and asthma risk: a systematic review and meta-analysis. Eur Respir J 2011;38:295–302.

85. Azad MB, Kozyrskyj AL. Perinatal programming of asthma: the role of gut microbiota. Clin Dev Immunol 2012;2012:932072.

86. van Nimwegen FA, Penders J, Stobberingh EE, et al. Mode and place of delivery, gastrointestinal microbiota, and their influence on asthma and atopy. J Allergy Clin Immunol 2011;128:948–55.

87. Thavagnanam S, Fleming J, Bromley A, et al. A meta-analysis of the association between caesarean section and childhood asthma. Clin Exp Allergy 2008;38:629–33.

88. Salminen S, Gibson GR, McCartney AL, et al. Influence of mode of delivery on gut microbiota composition in seven year old children. Gut 2004;53: 1388–9.

89. Gronlund MM, Gueimonde M, Laitinen K, et al. Maternal breast-milk and intestinal bifidobacteria guide the compositional development of the *Bifidobacterium* microbiota in infants at risk of allergic disease. Clin Exp Allergy 2007;37:1764–72.

90. Tanaka S, Kobayashi T, Songjinda P, et al. Influence of antibiotic exposure in the early postnatal period on the development of intestinal microbiota. FEMS Immunol Med Microbiol 2009;56:80–7.

91. Jernberg C, Lofmark S, Edlund C, et al. Long-term ecological impacts of antibiotic administration on the human intestinal microbiota. ISME J 2007;1: 56–66.

92. Risnes KR, Belanger K, Murk W, et al. Antibiotic exposure by 6 months and asthma and allergy at 6 years: findings in a cohort of 1,401 US children. Am J Epidemiol 2011;173:310–8.

93. Kukkonen K, Savilahti E, Haahtela T, et al. Probiotics and prebiotic galacto-oligosaccharides in the prevention of allergic diseases: a randomized, double-blind, placebo-controlled trial. J Allergy Clin Immunol 2007;119:192–8.

94. Blumer N, Sel S, Virna S, et al. Perinatal maternal application of *Lactobacillus rhamnosus* GG suppresses allergic airway inflammation in mouse offspring. Clin Exp Allergy 2007;37:348–57.

95. Forsythe P. Probiotics and lung diseases. Chest 2011;139:901–8.

Difficult Childhood Asthma
Management and Future

Isabelle Tillie-Leblond, MD, PhD[a,b,*],
Antoine Deschildre, MD[b,c], Philippe Gosset, PhD[b],
Jacques de Blic, MD[d]

KEYWORDS

- Asthma • Severe • Child • Difficult

KEY POINTS

- Severe childhood asthma, refractory to treatment, includes different phenotypes. Genetics mainly contribute to disease expression, progression, and response to treatment. The gene-environment interactions involving certain gene polymorphisms are probably essential for creating its severity.
- The quality of care and monitoring of children with severe asthma is as important as the prescription drug, and is also crucial for differentiating between severe asthma and difficult asthma, so expertise is required.
- Further studies (genetic and proteomic data), performed in well phenotyped children with severe asthma, should improve knowledge of the mechanisms involved in frequent exacerbations, persistent obstruction, sudden-onset severe asthma and help the pediatric pulmonologist to choose the appropriate monitoring and treatment of the phenotype.

Severe asthma in children represents about 5% of asthmatics.[1] Diagnosis and management of severe asthma implies the definition of different entities, that is, difficult asthma and refractory severe asthma, but also the different phenotypes included in the term refractory severe asthma. A complete reevaluation by a physician expert in asthma is necessary, adapted for each child. Identification of mechanisms involved in different phenotypes in refractory severe asthma, may improve the therapeutic approach.

DEFINITION OF SEVERE CHILDHOOD ASTHMA

A wide variety of terms has been used by clinicians when referring to asthmatic children who have severe asthma: difficult-to-treat asthma, therapy-resistant asthma, difficult-to-control asthma, severe therapy-resistant asthma, severe refractory asthma and, more recently, problematic asthma.

The initial criteria for severe asthma in children were proposed in 1999 by the task force on

Conflict of interest: J.de B. has received grant research from GSK for immunohistopathologic analysis in severe asthma, honoraria for lectures and expert advice by CHIESI, GSK, MSD, and AstraZeneca. I.T.L. has received grant research from GSK for immunohistopathologic analysis in severe asthma, honoraria for lectures and expert advice by CHIESI, GSK, NOVARTIS, and AstraZeneca. A.D. has received honoraria for lectures and expert advises by NOVARTIS, GSK, and MSD.

[a] Pulmonary Department, University Hospital, Medical University of Lille, Hôpital Calmette, 1 Boulevard Leclercq, Lille Cedex 59037, France; [b] INSERM U 1019 Lung Infection and Innate Immunity, Université de Lille 2, Institut Pasteur, 1 rue du Professeur Calmette, BP 245, Lille Cedex 59019, France; [c] Unité de pneumopédiatrie, Centre de compétence des maladies respiratoires rares, Université Lille 2 et CHRU, Hôpital Jeanne de Flandre, Avenue Eugène Avinée, Lille 59037, France; [d] Service de pneumologie et allergologie pédiatriques, Centre de référence des maladies respiratoires rares, Hôpital Necker Enfants Malades, Assistance Publique des Hôpitaux de Paris; Université Paris Descartes, Paris 75015, France

* Corresponding author. Pulmonary Department, University Hospital, Medical University of Lille, Hôpital Calmette, 1 Boulevard Leclercq, 59037 Lille, Cedex, France.
E-mail address: i-tillie@chru-lille.fr

Clin Chest Med 33 (2012) 485–503
http://dx.doi.org/10.1016/j.ccm.2012.05.006
0272-5231/12/$ – see front matter © 2012 Elsevier Inc. All rights reserved.

difficult/therapy-resistant asthma.[2] A dose of beclomethasone or budesonide higher than 800 µg/d, or 400 µg/d of fluticasone was considered as reasonable threshold. In 2005, the American Thoracic Society (ATS) workshop reviewed by Wenzel[3] defined severe asthma in adults by the presence of one major criterion, namely, the need for high-dose inhaled corticosteroids or oral corticosteroids, and at least 2 of the following 7 minor criteria: (1) the need for a daily long-acting β2-agonist or leukotriene antagonist in addition to inhaled corticosteroids; (2) asthma symptoms requiring daily or near-daily use of a short-acting β2-agonist; (3) persistent airway obstruction, forced expiratory volume in 1 second (FEV_1) less than 80% predicted; (4) one or more emergency-care visits for asthma per year (5) 3 or more oral steroid "bursts" per year; (6) prompt deterioration with less than 25% reduction in oral or inhaled corticosteroid dose; (7) near-fatal asthma event in the past.[3]

More recently, in 2010, the Problematic Severe Asthma in Childhood Initiative Group has defined different categories of severe asthma.[4] Severe asthma should be considered in school-age children who, despite prescribed therapy with inhaled corticosteroid (ICS) (budesonide or equivalent 800 µg or more) with long-acting β-agonist (LABA) or leukotriene receptor antagonist, still have persistent chronic symptoms or exacerbations, or persistent airflow obstruction. Persistent chronic symptoms are defined if they occur most days (at least 3 times a week for ≥3 months) with poor quality of life. Acute exacerbations over the last year may require at least one admission to an intensive care unit, at least 2 hospital admissions, or at least 2 courses of oral steroids. Persistent airflow obstruction (following steroid trial) is defined by postbronchodilator FEV_1 less than 80% predicted value or Z score less than 1.96. The need for alternate-day or daily oral steroids, which is the last category, is extremely rare.

In preschool children, severe asthma should be considered when maximum treatment according to the recommended guidelines fails.

Severe asthma is a heterogeneous condition with different phenotypes:

- Persistence of symptoms or frequent exacerbations in a child with normal pulmonary function tests
- Persistence of symptoms or frequent exacerbations in a child associated with persistent airflow obstruction
- Persistent airflow obstruction in a child with few or no clinical symptoms

Severe or problematic asthma could also be split into 2 subcategories[5]:

- Difficult asthma, which should be reserved for asthma that remains uncontrolled because of persistent of poor compliance, aggravating factors, and comorbidities
- Severe refractory asthma, which should be reserved for children who are still uncontrolled despite optimum treatment of aggravating factors and comorbidities

Definition of severe asthma also implies 3 notions: (1) alternative diagnoses are excluded, (2) precipitating factors are correctly assessed, and (3) adherence to treatment is good.

DIAGNOSIS WORKUP EXPLORATIONS OF SEVERE ASTHMA IN CHILDREN

In a child referred for supposed severe asthma, explorations aim to confirm asthma, to detect precipitating factors and comorbidities, and to evaluate inflammation and airways remodeling,[5] constituting a main step in differentiating difficult from severe asthma.

Exclude Other Diagnoses to Differentiate Difficult Asthma from Severe Asthma

The first step is to arrive at the correct diagnosis.[5–7] **Box 1** summarizes the main alternative diagnoses. It should be noted that all these diseases may be associated with a true asthma.

The initial workup should include: inspiratory and expiratory chest radiographs; inspiratory and, if possible, expiratory low-dose high-resolution computed tomography (HRCT); nasal and exhaled nitric oxide; and, if sufficiently suspected: biopsy for primary ciliary dyskinesia, immunologic investigations with at least immunoglobulin (Ig)G, IgA, IgM measures, antibody response to vaccines, pHmetry, sweat test, and genotyping for cystic fibrosis. Vocal cord dysfunction, which is a possible comorbid condition in severe asthma, may induce inadequate overload treatment. Endoscopic visualization of an inappropriate adduction of the vocal cords during inspiration is the gold standard for the diagnosis.

Bronchoscopy may be part of this workup to exclude an anatomic or dynamic abnormality such as tracheal stenosis or tracheomalacia.

Not all of the workup is necessary for all children, and a focused approach based on history and physical examination is more appropriate.

Box 1
Alternative diagnoses of asthma in children

- Proximal airway obstruction
  - Inhaled foreign body
  - Tracheal or bronchial stenosis
  - Bronchopulmonary malformation
  - Benign or malignant tumor
  - Aortic arch abnormalities, pulmonary sling
  - Tracheomalacia, bronchomalacia
- Peripheral airway obstruction
  - Cystic fibrosis
  - Bronchopulmonary disease
  - Primary ciliary dyskinesia
  - Postinfectious (viral) obliterative bronchiolitis
- Recurrent aspirations
  - Tracheoesophageal fistula
  - Swallowing disorders
  - Gastroesophageal reflux
- Bronchiectasis
- Defect of host defense
- Chronic interstitial lung disease
- Extrinsic allergic alveolitis
- Eosinophilic lung
- Congenital heart disease (especially left to right shunt)
- Cardiac failure
- Vocal cord dysfunction
- Hyperventilation/panic attack

Precipitating Factors and Comorbidities in Difficult-To-Treat Asthma

Inappropriate use of drug-delivery devices and poor adherence to medication are certainly the most frequent contributing factors for poor control of asthma.[8]

Precipitating factors include environmental tobacco smoke and ongoing allergen exposure. Data suggest that, as with active smoking, exposure to passive smoking leads to steroid resistance. Allergen exposure may induce both acute exacerbation and persistent airway inflammation. A complete allergic workup is necessary. Comorbid food allergy in asthma seems to reduce asthma control, whereas comorbid asthma in food allergy increases the risk of severe reactions and anaphylaxis.

The other main comorbidities associated with severe asthma in children are ear/nose/throat problems, mainly rhinitis and chronic rhinosinusitis, and gastroesophageal reflux. Complete examination, nasofibroscopy and sinus computed tomography (CT) scan, and esophageal pH testing may be necessary. In children, the impact of obesity on the severity and control of asthma is not evident, as in adults. However, obesity is associated with more severe acute asthma and also with a diminished response to ICSs.

Evaluation of Inflammation and Remodeling by Indirect and Noninvasive Techniques in Severe Asthma

This step is certainly the most innovative part of the evaluation of severe asthma. For ethical and safety reasons, only few studies have been performed on children with asthma, and this is particularly true for studies involving bronchoscopy. In children, the use of invasive and direct techniques (ie, bronchoscopy, bronchoalveolar lavage [BAL], and biopsy) to clarify diagnosis and guide management is justified only in cases of refractory asthma (see later discussion). The development of noninvasive markers is necessary, given the ethical difficulties of conducting research in severe asthmatic children. These techniques include induced sputum, fractional exhaled nitric oxide (FE_{NO}), exhaled breath condensate, and HRCT scan.

Sputum induction is performed with hypertonic saline after pretreatment with a bronchodilator. The success rate is 60% to 90% and safety is good.[9–12] Normal sputum eosinophil percentage is assumed to be less than 3%.[11] In 38 children with difficult asthma, only one-third had abnormal sputum cytology, either eosinophils or neutrophils.[11,12]

To date, the best performing biomarker appears to be an inflammatory profile in sputum, but the practical difficulties of sputum induction, and technical variation in sputum analysis and processing limit the clinical application.

Extensive literature has been published on the value of FE_{NO} in asthmatic children. FE_{NO} is elevated in asthma, especially when eosinophilic inflammation is present. Recent ATS guidelines suggest that FE_{NO} may be useful for detecting eosinophilic airway inflammation, determining the likelihood of corticosteroid responsiveness, monitoring airway inflammation to determine the potential need for corticosteroids, and as a tool for nonadherence to corticosteroid.[13]

FE_{NO} and induced sputum have been used by Zacharasiewicz and colleagues[14] to predict the success or failure of reducing inhaled steroids in 40 children with stable asthma. Step-down was successful in all children who had no eosinophils in induced sputum, whereas increased FE_{NO} and elevated eosinophils were predictive of failed reduction.

Lex and colleagues[12] investigated the relationships between FE_{NO}, eosinophils in induced sputum, BAL, and bronchial subepithelium in a group of children with severe asthma. The investigators found significant correlations between eosinophils in the sputum and both BAL eosinophils and FE_{NO}, as well as between FE_{NO} and BAL eosinophils. However, they were not related to airway wall eosinophilia. Despite a good negative predictive value (89%), there was a poor positive predictive value (36%).

The measurement of FE_{NO} at different flows may allow partitioning of NO production to proximal and distal airways. In children with severe asthma, NO measurements were related to inflammation and several parameters of airway remodeling, suggesting that both subacute inflammation and remodeling influence NO output in refractory asthma.[15] At present, the clinical use of FE_{NO} routinely in severe asthma remains to be determined.

Condensate from exhaled breath (EBC) may reflect the composition of the airway lining fluid. EBC may be obtained in children even during exacerbation. However, no biomarkers have been validated for clinical use.[7]

HRCT is a noninvasive technique that may be valuable for quantifying airway remodeling in patients with severe asthma. It may also identify other diagnoses in asthma that are difficult to treat. In adults, evaluations of HRCT have shown that abnormalities of the airways, particularly the extent of bronchial wall thickening (BWT), correlate with lung functions, reticular basement membrane (RBM) thickness, and matrix metalloproteinase 9/tissue inhibitor metalloproteinase 1 production imbalance.[16,17]

In children with severe asthma, BWT was significantly higher than in control children.[18] Furthermore, bronchial thickening assessed by the BWT score on HRCT correlated with RBM thickening and NO production by the airway wall, but not with inflammatory markers determined by BAL or bronchial biopsy, or with pulmonary functions.[19]

The new generations of multislice CT scanners will allow higher definition and lower radiation exposure, and will probably give a better assessment of airway remodeling and efficacy of treatment in children with asthma. HRCT is not a routine procedure in children with severe asthma, and should be performed only if there is doubt as to the diagnosis. However, it could be incorporated in research protocols to determine correlation with airway structures.

In conclusion, the first steps in the exploration of severe asthma are to achieve the correct diagnosis (alternative or associated diagnosis) and to evaluate adherence to treatment, precipitating factors, and comorbidities. These first steps should be done systematically in all children presenting with difficult asthma.

The second level aims to evaluate the phenotype of severe asthma related to the clinical and/or functional features, and the patterns of airway inflammation and remodeling.

The techniques used, either direct and invasive or indirect and noninvasive, are not systematic but are reserved only for specialized units, whose staff are trained for techniques as well as analyses. Most of these techniques are still used for clinical or biological research.

When alternative diagnoses are excluded, comorbidities and environmental factors are evaluated, and adherence to treatment seems to have been obtained, difficult asthma is excluded. The diagnosis of severe childhood asthma refractory to treatment is probable.

PATHOPHYSIOLOGY OF SEVERE ASTHMA IN CHILDREN

Severe asthma in children displays heterogeneity and variability in its clinical and pathologic expression. Different phenotypes are described: persistent symptoms and/or frequent exacerbations, and/or persistent airway obstruction despite therapy, neutrophilic versus eosinophilic inflammation, and so forth. In addition, phenotypes can overlap and change over time. Although the pathophysiology is often detailed by concomitant and successive events, severe asthma results from many different pathways. The role of viral infection and allergen exposure is better known, but their implication and relationship with the severity is not well established.

Severe Asthma: An Early Determination

Cohort studies are in favor of an early onset of the severity. In cohort studies, severity was often defined by the appearance of an airway obstruction that persists in small and/or large airways. The greatest absolute loss of lung function seems to occur very early on in childhood.[20–22] In a cohort of children followed from birth until the age of 10 years, functional abnormalities associated with the risk of asthma existed in the first year of life.[23] Atopy plays a key role in the onset of asthma in children. Sensitization to perennial allergens developing in the first 3 years of life is associated with a loss of lung function at school age. This loss is increased with concomitant exposure to high levels of perennial allergens early on in life.[24] Cohort studies show that a combination of early sensitization and early lower respiratory tract infections (particularly human rhinovirus) in children is strongly associated with persistent asthma.[25–28] Holt and colleagues[29,30] suggest that the development of immune and inflammatory responses at the same time by these separate stimuli (allergen and virus) in the airways during a period of lung growth may perturb normal tissue-differentiation programs and result in disturbed respiratory function. Nevertheless, not all children exposed to these environmental factors develop a severe form of asthma. A combination of multiple environmental factors and genetic background (at risk or not) define the characteristics of the inflammatory and immune responses, with a particular important signature in resident cells such as epithelial cells. The nature of this host response is probably critical for the emergence of the disease and the development of a severe form of asthma. In children at risk of severe asthma, constitutional factors leading to an excessive remodeling process or persistent inflammation after rhinovirus infection, related to a defect in antioxidative response, an impaired phagocytosis function, or a deficiency in type I interferon (IFN) production, may play a role in the development of its severity.

Severe Asthma in Children and Cellular Infiltrate: Lack of Specificity

The presence of inflammatory cell infiltrate, mainly composed of eosinophils, neutrophils, and T lymphocytes, has been described in severe asthma in children, even if the role of resident cells (epithelial, fibroblasts, dendritic cells and macrophages) is central.

Most asthmatic children have eosinophilic airway inflammation.[31] Neutrophilia or a mixed cellularity is also often described.[11,32,33] BAL neutrophilia is a frequent pattern observed in preschool wheeze, whether or not associated with viral or bacterial infection.[34–36] The responsibility of exposure to passive smoking, infection, treatments, allergens, gastroesophageal reflux, endotoxins, and other environmental factors in influx of inflammatory cells is complex.[37] One hypothesis is that, in asthma, neutrophilic inflammation may precede eosinophilic inflammation.

In severe asthma in children, T-helper (Th)2-derived cytokines and eosinophils have been described.[31–33,38,39] Airway eosinophils may persist in difficult asthma in children, despite prednisolone therapy.[31] Noneosinophilic inflammation has also been reported.[11,40] In children, BAL neutrophilia may be correlated to the severity of asthma.[35,41] Persistence of bronchial eosinophilia does not mean uncontrolled asthma when mucosal eosinophilia persists in clinical remission of asthma.[42] The location of inflammatory infiltrate may be important. There are few data concerning the presence and the role of inflammatory cell microlocalization to structural cells (smooth muscle cells, glandular cells, airway nerves, and so forth) in severe childhood asthma. Mechanisms involved in their migration and their interactions with structural cells may play a role in bronchial hyperresponsiveness or the remodeling process, which could determine a factor of severity.[43] In severe asthma, eosinophils and neutrophils persist in bronchial biopsies, even under ICSs.[33] In severe asthma characterized by persistent airway obstruction, Th2 inflammation was associated with the presence of activated eosinophils and neutrophils in the epithelium in symptomatic children, whereas the inflammatory infiltrate was not found in paucisymptomatic asthmatic children.[33] This correlation does not exist with eosinophils and neutrophils in BAL or bronchial mucosa.[33] This study confirms that, as in adults, lumen and airway walls are different compartments.[12]

Balance of Th1/Th2?

Persistent airway obstruction was associated with a greater number of CD4$^+$ T cells in bronchial biopsies in difficult asthma under systemic corticosteroids, compared with controls in school-age children.[44]

After previous studies showed no difference in interleukin (IL-4), IL-5, and RANTES expression in bronchial biopsies between difficult asthma and controls in children,[44] Fitzpatrick and colleagues[32] recently described molecular phenotypes in children with severe asthma, based on cytokines, chemokines, BAL levels, and lysates from alveolar macrophages. In BAL, CXCL1, RANTES (CCL5), IL-12, IFN-γ, and IL-10 best characterized severe versus moderate asthma in children. In alveolar-macrophage lysate, a higher level of IL-6 was the strongest discriminator for severe asthma.[32] De Blic and colleagues[33] also showed an increase in Th1 cytokine levels in and paucisymptomatic (compared with symptomatic) children with severe asthma with persistent obstruction, whereas the IFN-γ/IL-4 balance was lower in symptomatic children. The high levels of IFN-γ in paucisymptomatic children suggest that this Th1 cytokine may modulate the local inflammatory response.[33] These studies clearly demonstrate that the classic

Th1/Th2 pattern is not so constant in children with severe asthma.

Location of Inflammation

Bronchial or luminal, but also proximal or distal bronchial inflammation may also influence symptoms and severity. Involvement of distal airways in severe asthma in children is difficult to assess. BAL by definition evaluates a part of both compartments. Even if it has been performed,[45] there are some concerns about the practice of rigid bronchoscopy and transbronchial biopsies to evaluate respiratory symptoms routinely. Cohort studies with evaluation of lung function showed early distal impairment.[23,24]

IMMUNE RESPONSE: DO PREFERENTIAL PATHWAYS LEAD TO THE SEVERITY OF ASTHMA?
Environmental Factors: Virus and Allergen

Interaction of dendritic cells with allergens in the airway mucosa generates a Th2 cytokine response and, according to the genetic and environmental cofactors present, may lead to asthma induction.[46] Immune mechanisms involved in sensitization and allergic asthma have largely been developed. Recent developments provide new hypotheses concerning the immune response to respiratory viral infection in allergic asthmatics.[29,30,47]

Frequent exacerbations are associated with a phenotype of severe asthma, and repeated exacerbations are associated with an accelerated decline of lung function. The role of viral respiratory tract infections in severe asthma is probably essential, complex, and still widely debated. Virus produces wheezing episodes during the first 3 years of life in almost 50% of children.[48] In children at risk, rhinovirus infection is associated with a high risk of asthma.[49] The most recent hypothesis is that respiratory infection by rhinovirus, occurring in atopic asthmatic children (in a Th2 environment), is responsible for an enhanced FcεRI expression on dendritic cells. Thus, dendritic cells may produce proinflammatory mediators in response to allergens at challenge sites via nuclear factor κB–dependent mechanisms. Moreover, this may result in an enhanced capacity to capture the allergen (through its recognition by specific IgE) and to present the epitopes to specific allergen Th2 lymphocytes.[50] This process probably results in an enhanced activation of Th2 lymphocytes responsible for the production of Th2 cytokines IL-4, IL-5, and so forth. Their production may decrease or downregulate Th1 response to viral infection (IFN-γ) and increase airway inflammation. Signaling issued

from the action of Th2 cytokines may enhance FcεRI expression on dendritic-cell precursors in bone marrow.[29,30] This concept needs to be confirmed, but represents an enticing reasoning. Genome-wide patterns of gene expression in sputum cells in children with asthma following an exacerbation showed that the activation of the Th1-like and IFN signaling pathways was decreased and was associated with airway obstruction.[47]

Virus-induced asthma/or wheezing episodes may also reveal a preexisting tendency toward asthma secondary to an impaired response to viral infection (decrease in type I IFN and viral clearance, increase in remodeling, and so forth).[27,51–53] There is a discrepancy in antiviral immune response in asthmatics compared with the healthy population. Increased risk of recurrent wheezing in the preschool and school-age years was associated with low concentrations of IFN-γ and IFN-λ (Th1 cytokine) in early life.[54–57] Respiratory viruses enter and replicate within airway epithelial cells. This step is the first toward initiating an innate and adaptive immune response. In reaction to rhinovirus, bronchial epithelial cells secrete proinflammatory cytokines and chemokines as well as an antiviral immune response.[58–60] Bronchial epithelial cells in asthmatics produced lower levels of type-I and type-III IFN (IFN-β and IFN-λ), which is associated with a higher level of rhinovirus replication.[53] Bullens and colleagues[61] showed that IFN-γ mRNA levels obtained from sputum cells correlated negatively with asthma symptoms in moderate to severe asthma, demonstrating a protective role for IFN-γ. The mechanisms behind deficient IFN-β and IFN-λ production in asthmatics remain unknown. It may result either from a polymorphism in its genes or their promoters, or from an excess of TGF-β secretion in asthmatic airways that mediates enhanced rhinovirus replication, potentially through its suppressive action on host type-I IFN responses.[62] Among mediators implicated in antiviral immunity, a recent study showed that IL-15 is reduced in BAL in asthmatics and in supernatants of macrophage stimulated by rhinovirus. This process may also play a role in virus-induced exacerbation in asthma.[63] In allergic mice, it has been shown that the immune response to respiratory viruses differs from that in control mice. Activation of pattern-recognition receptors such as Toll-like receptors (TLR)3 and TLR7/TLR8 as well as the RNA helicases are responsible for the innate response to respiratory viruses through the recognition of single-stranded and double-stranded RNA. The mobilization of these receptors is responsible for the antiviral response through the activation of an interferon regulatory factor

(IRF)3/IRF7-dependent pathway. In asthmatic patients, an alteration of the expression and/or function of these receptors, and of the downstream signaling pathway, may be suspected.

The role of bacteria as superantigens, an exacerbating factor and risk factor of asthma, is also debated. Colonization with *Streptococcus pneumoniae*, *Haemophilus influenzae*, *Moraxella catarrhalis*, or *Staphylococcus aureus* is associated with an increased risk of recurrent wheezing and asthma before the age of 5 years.[64] The role of bacteria in the maintenance of a local inflammation and in the induction of a specific immune response to allergens remains a matter of debate. A recent discovery undermining the concept of sterility of the lower respiratory tract has been published.[65] Bronchial airways are not sterile; they contain bacterial flora, like the intestine, even if the number is much lower. Children with severe therapy-resistant asthma have different flora with more proteobacteria and fewer *Prevotella* species. This status could be related to the treatment, but could also be involved in the modulation of the local immune response to environmental factors. In germ-free mice, it has been shown that the presence of commensal bacteria is critical for ensuring control of allergic inflammation.[66] This effect may be related to a defect in the maturation of the immune system in the intestine, as demonstrated in mice. However, the role of the lung microbiome is still unknown, but may be involved in the maintenance of local inflammation and in the induction of a specific immune response to environmental factors.

One may hypothesize that rhinovirus induces severe asthma in predisposed children. A persistent obstructive pattern is a phenotype of severe asthma. In children with asthma, rhinovirus was detected in 45% by in situ hybridization on bronchial biopsies. Abnormal lung function was detected in 86% of rhinovirus-positive children and in 58% of rhinovirus-negative children. Persistence of the virus in the respiratory tract is associated with the severity of asthma, associated with persistent obstruction.[67] Resident cells, such as myofibroblasts, infected by rhinovirus in asthmatics, are associated with an enhanced viral replication and chemokine release involved in neutrophil recruitment.[62] In some predisposed children, local airway inflammation triggered by viral infection may alter lung growth and tissue differentiation, leading to alteration of lung function that persists for long time.[68] The immune (innate) response to rhinovirus or RSV differs between individuals, particularly between children at risk and not at risk of asthma. An aberrant innate immune response to repeated rhinovirus infections may facilitate airway remodeling and severe asthma via epithelial cell alterations, and enhance viral replication and persistence of bronchial inflammation.

Additional genetic factors that regulate the response to oxidative stress after viral infection or other environmental triggers also contribute to the quality of response.

Oxidative Stress and Genetic Factors in Severe Childhood Asthma

Excessive formation of reactive oxygen species and imbalance between pro-oxidant and anti-oxidant mediators are associated with severe asthma and reduced lung function. Systemic superoxide dismutase (SOD) deficiency was shown to correlate with airway obstruction.[69] The diminished systemic SOD activity associated with environmental tobacco-smoke exposure showed a specific oxidant mechanism by which tobacco-smoke exposure may affect patients with asthma.[70] SOD inhibition increased bronchial epithelial cell death through the cleavage/activation of caspases, and the oxidation and nitration of MnSOD, identified in the asthmatic airway, correlated with asthma severity.[71] These findings link oxidative stress to reduced SOD activity and downstream events that characterize asthma, including apoptosis and shedding of the airway epithelium. Glutathione is a powerful antioxidant. Fitzpatrick and colleagues[72] showed that in children with severe asthma associated with persistent airway obstruction, BAL fluid has more oxidized glutathione, compared with controls or children without airflow obstruction. This finding was associated in children with severe asthma with alveolar macrophage dysfunction (phagocytosis) after microbial stimulus. This macrophage dysfunction may compromise innate immune function and the clearance in pathogens.[73] The transcription nuclear factor (erythroid-derived 2)–like 2 (Nrf2) plays a main role in glutathione homeostasis and antioxidant defense. Children with severe asthma have a global disruption of thiol redox signaling and control in both the airway and systemic circulation that is associated with posttranslational modification of Nrf2.[74] Of note, Nrf2 deficiency in mice leads to the development of a severe form of asthma after allergen sensitization, a process associated with enhanced oxidative stress.[75] Increasing epithelial lining fluid glutathione level, that is, by Nrf2 reactivation, may reverse or limit the decrease in lung function in severe asthma in children.

Polymorphisms of the gene encoding for the glutathione transferase T1 and M1 is associated with the loss in lung function in utero when the pregnant woman is a tobacco smoker.[76] In early life, even in utero, the combination of tobacco smoke and a deficiency of antioxidants may lead, in children at risk, to more severe asthma with obstruction.

REMODELING IN SEVERE CHILDHOOD ASTHMA

The occurrence of remodeling is probably the consequence of interaction between both genetic (and epigenetic) and environmental factors. Decline in lung function may be a feature of airway remodeling, leading to a severe form of asthma and nonresponders to steroids, even if there are no studies on which to base conclusions. Many questions remain unanswered. What is the relationship between inflammation and remodeling? What is the impact of early anti-inflammatory treatment on prevention of remodeling? Does it occur in the early phase of the disease or later on? Does it respond to a specific trigger, or a combination of multiples?

Airway remodeling includes wall thickening, extracellular matrix deposition (including collagen), smooth muscle hyperplasia and hypertrophy, myofibroblast proliferation, mucus metaplasia, epithelial goblet-cell metaplasia and hyperplasia, subepithelial fibrosis, and thickening of the subepithelial reticular layer. The relative importance of each component is not clearly defined. Moreover, the nature of lung remodeling and of its evolution has not been extensively explored in children.

The concept explaining that airway remodeling in asthma is a process in response to long-term, unresolved airway inflammation, and that it may occur when asthma is not treated or controlled effectively, is widely discussed. Uncontrolled chronic bronchial inflammation is insufficient to explain the modification of bronchial structures.[77] Chronic inflammation may initiate tissue injury and repair, although remodeling may occur alongside inflammation.

Most studies in severe childhood asthma showed no correlation between RBM thickening and clinical characteristics or lung-function tests.[77–80] RBM thickening appears before the age of 3 years, as demonstrated in wheezy preschool children.[81] Children younger than 6 years with asthma ("confirmed wheeze" preschool children) had increased epithelial loss, RBM thickening, and eosinophilia compared with controls, showing that remodeling occurs early on in life,[81] but these modifications were not associated with the duration of symptoms, duration of asthma, and duration of treatment.[77,78] RBM is ultrastructurally similar to normal.[82] RBM thickening does not permit differentiation between moderate and severe asthma in children.[33,77,78] In severe asthma with an obstructive pattern, RBM thickening in children with persistent symptoms was similar to that seen in paucisymptomatic children.[33,78]

Even if this remodeling process may have a protective effect, smooth muscles encircling central and distal airways and muscular shortening produce constriction and shortening of the airways.[83] One hypothesis is that structural alterations can lead to fixed airway obstruction resistant to treatment, a feature of severe asthma,[84] which could contribute to loss of lung function. Airway smooth muscle is increased in severe asthma in children, correlated with an acute bronchodilation response to β2 agonists and inversely correlated with the FEV_1 value.[78,85] Hyperplasia and hypertrophy are important processes regulating increased smooth muscle mass in asthma.[86] Myofibroblasts display a phenotype intermediate between fibroblasts and smooth muscle cells, express a smooth muscle action, and have the ability to secrete matrix proteins and chemokines that prolong eosinophil survival.[87] Vitamin D seems to be an important immune-regulatory molecule. A recent study showed an inverse correlation between airway smooth muscle mass and 25(OH)D vitamin levels in severe therapy-resistant asthma,[88] and this was associated with a lower FEV_1 value. It is difficult to make conclusions because of the low number of patients included in this study[88] and the widespread vitamin D deficiency in the general population.

Vascular changes were demonstrated by the number of CD31-positive vascular structures in bronchial mucosa, significantly increased in severe childhood asthma with persistent obstruction, compared with those with normal function tests.[78] The CD31 expression was negatively correlated with FEV_1 and forced expiratory flow at 25% to 75% of vital capacity (FEF_{25-75}), and did not correlate with inflammatory infiltrates in bronchial mucosa.[78] Increased vessel numbers were confirmed to correlate with the severity of asthma in childhood asthma.[89] Increased vessel numbers, vasodilatation, and edema contribute to airway-wall thickening,[90] and also help cellular infiltration when endothelial cells express adhesion molecules in asthma.[91] Their expression (including intercellular adhesion molecule 1 and vascular cell adhesion molecule 1 [CD54 and CD104]) was controlled by both proinflammatory (TNF-α and IL-1β) and Th2 cytokines (IL-4, IL-13).

The role of epithelial cells and fibroblasts is essential in the pathogenesis of asthma (**Fig. 1**). The airway epithelium has a key role in the innate immunity. Epithelial cells interact with environmental agents and inflammatory mediators. In genetically susceptible children, impaired epithelial cells react to virus, allergen, and pollutant exposure, and may lead to an impaired repair response. An exaggerated remodeling response may lead to fixed airway obstruction associated with a more severe disease.[92] Factors responsible for bronchial remodeling are complex when inflammation does not always precede structural changes, as demonstrated in early life.[89,93,94] Comparing postmortem bronchial specimens from nonasthmatic with moderately to severely asthmatic children aged 5 to 15 years, Fedorov and colleagues[95] showed that the lamina reticularis was thicker in asthmatic biopsies, with increased deposition of collagen III, when eosinophils did not differ between groups. There was an upregulation of epidermal growth factor receptor (EGFR) expression in the bronchial epithelium, as demonstrated in adult asthma, with minimal evidence of increased proliferation.[95] This study showed that stressed epithelium exists without significant eosinophilic inflammation. Early treatment by inhaled steroids in children has a poor effect on the natural history of asthma, and eosinophils may persist under treatment in severely asthmatic children.[31,96,97] Activation of the epithelial-mesenchymal trophic unit early in life, even in utero, may support this hypothesis in the absence of recruited inflammatory cells. The first abnormality in asthma may be a disorder of repair relating to a dysregulation of EGFR-mediated repair, and the inflammation may be secondary to the abnormal tissue-repair processes.[98] Airway inflammation and remodeling could also have parallel pathways. In children genetically predisposed to severe asthma, impaired immune response to environmental triggers associated with persistent inflammation of resident cells, particularly a damaged epithelium, could lead to severe asthma.[98] For example, enhanced surface expression and phosphorylation of EGFRs have been observed in severe childhood asthma, suggesting a key role played by epithelial injury in its severity. Proteases (included in some allergens such as dermatophagoides pteronyssimus) as

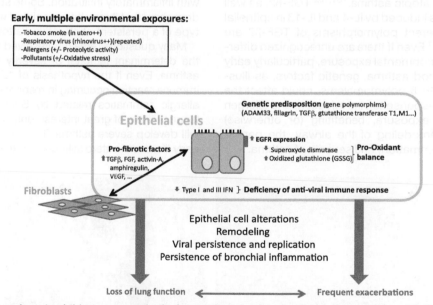

Fig. 1. Severe asthma in children: a central role for epithelial cells. The figure focuses on epithelial cell and its potential role in severe asthma. Early in life, bronchial epithelial cells are exposed to multiple environmental factors: tobacco smoke (in utero+++), respiratory virus (rhinovirus++, repeated episodes), allergens (+/− proteolytic activities), pollutants (+/− oxidatve stress). In asthma, EC have an increased expression of EGFR. Different gene polymorphisms seem to be associated with severe asthma (ADAM33, fillagrin, TGFβ, Glutathione transferase T1, M1...). Abnormal responses of EC to stress, in a predisposed genetic field, generate an excessive secretion of pro-fibrotic factors (TGFβ, FGF, Activin-A, VEGF, amphiregulin that interact with fibroblasts), a deficiency in anti-oxydant function and a deficiency in anti-viral immune response (a decrease in type I and III interferon that favors viral persistence and replication). This may lead to remodeling and enhanced and persistent bronchial inflammation and be an explanation for the frequent exacerbations, and the loss in lung function in refractory asthma in children.

well as tobacco smoke and pollutants generate reactive oxygen species and trigger the release of endogenous proteases. Proteases are implicated in damage to the airway epithelium. Impairment in antioxidant production, as demonstrated in severe asthmatic children,[72] associated with an enhanced surface expression and phosphorylation of EGFRs, may lead to a loss of integrity of the epithelium and be a factor in the severity of asthma in children.

Epithelial cells in reaction to stimuli are able to produce fibrogenic factors (growth factors) and inflammatory mediators. These factors may promote the transformation of fibroblasts in myofibroblasts. For example, TGF-β is produced and secreted by epithelial cells. TGF-β is involved in survival, proliferation, differentiation, and extracellular matrix regulation, and is particularly implicated in tissue repair and fibrosis.[99] Several genetic associations regarding the -509C>T polymorphism of TGF-β1 have been reported, and this polymorphism seems to contribute to the severity of asthma.[100] TGF-β2, a predominant isoform expressed in severe asthma, has an important role in regulating inflammation and remodeling in asthma, and may play a role in the development of childhood atopic asthma.[101,102] TGF-β2, as well as TGF-β1, is induced by IL-4 and IL-13 in epithelial cells.[101] Different polymorphisms of TGF-β2 are described.[101] Even if there are unrecognized differences in environmental exposure, particularly early on in childhood asthma, genetic factors, as illustrated by TGF-β polymorphisms, could affect the airway, the response to viral infection, and allergen or tobacco exposure, benefiting (or otherwise) excessive remodeling of the airway, the persistence of inflammation, and severity of asthma.

Another mediator that has been studied specifically in asthma is the ADAM33 (a disintegrin and metalloproteinase 33) polymorphism, implicated in airway caliber at the age of 3 and 5 years.[103]

Skin-barrier dysfunction is also being debated. Fillagrin gene variants are associated with a high risk of early-onset asthma, with a phenotype including acute severe asthma and recurrent wheeze but also with accelerated decline in lung function.[104–106] A recent cohort study conducted in Poland showed that fillagrin null variants were associated with the risk of atopic asthma (odds ratio [OR] 2.22, 95% confidence interval [CI] 1.24–3.96, P = .006),[107] revealing another potential factor of susceptibility to epithelial disease related to asthma.

There is a link between virus and remodeling. Rhinovirus infection of bronchial epithelial cells leads to upregulation of mediators implicated in airway remodeling: amphiregulin (a member of the EGF family), activin A (member of the TGF-β family), and vascular endothelial growth factor protein.[108] Fibroblasts have the ability to support rhinovirus replication and to promote inflammation through the secretion of IL-6 and IL-8.[109]

Remodeling in asthma may be initiated in early life, even in utero, and it can evolve in parallel with inflammatory infiltration. Some studies in children show that it may be associated with a phenotype of a persistent obstructive pattern (**Fig. 2**).

Many questions remain unresolved in identifying the determinant factor(s) of severity in childhood asthma. Even if the hypothesis of "ETMU" or the immune reaction occurring in response to a virus in allergic asthmatics related by Subrata and colleagues[30] are of great interest, only a few children will develop severe asthma. The role of triggers in early life, even in utero (allergen, protease, infection,

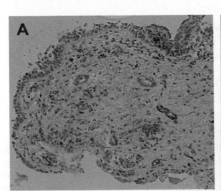
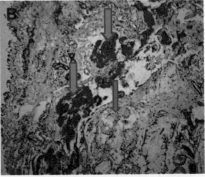

Fig. 2. (*A, B*) Diversity of airway remodeling in asthmatic children. Micrographs show indirect immunostaining (with fast *red*) obtained with antibody anti-alpha-smooth muscle actin mAb anti-SMA, clone asm-1 (Cymbus Biotech, Southampton, UK) on bronchial biopsies from children with severe asthma. In patient A (high magnification ×300), the airway epithelium is relatively untouched, and no hyperplasia of smooth muscle and mucous gland is detected. By contrast, in patient B (high magnification ×300) the airway epithelium is mainly desquamated, and a strong hyperplasia of mucous gland (*lower right*) and smooth muscle (in *red*) is observed. This appearance is associated with a different clinical profile, as reported in a previous article.[77]

tobacco smoke, pollutants, and so forth), particularly the combination of multiple environmental factors and the different modality of response related to genetic background (immune, antioxidant, repair process, epithelium junction, and so forth), probably act together to induce (or not) persistent inflammation and/or remodeling. Genetics mainly contribute to disease expression, progression, and response to treatment, and the gene-environment interactions are probably essential in creating severity (**Figs. 1 and 2**).[110–112]

SEVERE ASTHMA PHENOTYPES IN CHILDREN

The definition of severe asthma does not take into account phenotypic characteristics and heterogeneity illustrated by some cross-sectional evaluation of cohorts of school-age children with severe asthma, and this may lead to suboptimal or inappropriate treatment. A predominance of males, atopy (86%), long duration of asthma (first symptoms: 1.25 years), and a large frequency of comorbidities (eg, food allergy: 24%; gastroesophageal reflux: 75%) was observed among 102 children with severe asthma, who presented with an obstructive pattern (FEV_1 67% $\pm$ 19.2%), a partial response to corticosteroid testing, and an eosinophilic and/or neutrophilic profile on BAL.[113] Fitzpatrick and colleagues[114] (SARP cohort) phenotyped 161 children with severe asthma (ATS criteria) according to their clinical features and inflammatory biomarkers (cluster analysis). Four clusters were identified, very different from those of adult severe asthma: late-onset symptomatic asthma with normal pulmonary function test and less atopy, early-onset atopic asthma with normal pulmonary function test, early-onset atopic asthma with greater comorbidity and mild airflow limitation, early-onset atopic asthma with advanced airflow limitation, and the greatest symptoms and use of medication. Asthma duration, number of controller medications, and baseline lung function, but not atopy were predictors of cluster assignment. Konradsen and colleagues[115] evaluated the features of 54 children with severe asthma according to GA2LEN Task Force guidelines, and compared them with age-matched peers with controlled persistent asthma. Children with severe asthma more frequently had parents with asthma, came from families of a lower socioeconomic status, were less active, had more comorbidities (rhinoconjunctivitis), and more lung-function abnormalities (lower FEV_1 and higher bronchial hyperresponsiveness). This study highlighted the difference between asthma that is difficult to treat with asthma-identified aggravating factors (39%) and therapy-resistant asthma (61%).[115] All these studies emphasize that definitions of asthma severity proposed by current guidelines do not reflect real life. A more specific approach is needed with the aim of assessing all the characteristics of severe asthma, including the history of respiratory symptoms since birth, exposures during pregnancy, comorbidity, and aggravating factors. The risk of impairment associated with the disorder, as well as the response to treatments, is also characterized by different possibilities.

Description of Severe Asthma Phenotypes in Children

Phenotypes based on allergic profile and comorbidities, clinical features (symptoms, exacerbations), lung function, or inflammation have been described in children with severe asthma. Children's phenotypes may not be stable with age-related profiles, and may also vary over time. Furthermore, there is a possible overlap between the features of the different phenotypes.

- *Allergy.* Allergic sensitization is a main feature of severe asthma in children.[113–116] Persistence of a severe atopic dermatitis has been related to filaggrin mutations, and is associated with a more severe asthma and accelerated decline of lung function.[106] Food allergy (peanut and tree-nuts) is overrepresented in children with severe asthma (24% of the Brompton series),[113] and is associated with the risk of life-threatening asthma.[117] Indeed, acute asthma is a feature of food anaphylaxis, needing inhaled β2 agonists and epinephrine injection.[118] Finally, a high IgE level and multisensitization are frequent in severe asthma. Some sensitizations (molds, cockroaches) may be overrepresented.[119] Severe asthma with fungal sensitization described in adults is very rare in childhood, according to anecdotal case reports.[120]
- *Brittle asthma phenotype.* Most information comes from adult studies, but this phenotype is also observed in pediatric patients.[121] Type 1 is characterized by prolonged chaotic swings of peak flow and type 2 by a single catastrophic decrease in peak flow in the context of good control.
- *Exacerbating phenotype.* Recurrent exacerbations requiring general corticosteroids and/or health care characterize severe asthma and are usually virally induced.[122] In the SARP cohort, median oral

corticosteroid bursts and emergency-department visits for acute asthma exacerbations were significantly higher for the children with severe asthma than for those with moderate asthma, respectively 3 versus 1 and 3 versus 0.[114,116] Caroll and colleagues[123] describe a specific phenotype with isolated recurrent severe exacerbation requiring admission to the intensive care unit and sometimes assisted ventilation. This phenotype is also observed in preschool children, with personal or familial atopy.[124]

- *Pulmonary function abnormalities phenotype.* Pulmonary function abnormalities may be measured during early childhood and persist throughout the adult years.[125] Fixed obstruction with or without symptoms is also observed and may progress over time.[33,126] Decline in pulmonary function is also present in a subset of patients with mild to moderate asthma, as reported in 30% of the children in the CAMP study.[127] The clinical significance is not clear. However, these features may be associated with altered lung growth or specific airway remodeling, and possibly future asthma severity.

Inflammatory phenotypes also exist and are discussed in the pathophysiology section.[12,31,33,78,113,114,128] Cytology may be not sufficient, but the analysis of the nature of inflammation may improve the classification of severe asthma and the development of targeted treatments.

TREATMENT

The authors only consider the treatment of children uncontrolled under high-dose ICS (>400 µg/d fluticasone equivalent) and add-on therapies, long-acting β2-agonist (LABA) ± leukotriene receptor antagonist (LTRA), and an estimated correct medication adherence and inhaler technique. Allergic comorbidities, associated factors (gastroesophageal reflux, obesity, psychosocial condition), environment (allergens, tobacco, pollution) need also to be assessed and treated. Options can be divided into conventional treatments (ICS, oral corticosteroids [OCS], theophylline) with the new opportunity of biotherapy (omalizumab) and treatment not usually prescribed for asthma (macrolides, cytotoxics). Studies on daily lung-function monitoring or regular inflammation assessments have now been published. For all these options, pediatric data are lacking and the level of evidence for severe asthma in children remains poor. All these

treatment strategies require the supervision of a specialist pediatric pulmonologist. Bush and colleagues[129] (PSACI group) recently published a review on the pharmacologic treatment of severe, therapy-resistant asthma.

Conventional Treatment

Inhaled corticosteroids

It is assumed that 80% to 90% of the ICS effect is obtained with 100 to 250 µg fluticasone equivalent in children with mild to moderate asthma.[130] However, poor glucocorticoid responsiveness or corticoresistance is a feature of severe asthma,[129,131] enhanced by some comorbidities (tobacco-smoke exposure, being overweight). A trial with a high dose of ICS, up to 2000 µg/d, may be prescribed for 3 to 6 months.[132] Thereafter, if benefits are observed the dose should gradually be tapered under regular monitoring. Budesonide nebulizations (1 mg × 2/d) may be considered, particularly for the youngest.[133] To target the distal airways and enhanced deposition, extrafine particle treatment (beclometasone HFA, ciclesonide) is another option.[134] ICS are usually associated with LABA therapy. Concerns about LABA's safety have recently been debated. On the basis of 20 systematic reviews and databases, Rodrigo and Castro-Rodríguez[135] concluded that concomitant use of LABA with ICS is not associated with these serious side effects.

Systemic corticosteroids

Until recently, OCS was the final conventional step in treatment recommendations.[136] There is no evidence about which protocol should be used. After a period (2–4 weeks) with 0.5 to 1 mg/kg/d of prednisolone equivalent, the daily dose should gradually be tapered (alternate dosing), according to clinical and functional monitoring, to the lowest efficient dose (best patient control). Adverse effects are common and should be monitored and prevented (height, blood pressure, glucose metabolism, cataract, and osteoporosis). The same warning should be given for patients with frequent OCS bursts for severe exacerbations. A trial of intramuscular triamcinolone given either as a single dose or as repeated monthly injections has also been tested, as a test for the potential steroid effect or as an alternative to OCS for children who have poor compliance or pulmonary inflammation that is resistant to OCS.[137] There is no randomized controlled study to evaluate whether this strategy has additional benefits, or risks, compared with OCS.

Omalizumab

The anti-IgE treatment (omalizumab) is a new, expensive option for children age 6 years and older with atopic allergic uncontrolled severe asthma and the appropriate level of IgE (upper limit: 1500 UI/mL). There are no tests to predict the response, and the total IgE level is often over the recommended limit in children with severe asthma. Pediatric controlled studies were conducted in moderate to severe asthma and showed a significant reduction in severe exacerbation rates, ICS dosage, and improvement in the control and quality of life.[138–140] Busse and colleagues[141] also observed the attenuation of spring and autumn peaks of exacerbation in children under omalizumab. Response to treatment has been observed, even if the total IgE level was greater than 1500 UI/mL (personal data, AD/French cohort). Meta-analysis by Rodrigo and colleagues[142] (8 studies, including 2 on children, 3429 patients) confirmed the significant impact on exacerbations during the stable phase of ICS treatment (relative risk [RR] = 0.57, 95% CI 0.48–0.66, P = .0001) as well as the tapered phase (RR = 0.55, 95% CI 0.47–0.64, P = .0001). Impact on lung function is more controversial, but should be studied in the long term, as should the impact on asthma progression. Omalizumab was safe and well tolerated in pediatric studies, up to 1 year.[142] However, adverse effects have been described, including anaphylaxis, and first injections should be performed under medical supervision.[143] Consequently, Omalizumab is now a valid option in children with uncontrolled asthma and/or frequent exacerbations under optimal inhaled treatment or oral steroids.

Other Treatments

- *Theophylline.* The conclusion of the meta-analysis by Seddon and colleagues[144] on xanthines in asthmatic children was that they may have a role as add-on therapy in severe asthma not controlled by ICS, but that further studies (not done) are needed to incorporate the risk-benefit ratio. Theophylline is now prescribed at low doses (blood level at 5–10 mol/L) for the immunomodulatory properties that have been described.[144]
- *Anti-infective treatments.* Therapeutic trials of macrolides are being prescribed in some patients with refractory asthma who fail to respond to standard therapy. Along with direct antimicrobial activity against gram-positive cocci and atypical pathogens, macrolides also have immune-modifying effects and effects on bronchial cells, and on cells of innate immunity.[145] Chronic infection with *Chlamydia* and

Mycoplasma pneumoniae has been associated with severe asthma, as has nontuberculous mycobacteria.[146,147] However, no broad study confirms the role of macrolides in the treatment of severe asthma. Strunk and colleagues[148] were not able to demonstrate the role of azithromycin or montelukast as ICS-sparing agents in children with moderate to severe asthma controlled by medium ICS dose and LABA.

- *Cytotoxics.* These treatments have been tried in asthma that is resistant to conventional treatment or in asthma treated with OCS. Their side effects may outweigh the benefits and they need to be monitored.[149] Methotrexate and cyclosporine have been used with a small but significant effect in case series of children.[149,150] There are no pediatric data on azathioprine, anti–TNF-α, interferon-γ, or anti–IL-5 (mepolizumab).[151]

Monitoring Therapy

A few studies on lung-function telemonitoring in asthmatic patients have been published, mainly concerning the transmission of peak expiratory flow measures or the management program for asthma via the Internet.[152] A strategy based on daily home spirometry (FEV_1) with teletransmission to an expert medical center was applied in 50 children with severe uncontrolled asthma enrolled in a 12-month prospective study and randomized into 2 groups: treatment managed with daily home spirometry and medical feedback, and conventional treatment.[153] There was no significant difference in severe exacerbations, lung function (FEV_1, FEF_{25-75}), treatment outcome (daily ICS dose), or quality of life. These findings may highlight the weakness of the correlation between lung function and symptoms. The poor performance of this intensive management acts against telemonitoring with medical feedback, a position now supported by the latest ATS recommendations.[154]

Although asthma is an inflammatory disease, inflammation is not routinely assessed. FE_{NO} monitoring is easy, but was not more efficient than the conventional strategy in children with mild to moderate asthma (FE_{NO50}), and daily ICS dose may be higher.[155] Induced sputum cytology is another method of assessing bronchial inflammation. Fleming and colleagues[156] adopted this strategy in 55 children with severe asthma, randomized to either a conventional strategy or an inflammation strategy (first sputum eosinophilia and, if not obtained, FE_{NO}). Children were seen at 3-monthly intervals over a 1-year period. No improvement in the exacerbations rate or asthma control was observed. The investigators emphasize phenotypic variability (39% of children had at least one switch in phenotype over 1 year), the frequency of inflammation assessment, which is too low, and the use of FE_{NO} as a surrogate for sputum eosinophilia with the known nonconstant correlation between them. Development of biomarkers, which are easy to measure, is needed to optimize the choice of the treatment strategy according to the phenotype and to monitor the response to innovative therapy.

SUMMARY

Even if well defined, it is sometimes difficult to distinguish difficult from severe asthma in real life. When alternative diagnoses are excluded, comorbidities and environmental factors have been evaluated, and adherence to treatment seems to have been successful, difficult asthma is excluded. Severe asthma is probably determined early in life. Severe childhood asthma, refractory to treatment, includes different phenotypes. Genetics mainly contribute to disease expression, progression, and response to treatment. The gene-environment interactions involving certain gene polymorphisms are probably essential in creating its severity. An aberrant innate immune response to repeated rhinovirus infections may facilitate airway remodeling and severe asthma, via epithelial cell alterations, enhancing viral replication and persistence of bronchial inflammation. Additional genetic factors regulating the response to oxidative stress after viral infection or other environmental triggers also contribute to the quality of response. Different treatment strategies require the supervision of a specialist pediatric pulmonologist when the level of evidence remains poor. The quality of care and monitoring of children with severe asthma is as important as the prescription of drug. This factor is also crucial for differentiating between severe asthma and difficult asthma, and expertise is required. Further studies (genetic and proteomic data) performed in phenotypes of severe asthma in children should improve knowledge of the mechanisms involved in frequent exacerbations, persistent obstruction, and sudden-onset severe asthma, and help the pediatric pulmonologist to choose the appropriate monitoring and treatment for the phenotype.

REFERENCES

1. Lang A, Carlsen KH, Haaland G, et al. Severe asthma in childhood: assessed in 10 year olds in a birth cohort study. Allergy 2008;63:1054–60.

2. Chung KF, Godard P, Adelroth E, et al. Difficult/therapy-resistant asthma: the need for an integrated approach to define clinical phenotypes, evaluate risk factors, understand pathophysiology and find novel therapies. ERS Task Force on Difficult/Therapy-Resistant Asthma. European Respiratory Society. Eur Respir J 1999;13:1198–208.

3. Wenzel S. Severe asthma in adults. Am J Respir Crit Care Med 2005;172:149–60.

4. Hedlin G, Bush A, Lødrup Carlsen K, et al. Problematic severe asthma in children, not one problem but many: a GA2LEN initiative. Eur Respir J 2010; 36:196–201.

5. Bel EH, Sousa A, Fleming L, et al. Unbiased Biomarkers for the Prediction of Respiratory Disease Outcome (U-BIOPRED) Consortium, Consensus Generation. Diagnosis and definition of severe refractory asthma: an international consensus statement from the Innovative Medicine Initiative (IMI). Thorax 2011;66:910–7.

6. Iliescu C, Tillie-Leblond I, Deschildre A, et al. Difficult asthma in children. Arch Pediatr 2002;9: 1264–73.

7. Lødrup Carlsen KC, Hedlin G, Bush A, et al. PSACI (Problematic Severe Asthma in Childhood Initiative) group. Assessment of problematic severe asthma in children. Eur Respir J 2011;37:432–40.

8. de Groot EP, Duiverman EJ, Brand PL. Comorbidities of asthma during childhood: possibly important, yet poorly studied. Eur Respir J 2010;36:671–8.

9. Araújo L, Moreira A, Palmares C, et al. Induced sputum in children: success determinants, safety, and cell profiles. J Investig Allergol Clin Immunol 2011;21:216–21.

10. Jones PD, Hankin R, Simpson J, et al. The tolerability, safety, and success of sputum induction and combined hypertonic saline challenge in children. Am J Respir Crit Care Med 2001;164:1146–9.

11. Lex C, Payne DN, Zacharasiewicz A, et al. Sputum induction in children with difficult asthma: safety, feasibility, and inflammatory cell pattern. Pediatr Pulmonol 2005;39:318–24.

12. Lex C, Ferreira F, Zacharasiewicz A, et al. Airway eosinophilia in children with severe asthma: predictive values of noninvasive tests. Am J Respir Crit Care Med 2006;174:1286–91.

13. Dweik RA, Boggs PB, Erzurum SC, et al. American Thoracic Society Committee on Interpretation of Exhaled Nitric Oxide Levels (FENO) for Clinical Applications. An official ATS clinical practice guideline: interpretation of exhaled nitric oxide levels (FENO) for clinical applications. Am J Respir Crit Care Med 2011;184(5):602–15.

14. Zacharasiewicz A, Wilson N, Lex C, et al. Clinical use of noninvasive measurements of airway inflammation in steroid reduction in children. Am J Respir Crit Care Med 2005;171:1077–82.

15. Mahut B, Delclaux C, Tillie-Leblond I, et al. Both inflammation and remodeling influence nitric oxide output in children with refractory asthma. J Allergy Clin Immunol 2004;113:252–6.

16. Kasahara K, Shiba K, Ozawa T, et al. Correlation between the bronchial subepithelial layer and whole airway wall thickness in patients with asthma. Thorax 2002;57:242–6.

17. Vignola AM, Paganin F, Capieu L, et al. Airway re-modelling assessed by sputum and high-resolution computed tomography in asthma and COPD. Eur Respir J 2004;24:910–7.

18. Marchac V, Emond S, Mamou-Mani T, et al. Thoracic CT in pediatric patients with difficult-to-treat asthma. AJR Am J Roentgenol 2002;179:1245–52.

19. de Blic J, Tillie-Leblond I, Emond S, et al. High-resolution computed tomography scan and airway remodeling in children with severe asthma. J Allergy Clin Immunol 2005;116:750–4.

20. Spahn JD, Covar R. Clinical assessment of asthma progression in children and adults. J Allergy Clin Immunol 2008;121:548–57.

21. Taussig LM, Wright AL, Holberg CJ, et al. Tucson Children's Respiratory Study: 1980 to present. J Allergy Clin Immunol 2003;111:661–75.

22. Borrego LM, Stocks J, Leiria-Pinto P, et al. Lung function and clinical risk factors for asthma in infants and young children with recurrent wheeze. Thorax 2009;64:203–9.

23. Håland G, Carlsen KC, Sandvik L, et al. ORAACLE. Reduced lung function at birth and the risk of asthma at 10 years of age. N Engl J Med 2006;355:1682–9.

24. Illi S, von Mutius E, Lau S, et al, Multicentre Allergy Study (MAS) group. Perennial allergen sensitisation early in life and chronic asthma in children: a birth cohort study. Lancet 2006;368:763–70.

25. Oddy WH, de Klerk NH, Sly PD, et al. The effects of respiratory infections, atopy, and breast-feeding on childhood asthma. Eur Respir J 2002;19:899–905.

26. Holt PG, Rowe J, Kusel M, et al. Toward improved prediction of risk for atopy and asthma among preschoolers: a prospective cohort study. J Allergy Clin Immunol 2010;125:653–9.

27. Kusel MM, de Klerk NH, Kebadze T, et al. Early-life respiratory viral infections, atopic sensitization, and risk of subsequent development of persistent asthma. J Allergy Clin Immunol 2007;119:1105–10.

28. Lemanske RF Jr, Busse WW. Asthma: clinical expression and molecular mechanisms. J Allergy Clin Immunol 2010;125:S95–102.

29. Holt PG, Sly PD. Interaction between adaptive and innate immune pathways in the pathogenesis of atopic asthma: operation of a lung/bone marrow axis. Chest 2011;139:1165–71.

30. Subrata LS, Bizzintino J, Mamessier E, et al. Interactions between innate antiviral and atopic immunoinflammatory pathways precipitate and sustain asthma exacerbations in children. J Immunol 2009;183:2793–800.

31. Payne DN, Adcock IM, Wilson NM, et al. Relationship between exhaled nitric oxide and mucosal eosinophilic inflammation in children with difficult asthma, after treatment with oral prednisolone. Am J Respir Crit Care Med 2001;164:1376–81.

32. Fitzpatrick AM, Higgins M, Holguin F, et al. National Institutes of Health/National Heart, Lung, and Blood Institute's Severe Asthma Research Program. The molecular phenotype of severe asthma in children. J Allergy Clin Immunol 2010;125:851–7.

33. de Blic J, Tillie-Leblond I, Tonnel AB, et al. Difficult asthma in children: an analysis of airway inflammation. J Allergy Clin Immunol 2004;113:94–100.

34. Le Bourgeois M, Goncalves M, Le Clainche L, et al. Bronchoalveolar cells in children < 3 years old with severe recurrent wheezing. Chest 2002;122:791–7.

35. Marguet C, Jouen-Boedes F, Dean TP, et al. Bronchoalveolar cell profiles in children with asthma, infantile wheeze, chronic cough, or cystic fibrosis. Am J Respir Crit Care Med 1999;159:1533–40.

36. Stevenson EC, Turner G, Heaney LG, et al. Bronchoalveolar lavage findings suggest two different forms of childhood asthma. Clin Exp Allergy 1997;27:1027–35.

37. Starosta V, Kitz R, Hartl D, et al. Bronchoalveolar pepsin, bile acids, oxidation, and inflammation in children with gastroesophageal reflux disease. Chest 2007;132:1557–64.

38. Moore WC, Bleecker ER, Curran-Everett D, et al, National Heart, Lung, Blood Institute's Severe Asthma Research Program. Characterization of the severe asthma phenotype by the National Heart, Lung, and Blood Institute's Severe Asthma Research Program. J Allergy Clin Immunol 2007;119:405–13.

39. Miranda C, Busacker A, Balzar S, et al. Distinguishing severe asthma phenotypes: role of age at onset and eosinophilic inflammation. J Allergy Clin Immunol 2004;113:101–8.

40. Hauk PJ, Krawiec M, Murphy J, et al. Neutrophilic airway inflammation and association with bacterial lipopolysaccharide in children with asthma and wheezing. Pediatr Pulmonol 2008;43:916–23.

41. Just J, Fournier L, Momas I, et al. Clinical significance of bronchoalveolar eosinophils in childhood asthma. J Allergy Clin Immunol 2002;110:42–4.

42. Van den Toorn LM, Overbeek SE, de Jongste JC, et al. Airway inflammation is present during clinical remission of atopic asthma. Am J Respir Crit Care Med 2001;164:2107–13.

43. Siddiqui S, Hollins F, Saha S, et al. Inflammatory cell microlocalisation and airway dysfunction: cause and effect? Eur Respir J 2007;30:1043–56.

44. Payne DN, Qiu Y, Zhu J, et al. Airway inflammation in children with difficult asthma: relationships with airflow limitation and persistent symptoms. Thorax 2004;59:862–9.

45. Saglani S, Malmström K, Pelkonen AS, et al. Airway remodeling and inflammation in symptomatic infants with reversible airflow obstruction. Am J Respir Crit Care Med 2005;171:722–7.

46. Lambrecht BN, Hammad H. The role of dendritic and epithelial cells as master regulators of allergic airway inflammation. Lancet 2010;376:835–43.

47. Bosco A, Ehteshami S, Stern DA, et al. Decreased activation of inflammatory networks during acute asthma exacerbations is associated with chronic airflow obstruction. Mucosal Immunol 2010;3:399–409.

48. Stern DA, Morgan WJ, Halonen M, et al. Wheezing and bronchial hyper-responsiveness in early childhood as predictors of newly diagnosed asthma in early adulthood: a longitudinal birth-cohort study. Lancet 2008;372:1058–64.

49. Jackson DJ, Evans MD, Gangnon RE, et al. Evidence for a causal relationship between allergic sensitization and rhinovirus wheezing in early life. Am J Respir Crit Care Med 2012;185(3):281–5.

50. Maurer D, Fiebiger S, Ebner C, et al. Peripheral blood dendritic cells express Fc epsilon RI as a complex composed of Fc epsilon RI alpha- and Fc epsilon RI gamma-chains and can use this receptor for IgE-mediated allergen presentation. J Immunol 1996;157:607–16.

51. Singh AM, Moore PE, Gern JE, et al. Bronchiolitis to asthma: a review and call for studies of gene-virus interactions in asthma causation. Am J Respir Crit Care Med 2007;175:108–19.

52. Contoli M, Message SD, Laza-Stanca V, et al. Role of deficient type III interferon-lambda production in asthma exacerbations. Nat Med 2006;12:1023–6.

53. Wark PA, Johnston SL, Bucchieri F, et al. Asthmatic bronchial epithelial cells have a deficient innate immune response to infection with rhinovirus. J Exp Med 2005;201:937–47.

54. Message SD, Laza-Stanca V, Mallia P, et al. Rhinovirus-induced lower respiratory illness is increased in asthma and related to virus load and Th1/2 cytokine and IL-10 production. Proc Natl Acad Sci U S A 2008;105:13562–7.

55. Guerra S, Lohman IC, Halonen M, et al. Reduced interferon gamma production and soluble CD14 levels in early life predict recurrent wheezing by 1 year of age. Am J Respir Crit Care Med 2004; 169:70–6.

56. Martinez FD. Viral infections and the development of asthma. Am J Respir Crit Care Med 1995;151:1644–7.

57. Tang ML, Kemp AS, Thorburn J, et al. Reduced interferon-gamma secretion in neonates and subsequent atopy. Lancet 1994;344:983–5.

58. Schroth MK, Grimm E, Frindt P, et al. Rhinovirus replication causes RANTES production in primary bronchial epithelial cells. Am J Respir Cell Mol Biol 1999;20:1220–8.

59. Jackson DJ, Johnston SL. The role of viruses in acute exacerbations of asthma. J Allergy Clin Immunol 2010;125:1178–87.

60. Grünberg K, Sharon RF, Hiltermann TJ, et al. Experimental rhinovirus 16 infection increases intercellular adhesion molecule-1 expression in bronchial epithelium of asthmatics regardless of inhaled steroid treatment. Clin Exp Allergy 2000;30:1015–23.

61. Bullens DM, Decraene A, Dilissen E, et al. Type III IFN-lambda mRNA expression in sputum of adult and school-aged asthmatics. Clin Exp Allergy 2008;38:1459–67.

62. Thomas BJ, Lindsay M, Dagher H, et al. Transforming growth factor-beta enhances rhinovirus infection by diminishing early innate responses. Am J Respir Cell Mol Biol 2009;41:339–47.

63. Laza-Stanca V, Message SD, Edwards MR, et al. The role of IL-15 deficiency in the pathogenesis of virus-induced asthma exacerbations. PLoS Pathog 2011;7:e1002114.

64. Bisgaard H, Hermansen MN, Buchvald F, et al. Childhood asthma after bacterial colonization of the airway in neonates. N Engl J Med 2007;357: 1487–95.

65. Hilty M, Burke C, Pedro H, et al. Disordered microbial communities in asthmatic airways. PLoS One 2010;5:e8578.

66. Herbst T, Sichelstiel A, Schär C, et al. Dysregulation of allergic airway inflammation in the absence of microbial colonization. Am J Respir Crit Care Med 2011;184:198–205.

67. Malmström K, Pitkäranta A, Carpen O, et al. Human rhinovirus in bronchial epithelium of infants with recurrent respiratory symptoms. J Allergy Clin Immunol 2006;118:591–6.

68. Holt PG, Upham JW, Sly PD. Contemporaneous maturation of immunologic and respiratory functions during early childhood: implications for development of asthma prevention strategies. J Allergy Clin Immunol 2005;116:16–24.

69. Comhair SA, Ricci KS, Arroliga M, et al. Correlation of systemic superoxide dismutase deficiency to airflow obstruction in asthma. Am J Respir Crit Care Med 2005;172:306–13.

70. Comhair SA, Gaston BM, Ricci KS, et al. Detrimental effects of environmental tobacco smoke in relation to asthma severity. PLoS One 2011;6:e18574.

71. Comhair SA, Xu W, Ghosh S, et al. Superoxide dismutase inactivation in pathophysiology of asthmatic airway remodeling and reactivity. Am J Pathol 2005;166:663–74.

72. Fitzpatrick AM, Teague WG, Holguin F, et al. Airway glutathione homeostasis is altered in children with

severe asthma: evidence for oxidant stress. J Allergy Clin Immunol 2009;123:146–52.

73. Fitzpatrick AM, Holguin F, Teague WG, et al. Alveolar macrophage phagocytosis is impaired in children with poorly controlled asthma. J Allergy Clin Immunol 2008;121:1372–8.

74. Fitzpatrick AM, Stephenson ST, Hadley GR, et al. Thiol redox disturbances in children with severe asthma are associated with posttranslational modification of the transcription factor nuclear factor (erythroid-derived 2)-like 2. J Allergy Clin Immunol 2011;127:1604–11.

75. Rangasamy T, Guo J, Mitzner WA, et al. Disruption of Nrf2 enhances susceptibility to severe airway inflammation and asthma in mice. J Exp Med 2005;202:47–59.

76. Gilliland FD, Gauderman WJ, Vora H, et al. Effects of glutathione-S-transferase M1, T1, and P1 on childhood lung function growth. Am J Respir Crit Care Med 2002;166:710–6.

77. Tillie-Leblond I, de Blic J, Jaubert F, et al. Airway remodeling is correlated with obstruction in children with severe asthma. Allergy 2008;63:533–41.

78. Payne DN, Rogers AV, Adelroth E, et al. Early thickening of the reticular basement membrane in children with difficult asthma. Am J Respir Crit Care Med 2003;167:78–82.

79. Barbato A, Turato G, Baraldo S, et al. Airway inflammation in childhood asthma. Am J Respir Crit Care Med 2003;168:798–803.

80. Kim ES, Kim SH, Kim KW, et al. Basement membrane thickening and clinical features of children with asthma. Allergy 2007;62:635–40.

81. Saglani S, Payne DN, Zhu J, et al. Early detection of airway wall remodeling and eosinophilic inflammation in preschool wheezers. Am J Respir Crit Care Med 2007;176:858–64.

82. Saglani S, Molyneux C, Gong H, et al. Ultrastructure of the reticular basement membrane in asthmatic adults, children and infants. Eur Respir J 2006;28:505–12.

83. Pascual RM, Peters SP. Airway remodeling contributes to the progressive loss of lung function in asthma: an overview. J Allergy Clin Immunol 2005;116:477–86.

84. Mauad T, Bel EH, Sterk PJ. Asthma therapy and airway remodeling. J Allergy Clin Immunol 2007;120:997–1009.

85. Regamey N, Ochs M, Hilliard TN, et al. Increased airway smooth muscle mass in children with asthma, cystic fibrosis, and non-cystic fibrosis bronchiectasis. Am J Respir Crit Care Med 2008;177:837–43.

86. Johnson PR, Roth M, Tamm M, et al. Airway smooth muscle cell proliferation is increased in asthma. Am J Respir Crit Care Med 2001;164:474–7.

87. Lazaar AL, Panettieri RA Jr. Airway smooth muscle as a regulator of immune responses and bronchomotor tone. Clin Chest Med 2006;27:53–69.

88. Gupta A, Sjoukes A, Richards D, et al. Relationship between serum vitamin D, disease severity, and airway remodeling in children with asthma. Am J Respir Crit Care Med 2011;184:1342–9.

89. Barbato A, Turato G, Baraldo S, et al. Epithelial damage and angiogenesis in the airways of children with asthma. Am J Respir Crit Care Med 2006;174:975–81.

90. Kanazawa H, Nomura S, Yoshikawa J. Role of microvascular permeability on physiologic differences in asthma and eosinophilic bronchitis. Am J Respir Crit Care Med 2004;169:1125–30.

91. Gosset P, Tillie-Leblond I, Janin A, et al. Expression of E-selectin, ICAM-1 and VCAM-1 on bronchial biopsies from allergic and non-allergic asthmatic patients. Int Arch Allergy Immunol 1995;106:69–77.

92. Holgate ST. The sentinel role of the airway epithelium in asthma pathogenesis. Immunol Rev 2011;242:205–19.

93. Baraldo S, Turato G, Bazzan E, et al. Noneosinophilic asthma in children: relation with airway remodelling. Eur Respir J 2011;38:575–83.

94. Malmström K, Pelkonen AS, Malmberg LP, et al. Lung function, airway remodelling and inflammation in symptomatic infants: outcome at 3 years. Thorax 2011;66:157–62.

95. Fedorov IA, Wilson SJ, Davies DE, et al. Epithelial stress and structural remodelling in childhood asthma. Thorax 2005;60:389–94.

96. Guilbert TW, Morgan WJ, Zeiger RS, et al. Long-term inhaled corticosteroids in preschool children at high risk for asthma. N Engl J Med 2006;354:1985–97.

97. Murray CS, Woodcock A, Langley SJ, et al. IFWIN study team. Secondary prevention of asthma by the use of Inhaled Fluticasone propionate in Wheezy INfants (IFWIN): double-blind, randomised, controlled study. Lancet 2006;368:754–62.

98. Holgate ST, Roberts G, Arshad HS, et al. The role of the airway epithelium and its interaction with environmental factors in asthma pathogenesis. Proc Am Thorac Soc 2009;6:655–9.

99. Blobe GC, Schiemann WP, Lodish HF. Role of transforming growth factor beta in human disease. N Engl J Med 2000;342:1350–8.

100. Pulleyn LJ, Newton R, Adcock IM, et al. TGFbeta1 allele association with asthma severity. Hum Genet 2001;109:623–7.

101. Hatsushika K, Hirota T, Harada M, et al. Transforming growth factor-beta(2) polymorphisms are associated with childhood atopic asthma. Clin Exp Allergy 2007;37:1165–74.

102. Balzar S, Chu HW, Silkoff P, et al. Increased TGF-beta2 in severe asthma with eosinophilia. J Allergy Clin Immunol 2005;115:110–7.

103. Simpson A, Maniatis N, Jury F, et al. Polymorphisms in a disintegrin and metalloprotease 33

(ADAM33) predict impaired early-life lung function. Am J Respir Crit Care Med 2005;172:55–60.

104. Rodríguez E, Baurecht H, Herberich E, et al. Meta-analysis of filaggrin polymorphisms in eczema and asthma: robust risk factors in atopic disease. J Allergy Clin Immunol 2009;123:1361–70.

105. van den Oord RA, Sheikh A. Filaggrin gene defects and risk of developing allergic sensitisation and allergic disorders: systematic review and meta-analysis. BMJ 2009;339:b2433.

106. Marenholz I, Kerscher T, Bauerfeind A, et al. An interaction between filaggrin mutations and early food sensitization improves the prediction of childhood asthma. J Allergy Clin Immunol 2009;123: 911–6.

107. Ponińska J, Samoliński B, Tomaszewska A, et al. Filaggrin gene defects are independent risk factors for atopic asthma in a Polish population: a study in ECAP cohort. PLoS One 2011;6: e16933.

108. Leigh R, Oyelusi W, Wiehler S, et al. Human rhinovirus infection enhances airway epithelial cell production of growth factors involved in airway remodeling. J Allergy Clin Immunol 2008;121: 1238–45.

109. Bedke N, Haitchi HM, Xatzipsalti M, et al. Contribution of bronchial fibroblasts to the antiviral response in asthma. J Immunol 2009;182:3660–7.

110. Ober C, Hoffjan S. Asthma genetics 2006: the long and winding road to gene discovery. Genes Immun 2006;7:95–100.

111. Yang IA, Holloway JW. Asthma: advancing gene-environment studies. Clin Exp Allergy 2007;37: 1264–6.

112. von Mutius E. Genes and the environment: two readings of their interaction. J Allergy Clin Immunol 2008;122:99–100.

113. Bossley CJ, Saglani S, Kavanagh C, et al. Corticosteroid responsiveness and clinical characteristics in childhood difficult asthma. Eur Respir J 2009;34: 1052–9.

114. Fitzpatrick AM, Teague WG, Meyers DA, et al, National Institutes of Health/National Heart, Lung, and Blood Institute Severe Asthma Research Program. Heterogeneity of severe asthma in childhood: confirmation by cluster analysis of children in the National Institutes of Health/National Heart, Lung, and Blood Institute Severe Asthma Research Program. J Allergy Clin Immunol 2011;127:382–9.

115. Konradsen JR, Nordlund B, Lidegran M, et al, Swedish Network of Pediatric Allergists, Severe Asthma Network. Problematic severe asthma: a proposed approach to identifying children who are severely resistant to therapy. Pediatr Allergy Immunol 2011;22:9–18.

116. Fitzpatrick AM, Gaston BM, Erzurum SC, et al. National Institutes of Health/National Heart, Lung,

and Blood Institute Severe Asthma Research Program. Features of severe asthma in school-age children: Atopy and increased exhaled nitric oxide. J Allergy Clin Immunol 2006;118:1218–25.

117. Roberts G, Patel N, Levi-Schaffer F, et al. Food allergy as a risk factor for life-threatening asthma in childhood: a case-controlled study. J Allergy Clin Immunol 2003;112:168–74.

118. Sampson HA, Muñoz-Furlong A, Campbell RL, et al. Second symposium on the definition and management of anaphylaxis: summary report—Second National Institute of Allergy and Infectious Disease/Food Allergy and Anaphylaxis Network symposium. J Allergy Clin Immunol 2006;117: 391–7.

119. O'Driscoll BR, Hopkinson LC, Denning DW. Mold sensitization is common amongst patients with severe asthma requiring multiple hospital admissions. BMC Pulm Med 2005;5:4.

120. Vicencio AG, Muzumdar H, Tsirilakis K, et al. Severe asthma with fungal sensitization in a child: response to itraconazole therapy. Pediatrics 2010; 125:e1255–8.

121. Ayres JG, Jyothish D, Ninan T. Brittle asthma. Paediatr Respir Rev 2004;5:40–4.

122. Dougherty RH, Fahy JV. Acute exacerbations of asthma: epidemiology, biology and the exacerbation-prone phenotype. Clin Exp Allergy 2009;39: 193–202.

123. Carroll CL, Schramm CM, Zucker AR. Severe exacerbations in children with mild asthma: characterizing a pediatric phenotype. J Asthma 2008;45: 513–7.

124. Bacharier LB, Phillips BR, Bloomberg GR, et al, Childhood Asthma Research and Education Network, National Heart, Lung, and Blood Institute. Severe intermittent wheezing in preschool children: a distinct phenotype. J Allergy Clin Immunol 2007; 119:604–10.

125. Phelan PD, Robertson CF, Olinsky A. The Melbourne Asthma Study: 1964-1999. J Allergy Clin Immunol 2002;109:189–94.

126. Fitzpatrick AM, Teague WG, National Institutes of Health/National Heart, Lung, and Blood Institute's Severe Asthma Research Program. Progressive airflow limitation is a feature of children with severe asthma. J Allergy Clin Immunol 2011;127:282–4.

127. Covar RA, Spahn JD, Murphy JR, et al, Childhood Asthma Management Program Research Group. Progression of asthma measured by lung function in the childhood asthma management program. Am J Respir Crit Care Med 2004;170:234–41.

128. He XY, Simpson JL, Wang F. Inflammatory phenotypes in stable and acute childhood asthma. Paediatr Respir Rev 2011;12:165–9.

129. Bush A, Pedersen S, Hedlin G, et al, PSACI (Problematic Severe Asthma in Childhood Initiative)

group. Pharmacological treatment of severe, therapy-resistant asthma in children: what can we learn from where? Eur Respir J 2011;38:947–58.

130. Holt S, Suder A, Weatherall M, et al. Dose-response relation of inhaled fluticasone propionate in adolescents and adults with asthma: meta-analysis. BMJ 2001;323:253–6.

131. Lex C, Payne DN, Zacharasiewicz A, et al. Is a two-week trial of oral prednisolone predictive of target lung function in pediatric asthma? Pediatr Pulmonol 2005;39:521–7.

132. Adams NP, Bestall JC, Jones P, et al. Fluticasone at different doses for chronic asthma in adults and children. Cochrane Database Syst Rev 2008; 4:CD003534.

133. de Blic J, Delacourt C, Le Bourgeois M, et al. Efficacy of nebulized budesonide in treatment of severe infantile asthma: a double-blind study. J Allergy Clin Immunol 1996;98:14–20.

134. Cohen J, Postma DS, Douma WR, et al. Particle size matters: diagnostics and treatment of small airways involvement in asthma. Eur Respir J 2011;37:532–40.

135. Rodrigo GJ, Castro-Rodríguez JA. Safety of long-acting {beta} agonists for the treatment of asthma: clearing the air. Thorax 2012;67(4):342–9.

136. Global Strategy for Asthma Management and Prevention, Global Initiative for Asthma (GINA) 2011. Available at: http://www.ginasthma.org/. Accessed May 26, 2012.

137. Panickar JR, Kenia P, Silverman M, et al. Intramuscular triamcinolone for difficult asthma. Pediatr Pulmonol 2005;39:421–5.

138. Milgrom H, Berger W, Nayak A, et al. Treatment of childhood asthma with anti-immunoglobulin E antibody (omalizumab). Pediatrics 2001;108:e36.

139. Lanier B, Bridges T, Kulus M, et al. Omalizumab for the treatment of exacerbations in children with inadequately controlled allergic (IgE-mediated) asthma. J Allergy Clin Immunol 2009;124:1210–6.

140. Lemanske RF Jr, Nayak A, McAlary M, et al. Omalizumab improves asthma-related quality of life in children with allergic asthma. Pediatrics 2002;110:e55.

141. Busse WW, Morgan WJ, Gergen PJ, et al. Randomized trial of omalizumab (anti-IgE) for asthma in inner-city children. N Engl J Med 2011;364: 1005–15.

142. Rodrigo GJ, Neffen H, Castro-Rodriguez JA. Efficacy and safety of subcutaneous omalizumab vs placebo as add-on therapy to corticosteroids for children and adults with asthma: a systematic review. Chest 2011;139:28–35.

143. Cox L, Platts-Mills TA, Finegold I, et al, American Academy of Allergy, Asthma & Immunology; American College of Allergy, Asthma and Immunology. American Academy of Allergy, Asthma & Immunology/American College of Allergy, Asthma and

Immunology Joint Task Force Report on omalizumab-associated anaphylaxis. J Allergy Clin Immunol 2007;120:1373–7.

144. Seddon P, Bara A, Ducharme FM, et al. Oral xanthines as maintenance treatment for asthma in children. Cochrane Database Syst Rev 2006;1: CD002885.

145. Rottier BL, Duiverman EJ. Anti-inflammatory drug therapy in asthma. Paediatr Respir Rev 2009;10: 214–9.

146. Metz G, Kraft M. Effects of atypical infections with Mycoplasma and Chlamydia on asthma. Immunol Allergy Clin North Am 2010;30:575–85.

147. Patel KK, Vicencio AG, Du Z, et al. Infectious Chlamydia pneumoniae is associated with elevated interleukin-8 and airway neutrophilia in children with refractory asthma. Pediatr Infect Dis J 2010; 29:1093–8.

148. Strunk RC, Bacharier LB, Phillips BR, et al, CARE Network. Azithromycin or montelukast as inhaled corticosteroid-sparing agents in moderate-to-severe childhood asthma study. J Allergy Clin Immunol 2008;122:1138–44.

149. Evans DJ, Cullinan P, Geddes DM. Cyclosporin as an oral corticosteroid sparing agent in stable asthma. Cochrane Database Syst Rev 2001;2:CD002993.

150. Davies H, Olson L, Gibson P. Methotrexate as a steroid sparing agent for asthma in adults. Cochrane Database Syst Rev 2000;2:CD000391.

151. Firszt R, Kraft M. Pharmacotherapy of severe asthma. Curr Opin Pharmacol 2010;10:266–71.

152. Rasmussen LM, Phanareth K, Nolte H, et al. Internet-based monitoring of asthma: a long-term, randomized clinical study of 300 asthmatic subjects. J Allergy Clin Immunol 2005;115:1137–42.

153. Deschildre A, Béghin L, Salleron J, et al. Home telemonitoring (FEV1) in children with severe asthma does not reduce exacerbations. Eur Respir J 2012; 39(2):290–6.

154. Reddel HK, Taylor DR, Bateman ED, et al, American Thoracic Society/European Respiratory Society Task Force on Asthma Control and Exacerbations. An official American Thoracic Society/European Respiratory Society statement: asthma control and exacerbations: standardizing endpoints for clinical asthma trials and clinical practice. Am J Respir Crit Care Med 2009;180:59–99.

155. Petsky HL, Cates CJ, Lasseron TJ, et al. A systematic review and meta-analysis: tailoring asthma treatment on eosinophilic markers (exhaled nitric oxide or sputum eosinophils). Thorax 2012; 67:199–208.

156. Fleming L, Wilson N, Regamey N, et al. Use of sputum eosinophil counts to guide management in children with severe asthma. Thorax 2012;67:193–8.

Treating According to Asthma Control: Does it Work in Real Life?

Helen K. Reddel, MB, BS, PhD, FRACP

KEYWORDS

- Asthma control • Guidelines • Exacerbations • Primary health care • Drug therapy • Adults

KEY POINTS

- Control-based asthma management, adjusting the patient's treatment upward or downward according to simple measures of control, has been incorporated in asthma guidelines for many years.
- This article reviews the evidence for its utility in adults, describes its strengths and limitations in real life, and proposes areas for further research, particularly about incorporation of future risk and identification of patients for whom phenotype-guided treatment would be effective and efficient.
- The strengths of control-based management include its simplicity and feasibility for primary care, and its limitations include the nonspecific nature of asthma symptoms, the complex role of β_2-agonist use, barriers to stepping down treatment, and the underlying assumptions about asthma pathophysiology and treatment responses.

WHAT IS CONTROL-BASED MANAGEMENT?

The concept of adjusting asthma treatment according to the patient's \ level of asthma control has been embedded in asthma guidelines for so long that it is easy to forget that this approach is somewhat unusual in other areas of clinical practice. With many chronic diseases, patient assessment and treatment is guided by disease severity, an intrinsic feature usually manifest at the initial presentation and correlated with the underlying pathologic condition. However, for asthma, information about airway pathology was not (and is still not) generally available to clinicians, so the initial concept of asthma severity was based on the patient's clinical features at presentation (ie, symptoms, reliever use, and airflow limitation).[1,2] Early studies had shown that

- Symptoms and airflow limitation could be temporarily relieved by the use of short-acting β_2-agonist medications (SABA).
- More sustained control of symptoms required longer-term treatment with inhaled corticosteroids (ICS).[3]
- Patients with more severe asthma at baseline, already using ICS or oral corticosteroids, generally responded to higher ICS doses[4,5] or the addition of long-acting β_2-agonist (LABA).[6]
- Once symptoms and airflow limitation were well controlled (ie, occurring only a couple of times a week), the ICS dose could be reduced to minimize the potential for side effects.[7]

These principles, initially empiric and consensus based but later formalized with extensive

Disclosure of interests: H.K.R. is Chair of the Science Committee of the Global Initiative for Asthma (GINA) and a member of the Steering Committee for the 2012 update of the *Australian Asthma Management Handbook*. She has participated in asthma advisory boards for AstraZeneca, GlaxoSmithKline, and Novartis; has received unrestricted research funding from AstraZeneca and GlaxoSmithKline; is a member of a data monitoring committee for AstraZeneca, GlaxoSmithKline, Merck, and Novartis; and has given continuing medical education presentations at symposia funded by AstraZeneca, GlaxoSmithKline, and Novartis.
Clinical Management Group, Woolcock Institute of Medical Research, PO Box M77, Missenden Road Post Office, New South Wales 2050, Australia
E-mail address: hkr@med.usyd.edu.au

Clin Chest Med 33 (2012) 505–517
http://dx.doi.org/10.1016/j.ccm.2012.06.005
0272-5231/12/$ – see front matter © 2012 Elsevier Inc. All rights reserved.

chestmed.theclinics.com

randomized controlled trials and meta-analyses, still largely form the basis for current clinical practice recommendations, including from the Global Initiative for Asthma (GINA),[8] the National Heart Lung and Blood Institute's Expert Panel 3 Report,[9] and the British Thoracic Society/Scottish Intercollegiate Guidelines Network (BTS/SIGN).[10] The current recommended treatment steps for adults are:

- As-needed SABA
- Low-dose ICS
- Low-dose ICS/LABA
- Moderate-high dose ICS/LABA
- Add-on prednisone or other agents.

At each level, the guidelines also provide options for alternative medications to allow for patient preference, side effects, and cost.

From the start, the concept of control-based management also included:

- Short-term management of worsening asthma, with patients adjusting their medications according to a written asthma action plan based on worsening symptoms or lung function and returning to pre-exacerbation treatment levels once asthma was controlled
- Management of asthma within a framework of a good patient-doctor relationship, self-management education, and regular review.

Although evidence-based medicine places a high value on systematic reviews of good-quality randomized controlled trials, it is now recognized that:

- Only a small minority of community patients would have satisfied the entry criteria for the major studies on which asthma guidelines are based.[11]
- Substantial heterogeneity occurs in responses to ICS and other medications, with patients with similar clinical characteristics at baseline having widely differing responses to treatment.[12–14]
- Treatment strategies may have different effects on clinical measures of control and on exacerbations.[15]
- Finally, with sputum induction and bronchial biopsies more readily available, it was found that variation in treatment response could be at least partly attributed to heterogeneity in the underlying inflammatory processes.[16,17]

As a result, asthma, rather than being considered as a single disease, is gaining recognition as a syndromic descriptor for a group of conditions with similar clinical manifestations but different pathophysiologic mechanisms and responses to treatment,[18,19] as occurred with arthritis.

The assessment of asthma was recently reviewed to develop standardized definitions and criteria for asthma control, severity, and exacerbations for use in clinical trials and clinical practice.[20,21] The diversity of underlying pathophysiological phenotypes was emphasized; the assessment of asthma control was expanded from current clinical features, such as symptoms, airway obstruction, and impaired activity, to also include the assessment of patient's risks of adverse events, such as exacerbations, accelerated lung function decline, and side effects. These two components were named *current clinical control* and *future risk*.[20] Future risk was incorporated in recognition that symptoms were a superficial marker of asthma control in that they could be suppressed by LABA monotherapy while exacerbations remained uncontrolled, and that there were other predictors of future risk, such as smoking, low lung function, and airway eosinophilia, which were independent of the level of symptoms.[20]

The present article reviews the evidence for the utility of control-based asthma management in adults, describes the strengths and limitations of this approach in real life, and proposes areas for further research to improve its utility and to identify patients and populations for whom control-based management is appropriate.

EVIDENCE ABOUT CONTROL-BASED MANAGEMENT IN REAL LIFE

The first clinical practice guidelines for asthma were published in Australia in 1989.[2] They recommended the adjustment of treatment based on lung function and "severity", which was similar to the present assessment of asthma "control". A similar approach was taken in Canada the following year, with both countries undertaking intensive dissemination activities.[22] At the time, evidence-based medicine was in its infancy, so the guidelines were largely consensus based, and there were no formal studies comparing control-based management with the previous more ad hoc approach.

Assessing the impact of the control-based strategy in real life is difficult because it was intended to be part of a package of asthma care and education and to include both stepping up and stepping down. By contrast, most research evidence comes from closely monitored randomized controlled trials with a single-step treatment change at randomization. Planning clinical trials to examine medication adjustment strategies is challenging because the cumulative effect of algorithmic interventions can magnify any design flaws.[23]

Pre-Post Studies in Real Life

- Ecological evidence for the impact of control-based management may be suggested by the dramatic decrease in asthma mortality in countries, such as Australia and Canada, in the 20 years after the publication of their asthma guidelines despite increasing asthma prevalence.[24,25]
- In 1994, Finland adopted a comprehensive 10-year asthma-management program incorporating systematic implementation strategies, which achieved remarkable national penetration across all levels of health care. Again, hospitalizations and deaths caused by asthma were halved despite and increase in asthma prevalence, and there was a decrease in asthma-related costs.[26]
- In 1998 to 2000, the International Union Against Tuberculosis and Lung Disease (IUATLD) conducted asthma-management studies in 9 countries, using a control-based algorithm customized for developing countries. Over 1 year of follow-up, the proportion of patients with poorly controlled asthma decreased from 43% to 16%.[27]

However, evidence that the control-based approach to asthma management has not been (sufficiently) successful in real life comes from the many cross-sectional studies that have shown that a high proportion of patients, even in countries with well-established guidelines and ready access to controller medications, still experience frequent symptoms and interference with daily activities and many still require urgent health care for asthma.[28] From administrative datasets, too, comes evidence that prescribing and/or dispensing of controller medications are inconsistent with control-based guidelines. For example, according to control-based management, most patients should be started on low-dose ICS, and most should achieve good asthma control when this is taken regularly. However, in Australia, most ICS is dispensed as moderate/high potency ICS/LABA and only 9% of ICS recipients aged 15 to 34 years have dispensing rates consistent with daily use.[24] In a US claims database, patients with mild persistent asthma were more often initiated on more expensive treatments than on the low-dose ICS recommended by guidelines.[29]

Control-Based Management Versus Usual Care in Real Life

Because control-based management has been recommended by clinical practice guidelines for more than 20 years, the outcomes of studies that compare guidelines-based management with usual care reflect the extent to which guidelines have been adopted in clinical practice as well as the effectiveness of the control-driven regimen itself. For example, a cohort analysis from a large managed care organization showed that patients with uncontrolled asthma (n = 7177) had better asthma control, as indicated by reduced reliever use, if their treatment was stepped up in accordance with guidelines than those with no step-up; however there was no significant difference between groups in exacerbation rates.[30]

In several intervention studies, practical tools have increased the implementation of a control-based approach, with improved outcomes compared with usual care. For example:

- In Spain, a GINA-based management system with computerized decision support led to improved quality of life and reduced health care utilization and was cost-effective, compared with usual care.[31]
- In a US managed care organization with existing control-based processes for managing asthma, protocolized implementation of stepped-care guidelines by trained care managers, using customized worksheets and educational tools, led to significant improvements in medication adherence, asthma control and asthma-related quality of life, and a significant reduction in health care utilization compared with usual care within the same organisation.[32] Medication adherence was even higher when care managers used a shared decision-making process for medication choices,[32] emphasizing the importance of patient-clinician communication in the implementation of control-based management.

Control-Based Management Versus Inflammation-Guided Management

It might be expected that treatment guided by biomarkers which reflect the nature of underlying airway inflammation would improve overall outcomes. Studies comparing control-based management with inflammation-guided management are dealt with in detail by Nair and colleagues elsewhere in this issue, but the key issues for clinical practice are summarized below.

Sputum-guided management

The pivotal studies of sputum-guided treatment showed a halving of severe exacerbations and similar levels of current asthma control compared with control-based treatment.[33] However, the results are not directly applicable to real-life clinical practice because the studies involved very selected populations and research sites. Patients with moderate-severe asthma were recruited through specialist chest clinics with existing research expertise in sputum cell counting, and who were generally excluded if they were thought to have adherence problems or comorbidities, were current smokers, or had a significant smoking history. There was some variation between these studies in the details of the sputum-based and control-based algorithms, and there was a delay of 1 to 7 days between the patient visit and the treatment decision.

Now that the evidence for the efficacy of sputum-guided treatment has been established in these rigorously conducted studies, further research is needed to investigate its feasibility, cost-effectiveness, and acceptability to patients and clinicians within more general secondary care. In post hoc analysis of one study,[34] the advantages of sputum-guided treatment were seen in patients with discordant symptoms and eosinophilic inflammation, with lower ICS doses achieved in those with high symptoms but low inflammation, and fewer severe exacerbations in those with few symptoms but marked sputum eosinophilia.[35]

Fractional concentration of exhaled nitric oxide–guided treatment

There has been considerable interest in the use of the fractional concentration of exhaled nitric oxide (FeNO) as a more feasible surrogate marker of eosinophilic airway inflammation. However, the overall results of studies comparing FeNO-guided treatment with control-based treatment in children and adults have not been as convincing as for sputum-guided treatment, with meta-analysis failing to show an overall benefit either in clinical control or exacerbation rates.[36] Wide variation was seen between studies in the selection of patients and the design of the FeNO and control algorithms, including in the extent to which the control algorithm reflected guideline recommendations.

Gibson[23] recently highlighted several methodological issues that likely contributed to the lack of difference between the FeNO-based and control-based algorithms in these studies. These issues included the narrow range of patient ICS doses at entry, the use of 1 rather than 2 FeNO cut points, and the low probability that the selected algorithms within most of the studies would result in different treatment decisions. The implementation of these methodological principles in a subsequent algorithm study of pregnant women with asthma led to striking reductions in exacerbation rates, and lower ICS doses, with FeNO-guided compared with a control-based algorithm, although

the latter differed in several respects from current guidelines, although the latter differed in several respects from current recommendations.[37] Given the ease of measurement of FeNO and the rapidity with which results are obtained, further studies are awaited with interest.

As with sputum-guided treatment, it will be important to identify the patients and settings in which FeNO-guided management gives better outcomes than control-based management.

STRENGTHS OF CONTROL-BASED MANAGEMENT IN REAL LIFE

The major strengths of control-based management for real-life application are its simplicity, feasibility, and patient-centered approach.

The control-based strategy for medication adjustment is feasible for use in primary and secondary care:

- It can be implemented across broad populations, including in developing countries,[26,27,38] because it involves only a few simple questions about clinical features and the patient's risk factors for longer-term adverse outcomes.
- The measurement of forced expiratory volume in the first second of expiration (FEV_1) or peak flow is a component of the assessment of asthma control when available and is readily accessible (although currently underutilized) in primary care.
- Medication decisions can be made immediately during consultations without the need for specialized equipment, personnel, or processing.

Because a patient's individual experience of asthma is largely driven by their symptoms,[39] the concept of adjusting treatments based on symptoms can emphasize that the approach is patient-centered. Several studies have shown that patients taking maintenance controller treatment already adjust their usage in response to symptoms, although the reported level of use is less than that needed for good asthma control.[40,41]

LIMITATIONS OF CONTROL-BASED MANAGEMENT IN REAL LIFE

Despite, or perhaps because of, its simplicity, control-based management has some important limitations in real life. These limitations may not be sufficient to influence group mean results in a research study but are relevant to the management of individual patients in clinical practice.

Incorrect Diagnosis of Asthma

Integral to the concept of control-based management is the assumption that the diagnosis of asthma has been confirmed, because symptoms not caused by bronchoconstriction or airway inflammation are unlikely to respond to conventional asthma pharmacotherapy. However, studies of community-based populations in Sweden,[42,43] the Netherlands,[44] and Canada[45] report that objective evidence of asthma cannot be found in 24% to 34% of patients with a reported diagnosis of asthma.

High rates of overdiagnosis may be partly attributable to the success of previous public and medical awareness campaigns, encouraging clinicians to think of asthma for patients with respiratory symptoms[22,46]; however, the situation is worsened by barriers to use of spirometry in primary care.[47,48] Only 43% of Canadian patients with a new diagnosis of asthma had undergone spirometric testing in the 3.5 years around the time of diagnosis.[49]

Correct diagnosis of asthma is crucial because, in patients with respiratory symptoms, control-based management would otherwise promote a progressive increase in medication, with patients eventually likely labeled as having severe refractory asthma.

Heterogeneity in Inflammatory Profile

The stepwise treatment options recommended in current guidelines were based on the assumption from group mean data that asthma is usually characterized by eosinophilic inflammation, which in turn causes airway hyperresponsiveness, thence bronchoconstriction, and symptoms, and that an ICS-based strategy would be most effective. Alternative medication options are offered at each step but their selection is described as depending on patient preference, side effects, or cost. Although each medication change is regarded as a therapeutic trial, failure to respond usually prompts a step-up to the next level rather than trial of one of the other medication options at the same level.

However, as described previously, one of the most striking advances in asthma in recent years has been in the growing awareness of heterogeneity in the relationship between symptoms and eosinophilic airway inflammation, and in the existence of other inflammatory phenotypes with different response profiles to ICS. As yet, inflammometry (inflammation-guided treatment) is only available in specialized centers.

Reliance on Symptoms

Asthma symptoms are nonspecific

Even once the diagnosis of asthma has been confirmed, it cannot be assumed that all subsequent respiratory symptoms are also caused by asthma. It is important in clinical practice to consider the possibility that new respiratory symptoms may be caused by a comorbidity, such as sinusitis, deconditioning, obesity, or vocal cord dysfunction, before stepping up the patient's asthma treatment. In the past, patients were considered to be mislabeling asthma symptoms if lung function was not reduced at the time,[50] but, with reduced reliance on the assessment of lung function in clinical practice, clinicians now have fewer tools for distinguishing asthma from non-asthma symptoms.

Symptom perception is variable

Substantial variation is seen between patients in their ability to perceive airflow limitation and, hence, in their level of symptoms. Contributing factors include age, baseline lung function, airway hyperresponsiveness, and airway inflammation.[51,52] The ability to identify bronchoconstriction improves with improved asthma control.[51]

The extent of symptoms experienced for a given level of lung function may also vary according to the patient's level of physical activity. Patients with a sedentary lifestyle are unlikely to experience exercise-induced bronchoconstriction and may not experience day-to-day symptoms until moderate to severe airflow limitation is present.

The no-symptoms-no-asthma belief

Core to the concept of control-based management is that patients who respond to treatment with ICS should continue to take them every day even if they have no symptoms, because the treatment is for control rather than for a cure. Patients may perceive this to be inconsistent with the use of symptoms to guide treatment. The no-symptoms-no-asthma belief, in which asthma is perceived and managed by patients as an acute episodic condition rather than a chronic disease, is associated with worse asthma control and greater need for prednisone courses.[53]

Subjective measures of control may respond to placebo treatment

The importance of monitoring both subjective and objective measures of asthma control has been highlighted by recent studies that have shown significant effects of placebo or sham interventions on symptoms in patients with mild asthma, without significant effects on lung function.[54,55]

β_2-Agonist Use as a Measure of Asthma Control

Factors affecting usage of β_2-agonist

The frequency of reliever use is likely to be affected by the patient's level of physical activity, by doses taken before exercise, by psychological dependence, and by the use of LABA. As expected, β_2-agonist use typically decreases after the addition of LABA to maintenance ICS treatment; however, cessation of LABA does not necessarily lead to an increase in SABA use,[56,57] suggesting a contribution of tachyphylaxis or habitual use of SABA, which may impact the assessment of asthma control in these patients.

Adverse effects of excess β_2-agonist

Guidelines recommend that rapid-acting β_2-agonist should be used as needed for relief of symptoms and bronchoconstriction, including acute severe asthma. Less well known, particularly in primary care, is that the regular or frequent use of SABA is associated with increased symptoms, bronchial reactivity, airway inflammation, and risk of exacerbations compared with placebo or twice-daily LABA.[58] One of the most difficult aspects of the assessment of asthma control in clinical practice is to identify when β_2-agonist use, rather than being an *indicator* of poor asthma control, is *contributing* to poor asthma control. Clinical pointers may include the long-term use of high SABA dosages (eg, albuterol 8+ puffs per day or daily use of nebulizer); well-preserved lung function despite very frequent symptoms and β_2-agonist use; and a lack of improvement in lung function with the administration of extra SABA (although this can also be seen during viral exacerbations[59]). Improved asthma control has been seen in around one-third of patients when strategies are implemented to reduce β_2-agonist exposure.[60,61]

Instability of Control Measures in Poorly Controlled Asthma

Patients with untreated asthma demonstrate substantial variability in measures of asthma control from week to week. For example, in a 12-week study in which patients at baseline had daily symptoms consistent with uncontrolled asthma, those who received as-needed SABA alone had symptoms and reliever use consistent with well-controlled asthma in 18% and 30% of the study weeks, respectively.[62] The need for preventer treatment may, therefore, be underestimated if it is based on the short-term assessment of asthma control. However, after patients commence regular preventer treatment, week-to-week variability in control measures is substantially reduced.[63]

Patient Understanding of Control

Many studies have reported that patients overestimate their level of asthma control, based on the discordance between patient-reported asthma control and the guidelines-based assessment of control.[28] However, this is more likely to indicate that patients attribute a different meaning to control, such as self-control or the ease with which they can relieve their symptoms with SABA, compared with the medical usage of the term.[20,64] Similar differences are seen in the medical and lay usage of the term shock.

Patient-reported level of control is included in the Asthma Control Test (ACT).[65] It has been suggested that the discordance between responses to this item and the 4 clinical items might serve as a red flag to identify patients who would benefit from further education about their disease[65]; however, the impact that this might have on subsequent ACT scores has not been evaluated.

Barriers to Stepping Down Asthma Treatment

Control-based management is predicated on regular review by the clinician, with stepwise increases in treatment when asthma control is worse and stepwise decreases when symptoms improve. However, in a review of more than 2000 visits by 397 patients in a community population over 2 years, 85% of medication changes were a step-up and only 13% were a step-down. A contributory factor is that patients often fail to attend for scheduled follow-ups or review visits; in the same study, there were 2.3 times as many visits for acute asthma problems as for asthma evaluations or follow-up.[66]

Despite evidence that step-down can be performed safely once asthma is well controlled,[67] clinicians seem to be reluctant to reduce even high-intensity treatment,[68] presumably because of the potential for destabilizing patients. Both the patient's and the physician's personality may contribute to overtreatment in asthma.[69] In addition, there are few barriers for the physician to maintaining high doses, given the low side-effect profile of ICS. This factor contrasts with conditions, such as diabetes or hypertension, whereby overtreatment can have serious adverse effects. Nevertheless, patient-reported side effects increase with increasing ICS dose[70] and are associated with lower medication adherence.[71]

Other Factors Contributing to Poor Asthma Control

Teaching materials about asthma guidelines often focus on the key table or figure that summarizes the recommended stepwise changes in medications and doses that should be followed in response to worsening asthma control. This approach omits some of the most important components of asthma management, which are usually emphasized in the accompanying text, particularly the need to establish a patient-doctor partnership and to assess common factors, such as adherence and inhaler technique, before considering a step-up in asthma medication.[72]

Poor inhaler technique

Poor technique with respiratory devices is so common that, for practical purposes, inhaler technique should be considered to be incorrect until proven otherwise. Poor technique, regardless of inhaler type, is associated with poor asthma control and an increased risk of hospitalization, emergency department visits, and need for systemic corticosteroids.[73] Sadly, most health professionals are also unable to demonstrate correct inhaler technique,[74] showing errors similar to those demonstrated by patients.[75] Increasing the prescribed dose of an inhaled medication is unlikely to be effective if patients are unable to use the relevant inhaler correctly.

Poor adherence

Poor adherence, likewise, is so common in asthma that it is to be considered almost the norm. Although there is evidence that patients self-reporting less-than-perfect adherence can be believed,[71,76] clinicians have difficulty in identifying patients who, through embarrassment or fear, deliberately conceal poor adherence.[77]

HOW CAN CONTROL-BASED MANAGEMENT BE IMPROVED?
Improve the Diagnosis of Asthma

Improving the diagnosis of asthma should reduce the number of patients who seem to fail control-based management, but this is not a simple task. There is no gold standard for the diagnosis of asthma and, like most other chronic diseases, it does not seem to be dichotomous, with the most typical features of symptoms and variable lung function existing on a continuum.[78] Wheezing, shortness of breath, cough, and chest tightness may occur with many other conditions. Strategies that may assist with asthma diagnosis are:

- A useful tool provided by the BTS/SIGN guidelines is a list of simple features that increase or decrease the probability that patients with respiratory symptoms have asthma.[10]
- Increasing the availability of good-quality spirometry in primary care is essential for improving the quality of diagnosis[79]; this may include providing online diagnostic

and technical support, or centralized spirometry services.

Improve Implementation of Control-Based Management

Provide access to basic medications
Most of the benefit of ICS is obtained at low daily doses,[80,81] but these medications are not currently available widely in all countries. The Asthma Drug Facility of the IUATLD provides generic ICS at low cost to developing countries in conjunction with simple documentation of process measures and clinical outcomes.[82]

Reinforce existing components of control-based management
Simple tools, such as Asthma Control Questionnaire (ACQ)[83] and ACT, can standardize the assessment of asthma control from visit to visit; they can be completed on paper in the waiting room, online,[84,85] or by telephone.[86] For an individual patient, a change in ACT score of 3 is regarded as clinically important.[87]

Guidelines emphasize the importance of confirming that symptoms are caused by asthma and that inhaler technique and adherence are satisfactory before considering a step-up in treatment but these basic steps are often overlooked. The dissemination of simple tools may help. For example:

- Inhaler technique assessment and training takes an average of only 2.5 minutes and is effective in improving asthma control.[88,89]
- Brief questionnaires can screen for poor adherence,[71,90] and shared decision-making can improve adherence.[32]
- Automated text messaging can reduce no-shows with follow-up visits.[91]

Tools for integrating future risk assessment
In recent years, GINA reports[8] have emphasized that clinicians should not rely only on the assessment of the patient's current control status but should also consider their future risk.[20] Because this concept is unfamiliar, it may be helpful to develop simple tools for primary care to assist clinicians in identifying patients who report few symptoms but who should have their treatment stepped up and patients with frequent symptoms who should have further investigations or whose treatment should be reduced or modified. For example:

- Patients with asthma who continue to smoke may be considered for treatment with higher ICS doses[92] or a leukotriene receptor antagonist.[93]

- Patients with frequent β_2-agonist use may benefit from breathing exercises[94] or transfer to an alternative bronchodilator.[60]

Improve the Control Algorithm

More frequent control-based adjustments

Current control-based guidelines recommend that maintenance treatment should be reviewed at intervals of approximately 1 to 3 months. More frequent adjustment of inhaled controller medication may possibly lead to improved outcomes and may be better matched to patient preferences.[40] This concept is supported by 2 approaches to patient-driven control-based management that have been evaluated in recent years.

- The first approach is the prescription of ICS and rapid-acting LABA both as a low-dose maintenance treatment, which is adjusted at intervals by the clinician according to asthma control in the conventional manner, and as reliever medication, which is adjusted by patients in response to asthma symptoms. This regimen is incorporated into asthma guidelines as one option for patients whose asthma is inadequately controlled on step 2 therapy (low-dose ICS). Compared with conventional maintenance therapy, this strategy with low-dose budesonide/formoterol leads to similar or better levels of current asthma control, together with reduced exacerbation rates or lower ICS doses.[95,96] The reduction in exacerbation rates relative to overall ICS dose, including during reported colds,[97] may be related to more frequent adjustments of ICS/LABA dose.
- The second approach is again driven by patients, this time using weekly ACQ.[83] Van der Meer and colleagues[98] showed that asthma education with an internet-based algorithm for monthly patient-driven adjustment of controller medication, led to improved asthma control and lung function and similar exacerbation rates compared with usual care.

Clarify the role of spirometry

Some, but not all, control assessment tools include the assessment of lung function.

- Lung function is 1 of 5 criteria in the GINA[8] and National Asthma Education and Prevention Program Expert Panel Report 3 (EPR3)[9] control classifications (GINA: FEV$_1$ [or peak expiratory flow]: ≥80% or <80%

predicted or best; EPR3: >80%, 60%–80%, and <60% predicted or best).
- In the ACQ,[83] prebronchodilator FEV$_1$ is equally weighted with 6 symptom-related components. At a population level, the inclusion of FEV$_1$ in ACQ does not add significantly to the assessment of asthma control.[99]

Spirometry correlates poorly with symptom-based measures of asthma control,[100] so it may be more useful in asthma monitoring as an independent measure both for identifying patients at risk of exacerbations[101] and, when discordant with symptoms, by alerting the clinician to the possibility of alternative diagnoses.

Research to Improve Control-Based Management

Research is essential to improve the quality of asthma care. Further research will provide opportunities to improve asthma outcomes, particularly in primary care where most asthma is managed and where effective, efficient, and low-cost treatment is an important goal.

Carry out pragmatic research in community-based populations

Clinical practice guidelines for asthma are based largely on regulatory studies, with rigorous inclusion/exclusion criteria and a closely monitored environment. However, the generalizability of these studies is limited because a median of only 4% (range 0%–36%) of community patients with doctor-diagnosed asthma and variable airflow limitation would meet the eligibility criteria for major clinical asthma trials.[11] To clarify the role of control-based management, further research is needed in broad community-based populations. Pragmatic study designs can also markedly improve generalizability without sacrificing quality.[102]

Investigate cut points for control-based management

The schemas for control-based management were developed from consensus, and further research is needed to clarify the most appropriate control cut points for changing treatment[103] because repeated application of any guideline or algorithm with inappropriate cut points will magnify problems regardless of the treatment approach.[23] At present, a step-up is considered if asthma is "Partly Controlled" (GINA,[8]) or "Not Well Controlled" (EPR3,[9]); but in a retrospective analysis, the average ACQ score for patients with Partly Controlled asthma was 0.75,[104] a level at which most physicians would not increase asthma treatment.[105]

Analyze responder variation

In the past, the analysis of clinical trial results was often limited to group mean responses and these formed the basis for treatment guidelines on the assumption that they would be relevant to most patients. However, this approach often concealed substantial heterogeneity in individual responses.[12] Progress can be made through analysis of variation in response in asthma studies using simple baseline characteristics, such as age, gender, lung function, atopy, and smoking status, as well as more specialized biomarkers.[14]

For research about responder analysis to be reliable, it should be planned prospectively, and standardized measures should be recorded for all patients at baseline.[21] Utility for primary care is improved by examining the predictive ability of simple and deep phenotyping and in broad rather than highly selected populations.

Identify patients for whom control-based management is not appropriate

The identification of phenotypic clusters of patients with different treatment responses is one of the most exciting areas of asthma research at present because it provides the potential for better customization of asthma management and greater efficiency in the use of health resources. Although several randomized controlled trials have demonstrated better outcomes, a lower risk of side effects, or lower costs with phenotype-guided treatment compared with control-guided treatment, even the most enthusiastic supporters do not expect that this approach will be appropriate or necessary for all patients and all health care settings. For example, sputum-guided treatment was most effective in patients for whom symptoms were not a reliable indicator of eosinophilic inflammation; such discordance was found in about 60% of patients with treatment-resistant asthma recruited from secondary care but only about 15% of patients recruited from primary care.[35] Similar analysis is needed with other large databases to identify patients for whom control-based treatment would be appropriate and those for whom referral for phenotype-guided treatment would be more effective and efficient. Recently-published guidelines suggest that FeNO may be particularly useful in managing patients with respiratory symptoms due to comorbidities such as anxiety.[106]

Develop practical tools for patient-centered implementation of asthma care

As already reported, asthma outcomes have improved substantially compared with usual care when control-based management is actively implemented in clinical practice. This finding suggests that, in parallel with the research described previously, more work is needed to improve the dissemination and implementation of asthma guidelines within primary care.

Clinicians are more likely to adopt guidelines when the recommendations are clearly presented and explained, when they are integrated into existing practice routines and software, and when system barriers are addressed.[107,108] Patients are more likely to be adherent with the resulting treatment recommendations when they understand the reasons for treatment and are involved in the decision-making process.[32]

SUMMARY

In summary, control-based management (ie, adjusting the patient's asthma treatment upwards or downwards according to simple measures of control) has been incorporated in asthma guidelines, in concept if not in name, for the past 20 years. As a result, it is difficult to obtain evidence about its effectiveness in real life. However, when this approach has been actively disseminated and implemented, asthma outcomes have improved at a population level in both developed and developing countries. The advantages of this approach include its simplicity and feasibility for implementation. Its limitations include the lack of specificity of asthma symptoms; the complex role of β_2-agonist use; barriers to stepping down treatment; and the underlying assumption that, in most patients, symptoms will be concordant with eosinophilic airway inflammation and, therefore, responsive to ICS. Potential improvements include increasing the frequency of dose adjustment and use of Internet or telephone-based support. More research is needed in community-based populations to identify the patients for whom control-based management is appropriate and those for whom phenotype-guided treatment will lead to more effective and efficient treatment. The broadening of the definition of asthma control in recent years to include an assessment of future risk, independent of the patient's level of symptoms, provides a mechanism for incorporating feasible elements of phenotype-guided treatment into control-based asthma management.

ACKNOWLEDGMENTS

The contribution of D. Robin Taylor to the discussion of these concepts is appreciated.

REFERENCES

1. National Asthma Education Program. Expert panel report on diagnosis and management of asthma.

Washington, DC: National Institutes of Health. NIH Publication No. 92–2113a; 1992.

2. Woolcock A, Rubinfeld AR, Seale JP, et al. Thoracic Society of Australia and New Zealand. Asthma management plan, 1989. Med J Aust 1989; 151(11–12):650–3.

3. Juniper EF, Kline PA, Vanzieleghem MA, et al. Effect of long-term treatment with an inhaled corticosteroid (budesonide) on airway hyperresponsiveness and clinical asthma in nonsteroid-dependent asthmatics. Am Rev Respir Dis 1990;142:832–6.

4. Toogood JH, Lefcoe NM, Haines DS, et al. A graded dose assessment of the efficacy of beclomethasone dipropionate aerosol for severe chronic asthma. J Allergy Clin Immunol 1977; 59(4):298–308.

5. Busse WW, Chervinsky P, Condemi J, et al. Budesonide delivered by Turbuhaler® is effective in a dose-dependent fashion when used in the treatment of adult patients with chronic asthma [Erratum appears in J Allergy Clin Immunol 1998;102:511]. J Allergy Clin Immunol 1998;101:457–63.

6. Fitzpatrick MF, Mackay T, Driver H, et al. Salmeterol in nocturnal asthma: a double blind, placebo controlled trial of a long acting inhaled beta 2 agonist. BMJ 1990;301(6765):1365–8.

7. Juniper EF, Kline PA, Vanzieleghem MA, et al. Reduction of budesonide after a year of increased use: a randomized controlled trial to evaluate whether improvements in airway responsiveness and clinical asthma are maintained. J Allergy Clin Immunol 1991;87:483–9.

8. Global Initiative for Asthma. Global strategy for asthma management and prevention. 2011. Available at: www.ginasthma.com. Accessed July 1, 2012.

9. National Heart Lung and Blood Institute National Asthma Education and Prevention Program. Expert panel report 3: guidelines for the diagnosis and management of asthma. 2007. Available at: http://www.nhlbi.nih.gov/guidelines/asthma/asthgdln.htm. Accessed July 1, 2012.

10. British Thoracic Society, Scottish Intercollegiate Guidelines Network. British guideline on the management of asthma. 2011. Available at: http://www.brit-thoracic.org.uk/guidelines/asthma-guidelines.aspx. Accessed December 1, 2011.

11. Travers J, Marsh S, Williams M, et al. External validity of randomised controlled trials in asthma: to whom do the results of the trials apply? Thorax 2007;62(3):219–23.

12. Malmstrom K, Rodriguez-Gomez G, Guerra J, et al. Oral montelukast, inhaled beclomethasone, and placebo for chronic asthma. A randomized, controlled trial. Montelukast/beclomethasone study group. Ann Intern Med 1999;130(6):487–95.

13. Szefler SJ, Martin RJ, King TS, et al. Significant variability in response to inhaled corticosteroids for persistent asthma. J Allergy Clin Immunol 2002;109(3):410–8.

14. Szefler SJ, Martin RJ. Lessons learned from variation in response to therapy in clinical trials. J Allergy Clin Immunol 2010;125(2):285–92.

15. Gibson PG, Powell H, Ducharme FM. Differential effects of maintenance long-acting beta-agonist and inhaled corticosteroid on asthma control and asthma exacerbations. J Allergy Clin Immunol 2007;119(2):344–50.

16. Pavord ID, Brightling CE, Woltmann G, et al. Non-eosinophilic corticosteroid unresponsive asthma. Lancet 1999;353(9171):2213–4.

17. Berry M, Morgan A, Shaw DE, et al. Pathological features and inhaled corticosteroid response of eosinophilic and non-eosinophilic asthma. Thorax 2007;62(12):1043–9.

18. Bel EH. Clinical phenotypes of asthma. Curr Opin Pulm Med 2004;10(1):44–50.

19. Wenzel SE. Asthma: defining of the persistent adult phenotypes. Lancet 2006;368(9537):804–13.

20. Taylor DR, Bateman ED, Boulet LP, et al. A new perspective on concepts of asthma severity and control. Eur Respir J 2008;32:545–54.

21. Reddel HK, Taylor DR, Bateman ED, et al. An official American Thoracic Society/European Respiratory Society statement: asthma control and exacerbations: standardizing endpoints for clinical asthma trials and clinical practice. Am J Respir Crit Care Med 2009;180(1):59–99.

22. Bauman A, Antic R, Rubinfeld A, et al. "Could it be asthma?": the impact of a mass media campaign aimed at raising awareness about asthma in Australia. Health Educ Res 1993;8(4):581–7.

23. Gibson PG. Using fractional exhaled nitric oxide to guide asthma therapy: design and methodological issues for ASthma TReatment ALgorithm studies. Clin Exp Allergy 2009;39(4):478–90.

24. Australian Centre for Asthma Monitoring. Asthma in Australia 2011. Australian Institute of Health and Welfare, Canberra; 2011. Available at: www.asthmamonitoring.org. Accessed July 1, 2012.

25. Public Health Agency of Canada. Life and breath: respiratory disease in Canada. 2007. Available at: http://www.phac-aspc.gc.ca/publicat/2007/lbrdc-vsmrc/pdf/PHAC-Respiratory-WEB-eng.pdf. Accessed December 1, 2011.

26. Haahtela T, Tuomisto LE, Pietinalho A, et al. A 10 year asthma programme in Finland: major change for the better. Thorax 2006;61(8):663–70.

27. Ait-Khaled N, Enarson DA, Bencharif N, et al. Treatment outcome of asthma after one year follow-up in health centres of several developing countries. Int J Tuberc Lung Dis 2006;10(8):911–6.

28. Rabe KF, Adachi M, Lai CK, et al. Worldwide severity and control of asthma in children and

adults: the global asthma insights and reality surveys. J Allergy Clin Immunol 2004;114(1):40–7.

29. Colice GL, Yu AP, Ivanova JI, et al. Costs and resource use of mild persistent asthma patients initiated on controller therapy. J Asthma 2008;45(4):293–9.

30. Zeiger RS, Schatz M, Li Q, et al. Step-up care improves impairment in uncontrolled asthma: an administrative data study. Am J Manag Care 2010;16(12):897–906.

31. Plaza V, Cobos A, Ignacio-Garcia JM, et al. Cost-effectiveness of an intervention based on the Global INitiative for Asthma (GINA) recommendations using a computerized clinical decision support system: a physicians randomized trial. Med Clin (Barc) 2005;124(6):201–6 [in Spanish].

32. Wilson SR, Strub P, Buist AS, et al. Shared treatment decision making improves adherence and outcomes in poorly controlled asthma. Am J Respir Crit Care Med 2010;181(6):566–77.

33. Petsky HL, Kynaston JA, Turner C, et al. Tailored interventions based on sputum eosinophils versus clinical symptoms for asthma in children and adults. Cochrane Database Syst Rev 2007;2: CD005603.

34. Green RH, Brightling CE, McKenna S, et al. Asthma exacerbations and sputum eosinophil counts: a randomised controlled trial. Lancet 2002;360(9347):1715–21.

35. Haldar P, Pavord ID, Shaw DE, et al. Cluster analysis and clinical asthma phenotypes. Am J Respir Crit Care Med 2008;178(3):218–24.

36. Petsky HL, Cates CJ, Li A, et al. Tailored interventions based on exhaled nitric oxide versus clinical symptoms for asthma in children and adults. Cochrane Database Syst Rev 2009;4:CD006340.

37. Powell H, Murphy VE, Taylor DR, et al. Management of asthma in pregnancy guided by measurement of fraction of exhaled nitric oxide: a double-blind, randomised controlled trial. Lancet 2011;378(9795):983–90.

38. Guarnaccia S, Lombardi A, Gaffurini A, et al. Application and implementation of the GINA asthma guidelines by specialist and primary care physicians: a longitudinal follow-up study on 264 children. Prim Care Respir J 2007;16(6):357–62.

39. Osman LM, McKenzie L, Cairns J, et al. Patient weighting of importance of asthma symptoms. Thorax 2001;56(2):138–42.

40. Partridge MR, van der Molen T, Myrseth SE, et al. Attitudes and actions of asthma patients on regular maintenance therapy: the INSPIRE study. BMC Pulm Med 2006;6:13.

41. Ulrik C, Backer V, Soes-Petersen U, et al. The patient's perspective: adherence or non-adherence to asthma controller therapy? J Asthma 2006;43(9):701–4.

42. Marklund B, Tunsäter A, Bengtsson C. How often is the diagnosis bronchial asthma correct? Fam Pract 1999;16(2):112–6.

43. Montnémery P, Hansson L, Lanke J, et al. Accuracy of a first diagnosis of asthma in primary health care. Fam Pract 2002;19(4):365–8.

44. Lucas AE, Smeenk FW, Smeele IJ, et al. Overtreatment with inhaled corticosteroids and diagnostic problems in primary care patients, an exploratory study. Fam Pract 2008;25(2):86–91.

45. Aaron SD, Vandemheen KL, Boulet LP, et al. Overdiagnosis of asthma in obese and nonobese adults. Can Med Assoc J 2008;179(11):1121–31.

46. Carman PG, Landau LI. Increased paediatric admissions with asthma in Western Australia—a problem of diagnosis? Med J Aust 1990;152(1):23–6.

47. O'Dowd LC, Fife D, Tenhave T, et al. Attitudes of physicians toward objective measures of airway function in asthma. Am J Med 2003;114(5):391–6.

48. Dennis SM, Zwar NA, Marks GB. Diagnosing asthma in adults in primary care: a qualitative study of Australian GPs' experiences. Prim Care Respir J 2010;19(1):52–6.

49. Gershon AS, Victor JC, Guan J, et al. Pulmonary function testing in the diagnosis of asthma: a population study. Chest 2012;141(5):1190-0–6.

50. Dirks JF, Schraa JC, Robinson SK. Patient mislabeling of symptoms: implications for patient-physician communication and medical outcome. Int J Psychiatry Med 1982;12(1):15–27.

51. Salome CM, Reddel HK, Ware SI, et al. Effect of budesonide on the perception of induced airway narrowing in subjects with asthma. Am J Respir Crit Care Med 2002;165(1):15–21.

52. Rosi E, Stendardi L, Binazzi B, et al. Perception of airway obstruction and airway inflammation in asthma: a review. Lung 2006;184(5):251–8.

53. Halm EA, Mora P, Leventhal H. No symptoms, no asthma: the acute episodic disease belief is associated with poor self-management among inner-city adults with persistent asthma. Chest 2006;129(3):573–80.

54. Wise RA, Bartlett SJ, Brown ED, et al. Randomized trial of the effect of drug presentation on asthma outcomes: the American Lung Association Asthma Clinical Research Centers. J Allergy Clin Immunol 2009;124(3):436–44.

55. Wechsler ME, Kelley JM, Boyd IO, et al. Active albuterol or placebo, sham acupuncture, or no intervention in asthma. N Engl J Med 2011;365(2):119–26.

56. Godard P, Greillier P, Pigearias B, et al. Maintaining asthma control in persistent asthma: comparison of three strategies in a 6-month double-blind randomised study. Respir Med 2008;102(8):1124–31.

57. Reddel HK, Gibson PG, Peters MJ, et al. Down-titration from high-dose combination therapy in asthma: removal of long-acting β2-agonist. Respir Med 2010;104(8):1110–20.

58. Taylor DR. The beta-agonist saga and its clinical relevance: on and on it goes. Am J Respir Crit Care Med 2009;179(11):976–8.

59. Reddel H, Ware S, Marks G, et al. Differences between asthma exacerbations and poor asthma control [Erratum in Lancet 1999;353:758]. Lancet 1999;353(9150):364–9.

60. Taylor DR, Hannah D. Management of beta-agonist overuse: why and how? J Allergy Clin Immunol 2008;122(4):836–8.

61. Taylor DR, Sears MR, Cockcroft DW. The beta-agonist controversy. Med Clin North Am 1996; 80(4):719–48.

62. Calhoun WJ, Sutton LB, Emmett A, et al. Asthma variability in patients previously treated with beta2-agonists alone. J Allergy Clin Immunol 2003; 112(6):1088–94.

63. Bateman ED, Bousquet J, Busse WW, et al. Stability of asthma control with regular treatment: an analysis of the Gaining Optimal Asthma controL (GOAL) study. Allergy 2008;63(7):932–8.

64. Aroni R, Goeman D, Stewart K, et al. Enhancing validity: what counts as an asthma attack? J Asthma 2004;41(7):729–37.

65. Nathan RA, Sorkness CA, Kosinski M, et al. Development of the Asthma Control Test: a survey for assessing asthma control. J Allergy Clin Immunol 2004;113(1):59–65.

66. Yawn BP, Wollan PC, Bertram SL, et al. Asthma treatment in a population-based cohort: putting step-up and step-down treatment changes in context. Mayo Clin Proc 2007;82(4):414–21.

67. Hawkins G, McMahon AD, Twaddle S, et al. Stepping down inhaled corticosteroids in asthma: randomised controlled trial. BMJ 2003;326(7399): 1115.

68. Diette GB, Patino CM, Merriman B, et al. Patient factors that physicians use to assign asthma treatment. Arch Intern Med 2007;167(13):1360–6.

69. Dirks JF, Horton DJ, Kinsman RA, et al. Patient and physician characteristics influencing medical decisions in asthma. J Asthma Res 1978;15(4): 171–8.

70. Foster JM, van Sonderen E, Lee AJ, et al. A self-rating scale for patient-perceived side effects of inhaled corticosteroids. Respir Res 2006;7:131.

71. Foster JM, Smith L, Bosnic-Anticevich SZ, et al. Identifying patient-specific beliefs and behaviours for conversations about adherence in asthma. Intern Med J 2011;42(6):e136–44.

72. Hancox RJ, Souëf PL, Anderson GP, et al. Asthma - time to confront some inconvenient truths. Respirology 2010;15(2):194–201.

73. Melani AS, Bonavia M, Cilenti V, et al. Inhaler mishandling remains common in real life and is associated with reduced disease control. Respir Med 2011;105(6):930–8.

74. Guidry GG, Brown WD, Stogner SW, et al. Incorrect use of metered dose inhalers by medical personnel. Chest 1992;101(1):31–3.

75. Basheti IA, Qunaibi E, Bosnic-Anticevich SZ, et al. Investigation of errors in accuhaler and turbuhaler technique by asthma patients and pharmacists from Jordan and Australia. Respir Care 2011; 56(12):1916–23.

76. Rand CS, Nides M, Cowles MK, et al. Long-term metered-dose inhaler adherence in a clinical trial. Am J Respir Crit Care Med 1995;152:580–8.

77. Simmons MS, Nides MA, Rand CS, et al. Unpredictability of deception in compliance with physician-prescribed bronchodilator inhaler use in a clinical trial. Chest 2000;118(2):290–5.

78. Marks GB. Identifying asthma in population studies: from single entity to a multi-component approach. Eur Respir J 2005;26(1):3–5.

79. Levy ML, Quanjer PH, Booker R, et al. Diagnostic spirometry in primary care: proposed standards for general practice compliant with American Thoracic Society and European Respiratory Society recommendations: a General Practice Airways Group (GPIAG) document, in association with the Association for Respiratory Technology & Physiology (ARTP) and Education for Health. Prim Care Respir J 2009;18(3):130–47.

80. Powell H, Gibson PG. Inhaled corticosteroid doses in asthma: an evidence-based approach. Med J Aust 2003;178(5):223–5.

81. Suissa S, Ernst P, Benayoun S, et al. Low-dose inhaled corticosteroids and the prevention of death from asthma. N Engl J Med 2000;343(5):332–6.

82. International Union Against Tuberculosis and Lung Disease. Asthma Drug Facility. Available at: http://www.globaladf.org/. Accessed December 1, 2011.

83. Juniper EF, O'Byrne PM, Guyatt GH, et al. Development and validation of a questionnaire to measure asthma control. Eur Respir J 1999;14:902–7.

84. Peters SP, Jones CA, Haselkorn T, et al. Real-world Evaluation of Asthma Control and Treatment (REACT): findings from a national Web-based survey. J Allergy Clin Immunol 2007;119(6): 1454–61.

85. Juniper EF, Langlands JM, Juniper BA. Patients may respond differently to paper and electronic versions of the same questionnaires. Respir Med 2009;103(6):932–4.

86. Kosinski M, Kite A, Yang M, et al. Comparability of the Asthma Control Test telephone interview administration format with self-administered mail-out mail-back format. Curr Med Res Opin 2009;25(3): 717–27.

87. Schatz M, Kosinski M, Yarlas AS, et al. The minimally important difference of the Asthma Control Test. J Allergy Clin Immunol 2009;124(4):719–723. e711.

88. Basheti IA, Reddel HK, Armour CL, et al. Improved asthma outcomes with a simple inhaler technique intervention by community pharmacists. J Allergy Clin Immunol 2007;119(6):1537–8.

89. Basheti IA, Armour CL, Bosnic-Anticevich SZ, et al. Evaluation of a novel educational strategy, including inhaler-based reminder labels, to improve asthma inhaler technique. Patient Educ Couns 2008;72(1):26–33.

90. Morisky DE, Green LW, Levine DM. Concurrent and predictive validity of a self-reported measure of medication adherence. Med Care 1986;24(1): 67–74.

91. Downer SR, Meara JG, Da Costa AC, et al. SMS text messaging improves outpatient attendance. Aust Health Rev 2006;30(3):389–96.

92. Tomlinson JE, McMahon AD, Chaudhuri R, et al. Efficacy of low and high dose inhaled corticosteroid in smokers versus non-smokers with mild asthma. Thorax 2005;60(4):282–7.

93. Lazarus SC, Chinchilli VM, Rollings NJ, et al. Smoking affects response to inhaled corticosteroids or leukotriene receptor antagonists in asthma. Am J Respir Crit Care Med 2007;175(8):783–90.

94. Slader CA, Reddel HK, Spencer LM, et al. Double-blind randomised controlled trial of two different breathing techniques in the management of asthma. Thorax 2006;61:651–6.

95. Demoly P, Louis R, Soes-Petersen U, et al. Budesonide/formoterol maintenance and reliever therapy versus conventional best practice. Respir Med 2009;103(11):1623–32.

96. Bateman ED, Reddel HK, Eriksson G, et al. Overall asthma control: the relationship between current control and future risk. J Allergy Clin Immunol 2010;125(3):600–8.

97. Reddel HK, Jenkins C, Quirce S, et al. Effect of different asthma treatments on risk of cold-related exacerbations. Eur Respir J 2011;38:584–93.

98. van der Meer V, Bakker MJ, van den Hout WB, et al. Internet-based self-management plus education compared with usual care in asthma: a randomized trial. Ann Intern Med 2009;151(2):110–20.

99. Juniper EF, O'Byrne PM, Roberts JN. Measuring asthma control in group studies: do we need airway calibre and rescue beta2-agonist use? Respir Med 2001;95(5):319–23.

100. Schatz M, Sorkness CA, Li JT, et al. Asthma Control Test: reliability, validity, and responsiveness in patients not previously followed by asthma specialists. J Allergy Clin Immunol 2006;117(3):549–56.

101. Osborne ML, Pedula KL, O'Hollaren M, et al. Assessing future need for acute care in adult asthmatics: the profile of asthma risk study: a prospective health maintenance organization-based study. Chest 2007;132(4):1151–61.

102. Zwarenstein M, Treweek S, Gagnier JJ, et al. Improving the reporting of pragmatic trials: an extension of the CONSORT statement. BMJ 2008; 337:a2390.

103. O'Byrne PM, Reddel HK, Colice GL. A pro-con debate: does the current stepwise approach to asthma pharmacotherapy encourage over-treatment? Respirology 2010;15(4):596–602.

104. O'Byrne PM, Reddel HK, Eriksson G, et al. Measuring asthma control: a comparison of three classification systems. Eur Respir J 2010;36:269–76.

105. Juniper EF, Bousquet J, Abetz L, et al. Identifying 'well-controlled' and 'not well-controlled' asthma using the Asthma Control Questionnaire. Respir Med 2006;100(4):616–21.

106. Dweik RA, Boggs PB, Erzurum SC, et al. American Thoracic Society Committee on Interpretation of Exhaled Nitric Oxide Levels for Clinical A: An official ATS clinical practice guideline: interpretation of exhaled nitric oxide levels (FENO) for clinical applications. Am J Respir Crit Care Med 2011; 184:602–15.

107. Grol R, Dalhuijsen J, Thomas S, et al. Attributes of clinical guidelines that influence use of guidelines in general practice: observational study. BMJ 1998;317:858–61.

108. Grol RP, Bosch MC, Hulscher ME, et al. Planning and studying improvement in patient care: the use of theoretical perspectives. Milbank Q 2007; 85(1):93–138.

Occupational Asthma
New Deleterious Agents at the Workplace

Catherine Lemiere, MD, MSc[a],*, Jacques Ameille, MD[b],
Piera Boschetto, MD, PhD[c], Manon Labrecque, MD, MSc[a],
Jacques-André Pralong, MD, MSc[d]

KEYWORDS

- Occupational asthma • Irritant-induced asthma • RADS • Occupational agents
- High-molecular-weight agents • Low-molecular-weight agents • Irritant agents

KEY POINTS

- This article summarizes the main new categories of occupational agents responsible for causing occupational asthma, with and without a latency period reported in the last 10 years.
- This article also reports examples of occupational agents for which the fabrication processing or use have influenced the outcome of occupational asthma.

INTRODUCTION

Occupational asthma (OA) refers to de novo asthma or the recurrence of previously quiescent asthma (ie, asthma as a child or in the distant past that has been in remission) induced by either sensitization to a specific substance, which is termed sensitizer-induced OA, or by exposure to an inhaled irritant at work, which is termed irritant-induced OA.

More than 400 distinct agents have been documented as causing OA.[1,2] The agents responsible for OA are classically divided according to their molecular weight. High-molecular-weight (HMW) agents (>10 kDa[3]) include proteins and microorganisms of animal and vegetable origins. Low-molecular-weight (LMW) agents include wood dust, drugs, metals, and other chemicals. The list of agents that cause OA is constantly growing[4] (www.asthme.csssst.qc.ca). The causes of irritant-induced asthma (IIA; OA without a latency period)

are also steadily increasing.[5] Ammonia, chlorine, and sulfur dioxide are the most frequent causes of IIA.

Many agents, especially LMW agents can have both sensitizing and irritant properties. For example, isocyanates can induce OA by an immunologic mechanism but, at higher concentrations, they have been reported to induce irritant-induced asthma.[6]

Publications continue to report new causes of OA. This article reviews the new causes of sensitizer-induced OA and IIA reported in the last 10 years. It describes how interventions such as surveillance programs or changes in the fabrication process can influence the incidence of OA.

ALLERGIC OA
Newly Identified HMW Agents

HMW agents encountered at the workplace are natural proteins, derived from animal or plant

Disclosures: Catherine Lemière, Jacques Ameille, Piera Boschetto, Manon Labrecque, and Jacques-André Pralong do not have any conflict of interest in relation to this article.

[a] Chest Department, Sacré-Coeur Hospital, Montreal, 5400 Gouin Ouest, Montreal, Quebec H4J 1C5, Canada; [b] AP-HP, Unité de pathologie professionnelle, Hôpital Raymond Poincaré, Université de Versailles, 104 Boulevard Raymond Poincaré, Garches 92380, France; [c] Department of Clinical and Experimental Medicine, University of Ferrara, Via Fossato di Mortara, 64B, Ferrara 44100, Italy; [d] Research Center, Sacre-Coeur Hospital, Montreal, Université de Montréal, 5400 Gouin Ouest, Montreal, Quebec H4J 1C5, Canada
* Corresponding author. Hôpital du Sacré-Coeur de Montréal, 5400 Gouin Ouest, Montreal, Quebec H4J 1C5, Canada.
E-mail address: catherine.lemiere@umontreal.ca

sources that induce classic immunoglobulin (Ig) E–mediated sensitization after months or years of exposure.[4] HMW agents act as complete antigens and cause an allergic or immunologic asthma by producing specific IgE antibodies. Some newly recognized HMW agents that induce OA are discussed in this article.

Laboratory animals

Small animals represent a frequent cause of OA in laboratory technicians and veterinarians. Proteins excreted in urine, especially those produced by male rats, are the most potent source of sensitization.[7] A new gerbil allergen (Meriones unguiculatus) of 23 kDa has been identified in the gerbil urine, epithelium, hair, and airborne samples. Partial characterization of this allergen suggests that it could be a lipocalin.[8] Inhalation of bovine serum albumin (BSA) powder, commonly used in research laboratories, has been shown to cause OA and rhinitis in a laboratory worker in whom an IgE-mediated response was shown.[9] The patient had a high serum-specific IgE level to BSA, and a 66-kDa IgE-binding component was detected within the BSA extract on immunoblot analysis. During a bronchial provocation test with a BSA solution, the patient experienced severe systemic reactions, including eye itching, conjunctivitis, rhinorrhea, nasal obstructions, sneezing, shortness of breath, and bronchospasm, with a 30% decrease in forced expiratory volume in 1 second (FEV_1), 52% of predicted, and decreased blood pressure.

Allergens derived from flour, cereal, and vegetable matter

Cereals and flour are the oldest and most commonly identified causes of OA.[1,4] Purified wheat proteins either in natural or recombinant forms have been implicated in the pathogenesis of baker's asthma. The thaumatinlike protein and lipid transfer protein 2G were identified to be newly identified allergens associated with baker's asthma in a group of 20 patients with baker's rhinitis, asthma, or both who had positive skin-prick test reactions and specific IgE antibodies to wheat flour.[10] The recombinant wheat lipid transfer protein (Tri a 14) has also recently been recognized as a potential novel tool for the diagnosis of baker's asthma.[11] The possibility of discriminating baker's asthma, wheat-induced food allergy, and grass pollen allergy was investigated by serologic tests based on microarrayed recombinant wheat seed and grass pollen allergens.[12] Recombinant wheat flour allergens, specifically recognized by patients suffering from baker's asthma, but not from patients with food allergy to wheat or pollen allergy, were identified.

The first known case of an IgE-mediated OA to malt has been reported in a machine operator in a malt manufacturing plant.[13] Pirson and colleagues[14] described a case of a patient employed in a factory producing inulin from chicory who developed rhinoconjunctivitis and asthma to the dust of dry chicory roots. A specific inhalation challenge (SIC) with dry chicory was performed and an acute rhinoconjunctivitis and an immediate asthmatic response was seen. This case documents occupational rhinoconjunctivitis and asthma caused by IgE sensitization to inhaled chicory allergens, including one identified for the first time as a 17-kDa Bet v 1 homologous protein.

In addition, the first case of IgE-mediated occupational allergy (rhinitis and asthma) to marigold flour has been reported.[15] Marigold flour has been largely used by the food additive industry as poultry feed colorant. The sensitization was confirmed by a skin-prick test, a nasal challenge test, and specific IgE determination.

Food and fishing industry

Various foods, food additives, and contaminants have been associated with OA.[16] In the commercial fishing industry, crustaceans are the main source of sensitization, followed by mollusks and fin fish.[17] Patients who are allergic to fish can suffer asthma attacks when they breathe airborne particles from fish. Rosado and colleagues[18] described the first case of OA caused by handling and exposure to aerosolized octopus allergens in a seafood processing worker. Immunoblotting revealed IgE-binding bands of 43 and 32 kDa that likely correspond with tropomyosin (38–40 kDa) as the culprit allergen. Three workers experienced symptoms of rhinoconjunctivitis and bronchial asthma while classifying fish by size at the same fish farm.[19] Although they could eat turbot, they were sensitized to this fish probably by inhalation. Parvalbumin was identified as the causal allergen in 1 of the cases. Simultaneous type I and type IV allergic reactions (asthma and contact dermatitis) caused by occupational contact with fish parasitized by Anisakis simplex have been reported.[20] A simplex is a nematode that is a parasite of several marine organisms during its life cycle. It is known as an accidental gastrointestinal parasite in subjects who had ingested raw fish, but it has also been suggested to be the cause of allergic reactions in subjects who frequently eat or manipulate parasitized fish.

Pests and arthropods

Molds have been identified as causal agents of OA in workers exposed to coffee grounds (Chrysonilia sitophila [asexual state of Neurospora *sitophila*])[21,22] as well as in a pork butcher worker (dry sausage mold, *Penicillium nalgiovensis*[23]). The case of an electric power company engineer who suffered from OA caused by caddis flies (Phryganeiae) has been reported and proved by using an extract of these insects in a SIC.[24] In addition, Skousgaard and colleagues[25] pointed out that *Amblyseius californicus*, a beneficial predatory mite present in microbiological pesticides, was able to induce IgE sensitization and OA among greenhouse workers. The different agents are summarized in **Table 1**.

Key Points

- HMW act through an IgE-dependent mechanism to induce OA.
- The identification of proteins responsible for the sensitization can help to improve diagnosis and management of OA.

Newly Identified LMW Agents

Given the high number of new chemicals produced each year, many workers are exposed to LMW agents (<10 kDa). They include drugs, wood dusts, metals, chemicals, and biocides. The literature reported 42 new LMW agents causing OA for the period 2000 to 2011, including 12 drugs, 11 wood species, 4 metals, 10 chemicals, and 5 biocides/fungicides.

Drugs

Antibiotics, and especially penicillin-derived antibiotics, have long been known to induce OA.[26] During recent years, several new antibiotics or their precursors have been reported as causes of OA. Choi and colleagues[27] reported the case of a man working in a pharmaceutical company and exposed to vancomycin powder. The diagnosis of OA was based on history and peak expiratory flow (PEF) monitoring. The postulated mechanism to explain OA was a direct histamine-releasing effect. Gomez-Olles and colleagues[28] reported a case of colistin-induced OA and rhinitis presenting an immediate asthmatic reaction during the SIC. A type I hypersensitivity reaction was associated with OA in workers exposed to thiamphenicol, 7-aminocephalosporanic acid (7-ACSA; an intermediate metabolite of the synthesis of ceftriaxone), and cefteram.[29–31] Two workers exposed to 7-ACSA developed an immediate asthmatic reaction but no reaction was noted when they were exposed to ceftriaxone.[29] A case of OA caused by 7-amino-3-thiomethyl-3-cephalosporanic acid confirmed by an immediate asthmatic reaction during the SIC has also been reported.[32]

Several other drug categories have been reported to cause OA. An antineoplastic drug, mitoxantrone, induced OA and rhinitis in a nurse, which was confirmed by the occurrence of a late asthmatic reaction during SIC.[33] Two cases of OA have been reported among anesthetic staff workers using sevoflurane and isoflurane,[34] 1 confirmed by a late asthmatic reaction during the SIC and the second by a positive methacholine challenge, an equivocal SIC for isoflurane, and a 14% decrease in FEV_1 after indirect exposure to sevoflurane. Klusackova and colleagues[35] reported 3 cases of OA caused by exposure to lasamide (a precursor of the diuretic furosemide) in a pharmaceutical plant; all 3 experienced an immediate asthmatic reaction during the SIC. Sastre and colleagues[36] reported a case of OA caused by 5-aminosalicylic acid (used to treat inflammatory bowel disease) with a late asthmatic reaction during the SIC. OA has been showed in a worker employed in a pharmaceutical company and exposed to aescin, the compound inducing an atypical asthmatic reaction during the SIC.[37] Drought and colleagues[38] reported 2 cases of OA caused by thiamine in cereal manufacture, the diagnosis being confirmed by late asthmatic reactions during the SIC.

Wood dusts

Most wood species reported as occupational sensitizers during the past years are exotic woods from Africa, Asia, or South America.[39–48] It is difficult to estimate the number of woodworkers exposed to such species worldwide. A recent meta-analysis of 19 studies estimated that the relative risk of developing OA in workers exposed to wood dust was 1.53 (95% confidence interval [CI] 1.25–1.87).[49] During the past 11 years, 11 new species have been reported to induce OA.[39–48] Except for sapele, the diagnosis has been confirmed by SIC showing immediate (n = 5), late (n = 3), and dual (n = 3) reactions. Specific IgE antibodies were positive for 4 wood species (cedro arana, angelim pedra, antiaris, and sapele),[39,41–43] confirming a type I allergic reaction, even if the nature of the chemical compound responsible for OA remains unknown. Specific IgG have been found in a worker exposed to falcate,[47] postulating the presence of another immune mechanism.

Metals

Metal salts are known to be respiratory sensitizers.[50] Most of them belong to the transition series. In the first series of transition metals, chromium, cobalt, and nickel are all known to induce OA.[51–53]

Table 1
Newly identified HMW agents

Agents	Allergen	Workplace	Diagnosis Tests	Symptoms	Reference
Laboratory animals					
M unguiculatus (gerbil allergen)	23 kDa protein, lipocalin?	Biologist, laboratory animals	SPT, nasal challenge and SIC	Rhinoconjunctivitis asthma	7
BSA	BSA, 66 kDa binding protein	Research laboratory	SIC	Rhinitis, asthma	8
Flour, cereals					
Flour	Thaumatinlike protein; lipid transfer protein 2G	Baker	SPT, specific IgE	Rhinitis, asthma	9
Malt	—	Malt manufacturing plant	SPT, SIC	Rhinitis, asthma, alveolitis	12
Chicory	17 kDa Bet v 1 homologous protein	Factory producing inulin from chicory	SPT, specific IgE SIC	Rhinoconjunctivitis asthma	13
Marigold flour	—	Food additive industry	SPT nasal challenge	Rhinitis, asthma	14
Food and fishing industry					
Octopus	Tropomyosin (38–40 kDa)	Seafood processing industry	SPT, specific IgE SIC	Rhinitis, asthma	17
Turbot	Parvalbumin	Fish farm	SPT, specific IgE, Serial PEF monitoring	Rhinoconjunctivitis, asthma	18
A simplex	—	Fish industry	SPT, specific IgE	Dyspnea and contact dermatitis	19
Pests and arthropods					
C sitophila (mold)	—	Coffee dispenser operators	Mycologic analysis, SPT serial PEF monitoring, specific IgE	Asthma	21
P nalgiovensis (mold)	—	Pork butcher industry	SPT; favorable outcome after removal from exposure	Asthma	22
Phryganeiae (caddis flies)	—	Electric power company engineer	SPT; SIC	Rhinoconjunctivitis, asthma	23
A californicus (mite)	—	Greenhouse workers	Specific IgE, SIC	Cutaneous rash, rhinoconjunctivitis, asthma	24

Abbreviations: PEF, peak expiratory flow; SPT, skin-prick tests.

Manganese belongs to the same series and has been reported to induce OA in a welder working in a train factory.[54] The diagnosis has been confirmed by an immediate asthmatic reaction during SIC. Iron also belongs to the first series of transition metals. Munoz and colleagues[55] reported 3 cases of OA induced by iron welding fumes. Air analysis during the SIC found a high number of metals and gases, many of them known to be respiratory irritants (such as O_3, NO_2, NO, and CO). Even if none of these components exceeded the threshold limit value in the laboratory, it is possible that they participated in the mechanism of OA. Sputum cell count analysis showed an increase in neutrophils.

In the second series of transition metals, palladium has been reported to cause OA.[56] In the same series, Merget and colleagues[57] reported a case of OA and rhinitis induced by rhodium salt and confirmed by an immediate asthmatic reaction during the SIC.

Apart from the metal salts, alloys are also known to induce OA. Hannu and colleagues[58] reported the case of a welder exposed to stellite, an alloy made of cobalt (60%), chromium (30%), tungsten, and carbon. A positive SIC confirmed the diagnosis of OA when the worker was exposed to stellite fumes but not when he was exposed to cobalt or chromium solutions. Therefore, it seems that the alloy was responsible of OA and not the individual metals, even if cobalt and chromium are known to induce OA.

Biocides and fungicides

Several biocides have been described as causes of OA. For example, glutaraldehyde[59] and chlorhexidine[60] are disinfectants frequently used in hospitals and known to be respiratory sensitizers. Two new agents used by hospital staff in endoscopic units have been reported as causes of OA, namely a peracetic acid–hydrogen peroxide mixture and orthophthalaldehyde.[61,62] Chlorine-releasing agents are another type of disinfectant commonly used in swimming pools. The role of theses agents was recently evoked in the pathogenesis of asthma in swimmers and children[63–65] but, to date, no study has produced a definite conclusion. Thickett and colleagues[66] reported the cases of 2 lifeguards and a swimming pool instructor (working in separate indoor swimming pools) who developed OA, confirmed by either SIC to nitrogen trichloride (belonging to the chloramine family) in 2 workers or by a positive poolside challenge test. Draper and colleagues[67] published 2 cases of OA in workers employed in fungicides manufacturing. They were exposed to fluazinam and chlorothalonil respectively and SIC induced late asthmatic reactions.

Various chemicals

Many different chemicals are able to induce OA. Various chemicals responsible for OA that have been identified in the last 10 years are summarized in **Table 2**.[68–77]

Key Points

- Forty-two new LMW agents have been identified in the last 10 years as causing OA.
- An effort should be made to identify agents responsible for OA to facilitate an effective prevention program.

New Processing or New Utilization of Known Sensitizers

Many new agents responsible for OA are reported annually. However, some agents have been known to cause OA for a long time but their use or processing have changed with time, inducing an increase or decrease in the number of OA cases associated with their exposure.

Latex

Evidence that natural rubber latex (NRL) was acting as an aeroallergen causing OA was first published in 1990.[78,79] During the late 1990s, latex became widely used, especially in health care settings because of the extensive use of gloves or other medical devices. This wide use of NRL has been associated with a large increase in positive NRL skin-prick tests among exposed working groups,[80–82] especially in health care settings. The number of annual new cases increased in Belgium from 1 in 1982 to 20 in 1998.[83] This increase was also reported in other countries such as Canada[84] or Germany.[85] Policies were established in the health care system for replacing powdered latex gloves (associated with a high level of airborne latex allergen) with nonpowdered gloves.[83–85] Furthermore, the protein and allergen content of NRL gloves declined in the mid to late 1990s.[86] These changes resulted in a substantial decrease in the number of cases of OA to latex[83–85,87] in the last decade. Although latex remains a potential sensitizer for causing OA, the numbers of cases seen in clinical practice have markedly decreased.

Enzymes

Proteolytic enzymes were introduced the mid-1960s in washing powder for increasing their cleaning efficacy.[88] The enzymes were proteases produced from the growth of *Bacillus subtilis*, termed subtilisins. As a results of their wide use, many reports of OA and sensitization caused by subtilisin exposure occurred.[89] Their use in a powered form was

Table 2
Newly identified LMW agents

Agents	Workplace	Diagnosis	Symptoms	Reference
Drugs				
Cefteram	Pharmaceutical company	SPT, specific IgE, SIC	Asthma	30
Colistin	Pharmaceutical company	SIC	Rhinitis, asthma	28
Vancomycin	Pharmaceutical company	PEF, histamine release test	Rhinitis, asthma	27
Lasamide and precursors	Pharmaceutical company	SIC	Rhinitis, asthma	35
Sevoflurane and isoflurane	Hospital, anesthetic staff	PEF, SIC	Rhinitis, asthma	34
Thiamphenicol	Pharmaceutical company	SPT, specific IgE, SIC	Rhinitis, asthma	31
Aescin	Pharmaceutical company	PEF, SIC	Rhinitis, asthma	37
Thiamine	Cereal manufacture	PEF, SIC	Asthma	38
7-ACSA	Pharmaceutical company	SPT, specific IgE, SIC	Rhinitis, asthma	29
7-TACA	Pharmaceutical company	SIC	Rhinitis, asthma	32
Mitoxantrone	Hospital, oncology staff	SIC	Rhinitis, asthma	33
5-ASA	Pharmaceutical company	SIC	Asthma	36
Wood Dusts				
Chengal	Carpentry	PEF, SIC	Rhinitis, asthma	44
Tali	Carpentry	PEF, SIC	Rhinitis, asthma	44
Jatoba	Carpentry	PEF, SIC	Rhinitis, asthma	46
Falcata	Wood furniture plant	Specific IgG, SIC	Asthma	47
Cedroarana	Carpentry	SPT, specific IgE, SIC	Rhinitis, asthma	42
Bethabara	Railway platform	SIC	Asthma	48
Angelim pedra	Carpentry	SPT, specific IgE, SIC	Rhinitis, asthma	39
Ipe	Wood work	SPT, SIC	Asthma	40
Antiaris	Door manufacture	SPT, specific IgE, SIC	Rhinitis, asthma	43
African cherry	Carpentry	SIC	Asthma	45
Sapele	Carpentry	Specific IgE, history	Rhinitis, asthma, dermatitis	41
Metals				
Rhodium	Electroplating plant	SPT, SIC	Rhinitis, asthma	57
Iron (fumes)	Welding	PEF, SIC	Asthma	55
Manganese	Welding	PEF, SIC	Asthma	54
Stellite	Machine manufacture	PEF, SIC	Asthma	58
Biocides and Fungicides				
PA-HP	Endoscopic unit	PEF, SIC	Rhinitis, asthma	61
Nitrogen trichloride	Swimming pool	PEF, SIC	Asthma	66
Orthophthalaldehyde	Endoscopic unit	History	Asthma, dermatitis	62

(*continued on next page*)

Table 2
(continued)

Agents	Workplace	Diagnosis	Symptoms	Reference
Fluazinam	Fungicides manufacture	PEF, SIC	Asthma	67
Chlorothalonil	Fungicide manufacture	PEF, SIC	Asthma	67
Various Chemicals				
Sodium disulfite	Lobster fishing	PEF, SIC	Asthma	74
Adipic acid flux	Soldering	PEF, SIC	Asthma	68
Dodecanedioic acid gel flux	Electronics company	PEF, SIC	Rhinitis, asthma	69
Tetramethrin	Insect extermination firm	SIC	Asthma	72
Uronium salts	Peptide synthesis laboratory	SPT, SIC	Rhinitis, asthma	71
Eugenol	Hairdressing salon	SIC	Rhinitis, asthma, dermatitis	75
3-Amino-5-mercapto-1,2,4-triazole	Production of herbicides	PEF	Rhinitis, asthma	70
Artificial flavor	Popcorn popping company	History	Asthma	73
Chlorendic anhydride	Mechanic work	SPT, specific IgE, PEF	Asthma, dermatitis	77
Reactive dye Synozol Red-K 3BS	Textile industry	Specific IgE, SIC	Rhinitis, asthma	76

Abbreviations: 7-ACSA, 7-aminocephalosporanic acid; 5-ASA, 5-aminosalicylic acid; PA-HP, peracetic acid-hydrogen peroxide; PEF, peak expiratory flow; SPT, skin prick tests; 7-TACA, 7-amino-3-thiomethyl-3-cephalosporanic acid.

discontinued but these enzymes were reintroduced in encapsulated form. The capsulated form of the enzyme was not associated with a recurrence of OA and allergy cases. However, subtilisin started to be used in the health care setting for cleaning and/or disinfection of medical instruments. A first case report of OA caused by subtilisin in a health care worker was published in 1996.[90] More recently, 2 cases of OA and 4 other cases of possible OA or rhinitis associated with the use of detergent enzymes for cleaning medical instruments were reported in health care settings.[91] The use of enzymes as cleaning agents should be monitored and considered as a potential cause of OA or allergy.

Isocyanates

Isocyanates have been the leading cause of OA caused by LMW agents for many years. There have been efforts to lower and monitor the threshold of exposures to isocyanates in the occupational environment and to improve protective measures for workers, such as efficient respirators. Efficient surveillance programs have been implemented.[92] Although isocyanates remain one of the most frequent LMW agents causing OA, there has been a decrease of the number of OA cases caused by isocyanates compared with the late 1980s. In Ontario, there has been a substantial decrease in the number of cases of OA caused by isocyanates in the late 1990s,[93] which is likely to be caused by the implementation of surveillance programs.

Key Point

- The change in the fabrication processing of occupational agents or the implementation of effective surveillance programs can influence and improve the outcome of OA.

IIA

IIA encompasses a spectrum of clinical presentations. The most typical form is represented by reactive airways dysfunction syndrome (RADS),[94] which refers to a type of OA without latency and immunologic sensitization, occurring after a single massive irritant exposure, causing severe airway injury and resulting in persistent airway inflammation and nonspecific bronchial hyperresponsiveness (NSBH). Comprehensive lists of agents associated with RADS have been published.[95] The 7 most frequently reported agents for work-related RADS were, in decreasing order: cleaning materials; chemicals not otherwise specified

(NOS); chlorine; solvents NOS; acids, bases, oxidizers NOS, smoke NOS; and diesel exhaust.[96]

In many cases, onset of asthma is not sudden and follows repeated low-dose exposure to 1 or more bronchial irritants. Various names have been proposed for this phenotype of IIA: low-dose RADS,[97] not-so-sudden IIA,[98] and low-intensity chronic exposure dysfunction syndrome (LICEDS).[2,95] The role of repeated exposure to occupational irritants in the pathogenesis of new-onset asthma has been shown or suggested by several epidemiologic studies or case reports.[95] These publications particularly concern workers exposed to chlorine gas in pulp mills and paper mills; meat wrappers; workers exposed to formaldehyde; aluminum smelters exposed to pot fume emissions containing gaseous fluorides, hydrofluoric acid, and sulfur dioxide (potroom asthma); or workers exposed to machining fluids.

More recently, the hypothesis of asthma induced by recurrent episodes of irritant gas exposure has been supported by an epidemiologic study showing that the incidence of adult-onset, physician-diagnosed asthma among sulfite mill workers reporting SO_2 gassing was 6.2 per 1000 person years, compared with 1.9 per 1000 person years among subjects not exposed to SO_2 and any gassing (hazard ratio 4.0, 95% CI 2.1–7.7).[99] However, the pathophysiologic mechanisms leading to IIA seem to be different from OA. For example, a single exposure to those irritants at low concentration does not induce an acute asthmatic reaction.

In the last 10 years, the most important findings concerning IIA and its causal agents have come from studies that described the health problems observed in rescue and recovery workers following the terrorist attack on the World Trade Center (WTC), and from additional data on OA in cleaners.

The WTC Tragedy and the Onset of IIA

It has been estimated that more than 50,000 people worked on the rescue and recovery effort that followed destruction of the WTC on September 11, 2001, including first responders such as firefighters, police officers, and paramedics but also operating engineers, iron workers, railway tunnel workers, telecommunication workers, and sanitation workers. WTC rescue and recovery workers were exposed to a complex mix of airborne contaminants. Collapse of the towers pulverized building materials and created a dense cloud of dust that was found to consist predominantly of coarse particles and contained cement, glass fibers, asbestos, lead, polycyclic aromatic hydrocarbons, polychlorinated biphenyls, and polychlorinated furans and dioxins.[100]

The WTC dust was highly alkaline (pH 9.0–11.0) and consequently irritant. Despite most particles being greater than 10 μm in diameter, the dust burden on day 1 was so high that a substantial number of particles in the respirable range was present and inhaled into the small airways, as shown by induced sputum analysis in firefighters exposed to WTC dust.[10,101] Prezant and colleagues[102] investigated the incidence of severe cough and NSBH in firefighters in the first 6 months after the WTC collapse, according to the level of exposure to WTC dust. Severe cough, defined as persistent cough that developed after exposure to the site, and accompanied by respiratory symptoms severe enough to require medical leave for at least 4 weeks, named WTC cough, occurred in 128 of 1636 (8%) firefighters who arrived at the scene during the collapse, on the morning of September 11, 2001 (high level of exposure); 187 of 6958 (3%) firefighters with moderate level of exposure (arrival after the collapse but within the first 2 days); and 17 of 1320 (1%) firefighters with a low level of exposure (arrival between days 3 and 7). A provocative concentration of methacholine inducing a 20% fall in FEV1 which is less than 16 mg/mL was found in 47 (24%) of 196 firefighters with WTC cough who performed a methacholine challenge test. The time of arrival at the WTC site predicted the presence of NSBH and the incidence of WTC cough. NSBH was found in about one-quarter of the firefighters with a high level of exposure, whether or not they had WTC cough. One month after the WTC tragedy, the prevalence of NSBH was much higher in the exposed firefighters (24.6%) compared with a control group of firefighters who were absent from the WTC site for at least the first 2 weeks (3.6%).[103]

There is evidence that RADS may be an outcome of injury by inorganic particulates.[104] Two recently published longitudinal studies have shown high cumulative incidence of asthma in subjects exposed to WTC dust.[105,106] The prolonged increased incidence of asthma after the WTC collapse is in accordance with clinician observations that the onset of asthma symptoms in many cases was slow, without a complete clinical expression until several months after leaving the WTC site.[18]

Cleaning Activities and IIA

Cleaners represent a significant proportion of workers in all industrialized countries, with diverse jobs ranging from domestic cleaning to cleaning offices, plants, and kitchens. Professional cleaners have emerged, in the last 10 years, as one of the high-risk groups for work-related asthma in industrialized nations.[95,107] The main airway irritants in cleaning products are bleach (sodium hypochlorite), hydrochloric acid, and alkaline agents (ammonia and sodium hydroxide), which are commonly mixed together.[108] Recent studies have suggested that respiratory irritants probably play a key role in the increased risk of asthma among cleaners.[109,110]

Key Points

- Exposure to inorganic particulates can induce various forms of occupational IIA (RADS and LICEDS).

- In cleaners, RADS seems to be predominantly related to inappropriate mixtures of bleach with either hydrochloric acid or ammonia, leading to the release of large amounts of chlorine gas or chloramines, respectively.

- Cleaning workers may also have an increased risk of new-onset asthma caused by prolonged low-to-moderate exposure to respiratory irritants.

SUMMARY

Many occupational agents can potentially cause OA through different pathophysiologic mechanisms. The list of those agents is constantly growing. The causal agent of OA should be identified because effective interventions can be implemented in the workplace. As shown with the examples of latex or isocyanates, appropriate changes in the fabrication process, or effective measures of prevention, can substantially decrease the incidence of OA.

REFERENCES

1. Malo J, Chan-Yeung M. Agents causing occupational asthma with key references. In: Bernstein IL, Chan-Yeung M, Malo JL, et al, editors. Asthma in the workplace. New York: Taylor & Francis; 2006. p. 825–66.
2. Tarlo SM, Balmes J, Balkissoon R, et al. Diagnosis and management of work-related asthma: American College Of Chest Physicians Consensus Statement. Chest 2008;134(Suppl 3):1S–41S.
3. Dykewicz MS. Occupational asthma: current concepts in pathogenesis, diagnosis, and management. J Allergy Clin Immunol 2009;123(3):519–28 [quiz: 29–30].
4. Malo JL, Chan-Yeung M. Agents causing occupational asthma. J Allergy Clin Immunol 2009;123(3): 545–50.
5. Lemière C, Malo J, Gautrin D. Nonsensitizing causes of occupational asthma. Med Clin North Am 1996;80:749–74.
6. Leroyer C, Perfetti L, Cartier A, et al. Can reactive airways dysfunction syndrome (RADS) transform into occupational asthma due to "sensitisation" to isocyanates? Thorax 1998;53:152–3.
7. Smith AM, Bernstein D. Occupational allergens. Clin Allergy Immunol 2008;21:261–71.
8. de las Heras M, Cuesta-Herranz J, Cases B, et al. Occupational asthma caused by gerbil: purification and partial characterization of a new gerbil allergen. Ann Allergy Asthma Immunol 2010;104(6):540–2.
9. Choi GS, Kim JH, Lee HN, et al. Occupational asthma caused by inhalation of bovine serum albumin powder. Allergy Asthma Immunol Res 2009;1(1):45–7.
10. Lehto M, Airaksinen L, Puustinen A, et al. Thaumatin-like protein and baker's respiratory allergy. Ann Allergy Asthma Immunol 2010;104(2):139–46.
11. Palacin A, Varela J, Quirce S, et al. Recombinant lipid transfer protein Tri a 14: a novel heat and proteolytic resistant tool for the diagnosis of baker's asthma. Clin Exp Allergy 2009;39(8):1267–76.
12. Constantin C, Quirce S, Poorafshar M, et al. Microarrayed wheat seed and grass pollen allergens for component-resolved diagnosis. Allergy 2009; 64(7):1030–7.
13. Miedinger D, Malo JL, Cartier A, et al. Malt can cause both occupational asthma and allergic alveolitis. Allergy 2009;64(8):1228–9.
14. Pirson F, Detry B, Pilette C. Occupational rhinoconjunctivitis and asthma caused by chicory and oral allergy syndrome associated with bet v 1-related protein. J Investig Allergol Clin Immunol 2009; 19(4):306–10.
15. Lluch-Perez M, Garcia-Rodriguez RM, Malet A, et al. Occupational allergy caused by marigold (*Tagetes erecta*) flour inhalation. Allergy 2009; 64(7):1100–1.
16. Cartier A. The role of inhalant food allergens in occupational asthma. Curr Allergy Asthma Rep 2010;10(5):349–56.
17. Lucas D, Lucas R, Boniface K, et al. Occupational asthma in the commercial fishing industry: a case series and review of the literature. Int Marit Health 2010;61(1):13–6.
18. Rosado A, Tejedor MA, Benito C, et al. Occupational asthma caused by octopus particles. Allergy 2009;64(7):1101–2.
19. Perez Carral C, Martin-Lazaro J, Ledesma A, et al. Occupational asthma caused by turbot allergy in 3 fish-farm workers. J Investig Allergol Clin Immunol 2010;20(4):349–51.
20. Barbuzza O, Guarneri F, Galtieri G, et al. Protein contact dermatitis and allergic asthma caused by *Anisakis simplex*. Contact Dermatitis 2009;60(4):239–40.

21. Heffler E, Nebiolo F, Pizzimenti S, et al. Occupational asthma caused by *Neurospora sitophila* sensitization in a coffee dispenser service operator. Ann Allergy Asthma Immunol 2009;102(2):168–9.

22. Francuz B, Yera H, Geraut L, et al. Occupational asthma induced by *Chrysonilia sitophila* in a worker exposed to coffee grounds. Clin Vaccine Immunol 2010;17(10):1645–6.

23. Talleu C, Delourme J, Dumas C, et al. Allergic asthma due to sausage mould. Rev Mal Respir 2009;26(5):557–9 [in French].

24. Miedinger D, Cartier A, Lehrer SB, et al. Occupational asthma to caddis flies (Phryganeiae). Occup Environ Med 2010;67(7):503.

25. Skousgaard SG, Thisling T, Bindslev-Jensen C, et al. Occupational asthma caused by the predatory beneficial mites *Amblyseius californicus* and *Amblyseius cucumeris*. Occup Environ Med 2010; 67(4):287.

26. Diaz Angulo S, Szram J, Welch J, et al. Occupational asthma in antibiotic manufacturing workers: case reports and systematic review. J Allergy (Cairo) 2011;2011:365683.

27. Choi GS, Sung JM, Lee JW, et al. A case of occupational asthma caused by inhalation of vancomycin powder. Allergy 2009;64(9):1391–2.

28. Gomez-Olles S, Madrid-San Martin F, Cruz MJ, et al. Occupational asthma due to colistin in a pharmaceutical worker. Chest 2010;137(5):1200–2.

29. Park HS, Kim KU, Lee YM, et al. Occupational asthma and IgE sensitization to 7-aminocephalosporanic acid. J Allergy Clin Immunol 2004; 113(4):785–7.

30. Suh YJ, Lee YM, Choi JH, et al. Heterogeneity of IgE response to cefteram pivoxil was noted in 2 patients with cefteram-induced occupational asthma. J Allergy Clin Immunol 2003;112(1):209–10.

31. Ye YM, Kim HM, Suh CH, et al. Three cases of occupational asthma induced by thiamphenicol: detection of serum-specific IgE. Allergy 2006;61(3):394–5.

32. Pala G, Pignatti P, Perfetti L, et al. Occupational asthma and rhinitis induced by a cephalosporin intermediate product: description of a case. Allergy 2009;64(9):1390–1.

33. Walusiak J, Wittczak T, Ruta U, et al. Occupational asthma due to mitoxantrone. Allergy 2002;57(5):461.

34. Vellore AD, Drought VJ, Sherwood-Jones D, et al. Occupational asthma and allergy to sevoflurane and isoflurane in anaesthetic staff. Allergy 2006; 61(12):1485–6.

35. Klusackova P, Lebedova J, Pelclova D, et al. Occupational asthma and rhinitis in workers from a lasamide production line. Scand J Work Environ Health 2007;33(1):74–8.

36. Sastre J, Garcia del Potro M, Aguado E, et al. Occupational asthma due to 5-aminosalicylic acid. Occup Environ Med 2010;67(11):798–9.

37. Munoz X, Culebras M, Cruz MJ, et al. Occupational asthma related to aescin inhalation. Ann Allergy Asthma Immunol 2006;96(3):494–6.

38. Drought VJ, Francis HC, Mc LNR, et al. Occupational asthma induced by thiamine in a vitamin supplement for breakfast cereals. Allergy 2005;60(9):1213–4.

39. Alday E, Gomez M, Ojeda P, et al. IgE-mediated asthma associated with a unique allergen from *Angelim pedra* (*Hymenolobium petraeum*) wood. J Allergy Clin Immunol 2005;115(3):634–6.

40. Algranti E, Mendonca EM, Ali SA, et al. Occupational asthma caused by Ipe (*Tabebuia* spp) dust. J Investig Allergol Clin Immunol 2005;15(1):81–3.

41. Alvarez-Cuesta C, Gala Ortiz G, Rodriguez Diaz E, et al. Occupational asthma and IgE-mediated contact dermatitis from sapele wood. Contact Dermatitis 2004;51(2):88–98.

42. Eire MA, Pineda F, Losada SV, et al. Occupational rhinitis and asthma due to cedroarana (*Cedrelinga catenaeformis* Ducke) wood dust allergy. J Investig Allergol Clin Immunol 2006;16(6):385–7.

43. Higuero NC, Zabala BB, Villamuza YG, et al. Occupational asthma caused by IgE-mediated reactivity to *Antiaris* wood dust. J Allergy Clin Immunol 2001; 107(3):554–6.

44. Lee LT, Tan KL. Occupational asthma due to exposure to chengal wood dust. Occup Med (Lond) 2009;59(5):357–9.

45. Obata H, Dittrick M, Chan H, et al. Occupational asthma due to exposure to African cherry (Makore) wood dust. Intern Med 2000;39(11):947–9.

46. Quirce S, Parra A, Anton E, et al. Occupational asthma caused by tali and jatoba wood dusts. J Allergy Clin Immunol 2004;113(2):361–3.

47. Tomioka K, Kumagai S, Kameda M, et al. A case of occupational asthma induced by falcata wood (*Albizia falcataria*). J Occup Health 2006;48(5): 392–5.

48. Yacoub MR, Lemiere C, Labrecque M, et al. Occupational asthma due to bethabara wood dust. Allergy 2005;60(12):1544–5.

49. Perez-Rios M, Ruano-Ravina A, Etminan M, et al. A meta-analysis on wood dust exposure and risk of asthma. Allergy 2010;65(4):467–73.

50. Malo JL. Occupational rhinitis and asthma due to metal salts. Allergy 2005;60(2):138–9.

51. Gheysens B, Auwerx J, Van den Eeckhout A, et al. Cobalt-induced bronchial asthma in diamond polishers. Chest 1985;88(5):740–4.

52. Malo JL, Cartier A, Doepner M, et al. Occupational asthma caused by nickel sulfate. J Allergy Clin Immunol 1982;69(1 Pt 1):55–9.

53. Novey HS, Habib M, Wells ID. Asthma and IgE antibodies induced by chromium and nickel salts. J Allergy Clin Immunol 1983;72(4):407–12.

54. Wittczak T, Dudek W, Krakowiak A, et al. Occupational asthma due to manganese exposure: a case

report. Int J Occup Med Environ Health 2008;21(1): 81–3.

55. Munoz X, Cruz MJ, Freixa A, et al. Occupational asthma caused by metal arc welding of iron. Respiration 2009;78(4):455–9.

56. Daenen M, Rogiers P, Van de Walle C, et al. Occupational asthma caused by palladium. Eur Respir J 1999;13(1):213–6.

57. Merget R, Sander I, van Kampen V, et al. Occupational immediate-type asthma and rhinitis due to rhodium salts. Am J Ind Med 2010;53(1):42–6.

58. Hannu T, Piipari R, Tuppurainen M, et al. Occupational asthma due to welding fumes from stellite. J Occup Environ Med 2007;49(5):473–4.

59. Corrado OJ, Osman J, Davies RJ. Asthma and rhinitis after exposure to glutaraldehyde in endoscopy units. Hum Toxicol 1986;5(5):325–8.

60. Waclawski ER, McAlpine LG, Thomson NC. Occupational asthma in nurses caused by chlorhexidine and alcohol aerosols. BMJ 1989; 298(6678):929–30.

61. Cristofari-Marquand E, Kacel M, Milhe F, et al. Asthma caused by peracetic acid-hydrogen peroxide mixture. J Occup Health 2007;49(2):155–8.

62. Fujita H, Ogawa M, Endo Y. A case of occupational bronchial asthma and contact dermatitis caused by ortho-phthalaldehyde exposure in a medical worker. J Occup Health 2006;48(6):413–6.

63. Bernard A, Nickmilder M, Voisin C. Outdoor swimming pools and the risks of asthma and allergies during adolescence. Eur Respir J 2008;32(4):979–88.

64. Bernard A, Nickmilder M, Voisin C, et al. Impact of chlorinated swimming pool attendance on the respiratory health of adolescents. Pediatrics 2009; 124(4):1110–8.

65. Goodman M, Hays S. Asthma and swimming: a meta-analysis. J Asthma 2008;45(8):639–47.

66. Thickett KM, McCoach JS, Gerber JM, et al. Occupational asthma caused by chloramines in indoor swimming-pool air. Eur Respir J 2002;19(5):827–32.

67. Draper A, Cullinan P, Campbell C, et al. Occupational asthma from fungicides fluazinam and chlorothalonil. Occup Environ Med 2003;60(1):76–7.

68. Moore VC, Burge PS. Occupational asthma to solder wire containing an adipic acid flux. Eur Respir J 2010;36(4):962–3.

69. Moore VC, Manney S, Vellore AD, et al. Occupational asthma to gel flux containing dodecanedioic acid. Allergy 2009;64(7):1099–100.

70. Hnizdo E, Sylvain D, Lewis DM, et al. New-onset asthma associated with exposure to 3-amino-5-mercapto-1,2,4-triazole. J Occup Environ Med 2004;46(12):1246–52.

71. Vandenplas O, Hereng MP, Heymans J, et al. Respiratory and skin hypersensitivity reactions caused by a peptide coupling reagent. Occup Environ Med 2008;65(10):715–6.

72. Vandenplas O, Delwiche JP, Auverdin J, et al. Asthma to tetramethrin. Allergy 2000;55(4):417–8.

73. Sahakian N, Kullman G, Lynch D, et al. Asthma arising in flavoring-exposed food production workers. Int J Occup Med Environ Health 2008;21(2):173–7.

74. Madsen J, Sherson D, Kjoller H, et al. Occupational asthma caused by sodium disulphite in Norwegian lobster fishing. Occup Environ Med 2004;61(10): 873–4.

75. Quirce S, Fernandez-Nieto M, del Pozo V, et al. Occupational asthma and rhinitis caused by eugenol in a hairdresser. Allergy 2008;63(1):137–8.

76. Jin HJ, Kim JH, Kim JE, et al. Occupational asthma induced by the reactive dye Synozol Red-K 3BS. Allergy Asthma Immunol Res 2011;3(3):212–4.

77. Keskinen H, Pfaffli P, Pelttari M, et al. Chlorendic anhydride allergy. Allergy 2000;55(1):98–9.

78. Baur X, Jager D. Airborne antigens from latex gloves. Lancet 1990;335(8694):912.

79. Lagier F, Badier M, Charpin D, et al. Latex as aeroallergen. Lancet 1990;2:516–7.

80. Lagier F, Vervloet D, Lhermet I, et al. Prevalence of latex allergy in operating room nurses. J Allergy Clin Immunol 1992;90:319–22.

81. Liss G, Sussman G, Deal K, et al. Latex allergy: epidemiological study of 1351 hospital workers. Occup Environ Med 1997;54:335–42.

82. Vandenplas O. Occupational asthma caused by natural rubber latex. Eur Respir J 1995;8:1957–65.

83. Vandenplas O, Larbanois A, Vanassche F, et al. Latex-induced occupational asthma: time trend in incidence and relationship with hospital glove policies. Allergy 2009;64(3):415–20.

84. Liss G, Tarlo S. Natural rubber latex-related occupational asthma: association with interventions and glove changes over time. Am J Ind Med 2001;40:347–53.

85. Latza U, Haamann F, Baur X. Effectiveness of a nationwide interdisciplinary preventive programme for latex allergy. Int Arch Occup Environ Health 2005;78:394–402.

86. Sussman G, Liss G, Deal K, et al. Incidence of latex sensitization among latex glove users. J Allergy Clin Immunol 1998;101:171–8.

87. Turjanmaa K, Kanto M, Kautiainen H, et al. Long-term outcome of 160 adult patients with natural rubber latex allergy. J Allergy Clin Immunol 2002; 110(Suppl 2):S70–4.

88. Hole A, Draper A, Jolliffe G, et al. Occupational asthma caused by bacillary amylase used in the detergent industry. Occup Environ Med 2000;57:840–2.

89. Pepys J, Longbottom J, Hargreave F, et al. Allergic reactions of the lungs to enzymes of Bacillus subtilis. Lancet 1969;1:1811–4.

90. Lemière C, Cartier A, Dolovich J, et al. Isolated late asthmatic reaction after exposure to a high-molecular-weight occupational agent, subtilisin. Chest 1996;110:823–4.

91. Adisesh A, Murphy E, Barber CM, et al. Occupational asthma and rhinitis due to detergent enzymes in healthcare. Occup Med (Lond) 2011; 61(5):364–9.

92. Labrecque M, Malo JL, Alaoui KM, et al. Medical surveillance programme for diisocyanate exposure. Occup Environ Med 2011;68(4):302–7.

93. Buyantseva LV, Liss GM, Ribeiro M, et al. Reduction in diisocyanate and non-diisocyanate sensitizer-induced occupational asthma in Ontario. J Occup Environ Med 2011;53(4):420–6.

94. Brooks S, Weiss M, Bernstein I. Reactive airways dysfunction syndrome (RADS). Persistent asthma syndrome after high level irritant exposures. Chest 1985;88:376–84.

95. Gautrin D, Bernstein I, Brooks S, et al. Reactive airways dysfunction syndrome and irritant-induced asthma. In: Bernstein IL, Chan-Yeung M, Malo JL, et al, editors. Asthma in the workplace. 3rd edition. New York: Taylor & Francis; 2006. p. 579–627.

96. Henneberger P, Derk S, Davis L, et al. Work-related reactive airways dysfunction syndrome cases from surveillance in selected US States. J Occup Environ Med 2003;45:360–8.

97. Kipen H, Blume R, Hutt D. Occupational and environmental Medicine Clinic. Low-dose reactive airways dysfunction syndrome. J Occup Med 1994;36:1133–7.

98. Brooks S, Hammad Y, Richards I, et al. The spectrum of irritant-induced asthma. Chest 1998;113:42–9.

99. Andersson E, Knutsson A, Hagberg S, et al. Incidence of asthma among workers exposed to sulphur dioxide and other irritant gases. Eur Respir J 2006;27:720–5.

100. Landrigan PJ, Lioy PJ, Thurston G, et al. Health and environmental consequences of the World Trade Center disaster. Environ Health Perspect 2004;112(6):731–9.

101. Fireman EM, Lerman Y, Ganor E, et al. Induced sputum assessment in New York City firefighters exposed to World Trade Center dust. Environ Health Perspect 2004;112(15):1564–9.

102. Prezant D, Weiden M, Banauch G, et al. Cough and bronchial responsiveness in firefighters at the World Trade Center site. N Engl J Med 2002;347: 806–15.

103. Banauch G, Alleyne D, Sanchez R, et al. Persistent hyperreactivity and reactive airway dysfunction syndrome in firefighters at the World Trade Center. Am J Respir Crit Care Med 2003;168:54–62.

104. Nemery B. Reactive fallout of World Trade Center dust. Am J Respir Crit Care Med 2003; 168(1):2–3.

105. Brackbill RM, Hadler JL, DiGrande L, et al. Asthma and posttraumatic stress symptoms 5 to 6 years following exposure to the World Trade Center terrorist attack. JAMA 2009;302(5):502–16.

106. Wisnivesky JP, Teitelbaum SL, Todd AC, et al. Persistence of multiple illnesses in World Trade Center rescue and recovery workers: a cohort study. Lancet 2011;378(9794):888–97.

107. Jaakkola J, Jaakkola M. Professional cleaning and asthma. Curr Opin Allergy Clin Immunol 2006;6: 85–90.

108. Quirce S, Barranco P. Cleaning agents and asthma. J Investig Allergol Clin Immunol 2010; 20(7):542–50 [quiz: 2p following 50].

109. Medina-Ramon M, Zock J, Kogevinas M, et al. Asthma, chronic bronchitis, and exposure to irritant agents in occupational domestic cleaning: a nested case-control study. Occup Environ Med 2005;62: 598–606.

110. Vizcaya D, Mirabelli MC, Anto JM, et al. A workforce-based study of occupational exposures and asthma symptoms in cleaning workers. Occup Environ Med 2011;68(12):914–9.

Corticosteroids
Still at the Frontline in Asthma Treatment?

Renaud Louis, MD, PhD[a],*, Florence Schleich, MD[a],
Peter J. Barnes, MD, PhD[b]

KEYWORDS

- Eosinophilic asthma • Corticosteroids • Inflammation • Mast cells • Asthma phenotypes

KEY POINTS

- Inhaled corticosteroids (ICS) have led to considerably improved asthma control and reduced asthma mortality in the Western world over the last 2 decades, particularly in combating T-helper type 2–driven inflammation featuring mast cell and eosinophilic airway infiltration.
- Their effect on innate immunity-driven neutrophilic inflammation is rather poor and their ability to prevent airway remodeling and accelerated lung decline is highly controversial.
- Although ICS remain pivotal drugs in asthma management, research is needed to find drugs complementary to the combination ICS/long-acting β2-agonist in refractory asthma and perhaps a new class of drugs as a first-line treatment in mild to moderate noneosinophilic asthma.

INTRODUCTION

There was a time when asthmatics had their symptoms treated with a regular short-acting bronchodilator and theophylline, while reserving the use of systemic corticosteroids for severe exacerbations and for chronic maintenance treatment of the most severe patients. The emergence of corticosteroids suitable for the inhaled route in the 1970s followed by convincing clinical trials during the late 1980s has dramatically changed the picture of asthma treatment. The class of inhaled corticosteroids (ICS) has rapidly demonstrated its superiority over other classes of drugs used in asthma.[1] The first Global Initiative for Asthma consensus in the early 1990s further highlighted the importance of the role of ICS in asthma treatment.[2] There is no doubt that the reduced mortality and morbidity of asthma observed since the 1990s is, in a large part, related to the regular use of ICS as the mainstay of asthma treatment. Yet some studies have pointed out the variability of the response to ICS in patients with asthma, suggesting that ICS administered alone might not be the best drug for all patients.[3]

FROM EARLY PROMISE TO THE TIME OF CERTITUDE

The first studies using inhaled hydrocortisone and prednisone in asthma were disappointing. It became apparent that this was because of the inappropriate chemical structure of prednisone, which has first to be metabolized to become pharmacologically effective, and the lack of topical activity of these corticosteroids. The chemical transformation of prednisone to increase both lipophilicity and interaction with glucocorticosteroid receptor made it possible to find compounds that were suitable for the inhaled route. Early studies in the 1970s used inhaled beclomethasone dipropionate and triamcinolone acetate in moderate to severe asthma and showed that these drugs were effective in improving lung function and reducing symptoms despite tapering oral corticosteroids.[4–6] The introduction of ICS dramatically and effectively changed the conventional approach to asthma therapy. The institution of ICS made it possible to replace, in most of the patients, the chronic use of oral corticosteroids, thereby avoiding side effects that were often

[a] Deparment of Pneumology, CHU Liege, GIGAI3 Research Group, University of Liege, Liege, Belgium;
[b] National Heart and Lung Institute, Imperial College, London, UK
* Corresponding author.
E-mail address: R.Louis@chu.ulg.ac.be

Clin Chest Med 33 (2012) 531–541
http://dx.doi.org/10.1016/j.ccm.2012.05.004
0272-5231/12/$ – see front matter © 2012 Elsevier Inc. All rights reserved.

severe and debilitating.[7] Furthermore, it soon seemed to be an inverse relationship between the rate of hospitalization for acute asthma exacerbation and the sales of ICS. In a cohort study of more than 13,000 patients with asthma, ICS were shown to be more effective than theophylline in reducing the hospitalization rate as long as they were taken regularly.[8] In a population-based epidemiologic study it was found that the regular use of low-dose ICS was associated with a reduced risk of death from asthma.[9]

The interest of ICS in the milder form of the disease was established later. The first pivotal study proving the superiority of ICS over β2-agonists as a maintenance treatment dates back to 1991. Haahtela and colleagues[10] demonstrated that the regular use of inhaled budesonide at the dosage of 1200 µg/d was by far superior to the regular use of terbutaline in improving the day-to-day peak expiratory flow rate and reducing asthma symptoms and as-needed relief bronchodilator usage. It is also by this time that the fundamental inflammatory nature of asthma was recognized even in the mildest form of the disease.[11] Asthma has then been regarded as a chronic airway inflammatory disease featuring eosinophil and mast cell airway wall infiltration as a consequence of a T-helper type 2 (Th2)–driven inflammatory process. The role of cytokines, such as interleukin 4 (IL-4) and IL-5, were highlighted as key cytokine in immunoglobulin E (IgE) synthesis from B cells and eosinophil survival respectively.[12] The role of chemokines for eosinophils, like eotaxin, was also demonstrated in asthma.[13] Regular treatment with ICS was shown to reduce the number of T-lymphocytes, eosinophils, and mast cells[14] and restore epithelial integrity[15] in bronchial biopsies. Numerous studies showed that regular treatment with ICS sharply and quickly reduces the percentage of eosinophils contained in the sputum from patients with asthma.[16–20] Therefore, corticosteroids were thought to be effective in asthma treatment because of their ability to repress the release of Th2 cytokine from lymphocytes[21] and eotaxin from epithelial cells,[22] thereby depleting airways from eosinophils and mast cells. More recently, it has been shown that corticosteroids are highly effective in inhibiting the transcription factor GATA3, which drives Th2 cells and the release of Th2 cytokines.[23] Therefore, ICS have been regarded as the perfect treatment of asthma leading to control for the peculiar airway inflammation while minimizing the systemic side effects because of their local action. Even in the mildest form of the disease, severe exacerbations may occur and ICS were shown to be extremely effective in preventing them.[24] This important property of ICS can lead us to think of this drug class as a disease-modifying drug in asthma. However, it soon appeared that ICS, even administrated at high doses, might not treat all facets of asthma or control all patients with asthma.

CORTICOSTEROIDS AND LOSS OF LUNG FUNCTION

Accelerated lung decline is a well-known feature of chronic obstructive pulmonary disease (COPD) and it is generally accepted that ICS fails to prevent it when patients continue to smoke.[25] The recognition that patients with asthma also have an accelerated lung function decline regardless of smoking[26,27] and despite regular treatment with ICS[24,28] has questioned the role of this class of drugs as a disease-modifying agent in asthma. In contrast to what has been shown for airway inflammation, it has been extremely difficult to convincingly demonstrate an effect of corticosteroids on airway remodeling. These effects require higher doses and sustained administration to show small changes in airway structure.[29,30] On the other hand, it has been demonstrated that in some young children, there is intense airway remodeling without any inflammation.[31,32] These observations led to the concept that airway inflammation and airway remodeling may be largely independent processes and, consequently, governed by different cytokine and growth factor networks, with corticoids being essentially active against the Th2 inflammatory component.[33] The recent observation that bronchoconstriction by itself may be a trigger for airway remodeling is of great importance because it may have potential significant implications for a treatment strategy to prevent lung function decrease.[34] In this view, it would seem logical to combine corticoids and long-acting-β2-agonist (LABA) at the early stages of asthmatic disease to maximize the bronchoprotecting effect and reduce the chance to evolve toward airway remodeling.

THE RECOGNITION OF REFRACTORY ASTHMA

The Gaining Optimal Asthma Control study showed that most patients with asthma can become largely asymptomatic when regularly treated by a combination ICS/LABA.[35] This therapeutic strategy also proved to be efficient in preventing asthma exacerbation in most patients. Yet a small fraction of patients with asthma, called patients with refractory or severe asthma, escape to that treatment. Severe or refractory asthma is generally thought to affect 1% to 5% of all patients with asthma and accounts for most asthma costs.[35–39] This phenotype is defined by inadequate asthma control despite a high dose of inhaled corticosteroids or the need for oral corticosteroids, often associated with other controller medication, such as LABA, leukotriene receptor antagonist, or theophylline.[40,41] By itself, this phenotype clearly points out the inability of corticosteroids to control disease expression in some patients with asthma. Early studies showed that these patients had consistent persistent eosinophilic or neutrophilic airway inflammation despite regular antiinflammatory treatment,[42–46] indicating that corticosteroids were unable to control the underlying airway inflammation. These studies have certainly contributed to the emergence of the concept of an eosinophilic versus neutrophilic asthma phenotype, a concept that has extended beyond the sole group of refractory asthma (see later discussion). In severe asthma, this concept has proved to be useful in asthma management. It was clearly demonstrated that persistent eosinophilic inflammation may still be responsive to an increase in the dose of inhaled or systemic corticosteroids in terms of lung function and symptom improvement[47] and chiefly in terms of the reduction of exacerbation.[48,49] These important studies point to a reduced sensitivity rather than to a real resistance to eosinophilic inflammation to corticosteroids. Reduced eosinophil apoptosis in induced sputum despite a high dose of inhaled corticosteroids was shown to be related to disease severity.[50] The molecular reason why severe eosinophilic inflammation may persist despite heavy treatment with corticosteroids remains unknown, but there are several molecular mechanisms for corticosteroid resistance in asthma.[51]

THE MOLECULAR CONCEPT OF CORTICOSTEROID RESISTANCE

It has been well demonstrated that corticosteroids have a positive interaction with $\beta2$-agonists at the molecular level. Indeed, corticosteroids increase the transcription of the $\beta2$-agonist receptor, resulting in increased expression of the receptor at the cell surface.[52,53] On the other hand, there is growing evidence to show that $\beta2$-agonists enhance the action of corticosteroids, particularly through enhancing the translocation of glucocorticoid receptor (GR), therefore, increasing the binding of GR to the glucocorticoid response element at the gene level.[54] However, patients with severe asthma have a poor response to corticosteroids, even when combined to $\beta2$-agonists, which necessitates the need for high doses and a few patients are completely resistant. Patients with asthma who smoke are also relatively corticosteroid resistant and require increased doses of corticosteroids for

asthma control.[55] Several molecular mechanisms have now been identified to account for corticosteroid resistance in severe asthma.[51] In smoking patients with asthma and patients with severe asthma, there is a reduction in activity and expression of the critical nuclear enzyme histone deacetylase-2, which prevents corticosteroids from switching off activated inflammatory genes.[56–58] In steroid-resistant asthma, other mechanisms may also contribute to corticosteroid insensitivity, including the reduced translocation of GR as a result of phosphorylation by p38 mitogen-activated protein (MAP) kinase[59] and abnormal histone acetylation patterns.[60] A proposed mechanism is an increase in GR-β, which prevents GR binding to DNA,[61] but there is little evidence that this would be sufficient to account for corticosteroid insensitivity because the amounts of GR-β are too low.[62] Th17 cells may be involved in driving neutrophilic inflammation in some patients with severe asthma and these cells seem to be largely corticosteroid resistant.[63,64]

COMPLEMENTARY TREATMENT TO CORTICOSTEROIDS IN REFRACTORY ASTHMA

Although abundantly used in COPD, tiotropium has been poorly validated in asthma treatment. A recent study conducted in patients with uncontrolled asthma, despite a moderate dose of inhaled beclomethasone, showed that tiotropium was at least equivalent to salmeterol in improving asthma lung function and symptoms.[65] Further studies focusing on patients with more severe asthma and looking at exacerbations as the major outcome are now warranted to validate the use of a long-acting anticholinergic in refractory asthma.

In those patients with refractory asthma, with moderately elevated total serum IgE and sensitization to a perennial allergen, omalizumab, a humanized monoclonal antibody against IgE, has proved to be effective in reducing the exacerbation rate and improving quality of life,[66,67] although part of the effect seen in clinical practice in quality-of life-improvement is likely to be caused by a placebo effect and a careful follow-up of patients inherent in the mode of drug administration.[68] Like for corticosteroids, the clinical benefit of omalizumab might be partly explained by a reduction of eosinophilic inflammation.[69,70] The major drawback of this currently available treatment is the high cost, which weakens the cost-effectiveness relationship.[71] Cost-effectiveness, however, depends on how hospitalization for exacerbation may be prevented; a drug that may reduce the hospitalization rate in high-risk patient is likely to be cost-effective.

Some studies indicate a continuous synthesis and release of Th2 cytokines, such as IL-4 and

IL-5, both at a systemic[72] and airway level[73] despite the regular treatment with inhaled corticoids. Yet there is no sign of reduced activity of corticosteroids in vitro to inhibit cytokine release from circulating leukocytes in those patients with refractory asthma.[72] The importance of IL-5 in driving the persistent systemic and airway eosinophilic inflammation has recently been demonstrated by the efficacy of mepolizumab, an anti–IL-5 monoclonal antibody, to further decrease eosinophilic inflammation in those patients with refractory asthma despite a high dose of corticosteroids.[74,75] The clinical relevance of the persistent eosinophilic inflammation is demonstrated by the reduction in the exacerbation rate and the improvement in quality of life observed in those patients receiving mepolizumab,[74] even if no effect is observed on airway caliber and bronchial hyperresponsiveness,[74] which is confirmatory of earlier studies with other anti–IL-5 antibodies.[76,77] Importantly, mepolizumab made it possible to taper and sometimes suppress the use of oral corticosteroids.[75] A recent 16-week study using reslizumab, a new monoclonal antibody against IL-5, has shown a significant improvement in forced expiratory volume in the first second of expiration in patients with moderate to severe eosinophilic asthma displaying prominent reversibility to a β2-agonist.[78]

Anti–tumor necrosis factor (TNF)-α is an established treatment in chronic inflammatory diseases, like Crohn disease or rheumatoid arthritis. Despite early promising pilot studies,[79–82] treatments that target TNF-α have generally proved to be disappointing in improving asthma control in patients with refractory asthma. This finding has been demonstrated with drugs, such as golimumab[83] and etanercept.[84]

The studies focusing on neutrophilic inflammation in refractory asthma have been limited so far. One study using clarithromycin has shown a significant reduction of sputum neutrophil count and sputum elastase together with an improved quality of life.[85] However, there was no improvement in asthma control or airway caliber. On the other hand, targeting neutrophils may theoretically prove to be a dangerous strategy in patients with refractory asthma by increasing their susceptibility to infections.[86] A recent study in COPD, another disease with prominent neutrophilic inflammation,[87,88] has shown a reduction of the exacerbation rate by regular treatment with azithromycin.[89] The mechanisms by which macrolide antibiotics might be effective remain elusive. Whether it is through antiinflammatory activity or by limiting airway colonization with typical or atypical bacterial pathogens remains to be investigated.[90] Clearly, in refractory asthma, further studies conducted on a longer-term period are needed to investigate the impact of macrolides on asthma exacerbation rate. Other treatments in development, mainly for COPD, also target neutrophilic inflammation, including antagonists against the chemokine receptor CXCR2, phosphodiesterase-4 inhibitors, and p38 MAP kinase inhibitors.[91]

Bronchial thermoplasty (BT) is an innovative non-pharmacologic treatment approach to reduce the bronchoconstrictor response in asthma. Although technically demanding, BT has been shown to improve asthma control and quality of life and to be safe in patients with moderate to severe asthma.[92–94] A recent multicenter study confirmed the ability of BT to improve control and quality of life in patients with refractory asthma and showed that BT resulted in a reduced severe exacerbation rate in the posttreatment period.[95]

EMERGENCE OF THE CONCEPT OF ASTHMA PHENOTYPE IN MILD TO MODERATE ASTHMA

The development of the technique of induced sputum has been a key step in the appearance of the concept of inflammatory phenotype in asthma. Although it confirmed the eosinophilic inflammation as a prominent feature of asthma,[96] which relates to disease severity,[43,50,72] it also showed that up to 50% of patients with asthma failed to exhibit this eosinophilic phenotype.[97,98] Almost half of them are characterized by intense neutrophilic inflammation[99] but the other half fails to show any abnormal granulocytic inflammation despite excessive lung function variability. The importance of these phenotypes is that the underlying molecular mechanisms are different. Although the eosinophilic phenotype is likely to reflect ongoing adaptive immunity in response to an allergen with Th2 cytokine IL-4, IL-5, and IL-13 playing a key role, the neutrophilic phenotype is thought to reflect innate immune system activation in response to pollutants or infectious agents.[100,101] Therefore, it is conceivable that the 2 phenotypes actually require different therapeutic molecular approaches.

Exhaled nitrous oxide (NO) is increased in patients with asthma[102] and particularly in those with eosinophilic inflammation.[103] A large-scale study conducted in routine has shown that a fractional exhaled NO threshold of around 40 ppb (measured at an exhaled flow of 50 mL/s) is predictive of eosinophilic inflammation in patients with asthma even though this threshold may be decreased by smoking and a high dose of ICS. The threshold was 27 ppb in smoking asthmatics and 28 ppb in those receiving at least 1000 μg/d of fluticasone (considered as high dose ICS). Moreover the threshold can be as low as 15 ppb in a non atopic smoking patient receiving high dose of ICS.[104] However, we lack an equivalent noninvasive marker for neutrophilic inflammation. The development of breath print by chromatography and mass spectrometry is a promising tool to approach these cellular phenotypes.

PREDICTING FACTORS OF CLINICAL RESPONSE TO CORTICOSTEROIDS

The results of large, randomized controlled clinical trials have perhaps masked for too long the fact that the response of ICS is variable in patients with asthma.[105] As pointed out earlier, the response to ICS is characterized by a high intraindividual repeatability and a high interindividual variability, with up to 40% of patients showing no short-term response to the treatment.[3] The presence of a persistent airway eosinophilic inflammation seems to be a good predicting factor for a short-term response to ICS.[105–109] Alternatively, a high exhaled NO level (>47 ppb according to the studies) is predictive of a good response to ICS in patients with chronic respiratory symptoms regardless of the disease label.[110] Furthermore, the presence of a Th2 cytokine profile in the airways seems to be needed to have rapid lung function improvement with ICS.[111] Even if a convincing response may be sometimes observed[112] in those with high exhaled NO (>33 ppb),[107] noneosinophilic asthma generally exhibits a limited response to ICS[113] and the response seems to be particularly poor in those patients exhibiting intense airway neutrophilic inflammation,[99] which is reminiscent of the inability of ICS to control airway inflammation in COPD.[114,115] A recent study has highlighted the importance of the genetic background in the improvement of lung function following chronic treatment with ICS. A functional variant of glucocorticosteroid transcript 1 gene was found to be associated with a decreased response to ICS in several randomized clinical trials.[116] In the studies published so far, the corticosteroid response has been assessed either by lung function or quality-of-life improvement over a short-term period (a few weeks). There is, however, a lack of evidence to support that denying treatment with ICS over a long-term period in some patients does not place them at risk of severe exacerbation. Clearly, new long-term prospective studies with asthma exacerbation as the main outcome are needed to clarify this important point.

CORTICOSTEROIDS IN CLINICAL PRACTICE

Like in many chronic diseases, poor compliance to maintenance treatment has been shown to be a major issue in asthma.[117] Poor inhalation technique is a further impediment in achieving a successful treatment with inhaled therapies in patients with asthma.[117] Because corticosteroids do not bring acute relief for asthma symptoms, it is likely to play a role in poor compliance. Although ICS have clearly demonstrated superior efficacy to leukotriene receptor antagonists with respect to most clinical outcomes in randomized controlled trials, a recent field study conducted in the United Kingdom has not confirmed this superiority in terms of asthma control.[118] The emergence of the SMART concept (Symbicort as a maintenance and relief therapy) has been an interesting paradigm that allows patients to inhale a dose of corticosteroids whenever he or she feels the need to use a rapid-acting bronchodilator. The concept that has been extensively validated in randomized controlled clinical trials[119] has also been shown to be valid in daily clinical practice.[120] The SMART approach has been shown to be particularly efficient in reducing the rate of severe asthma exacerbation.

NEW CLASS DRUG IN DEVELOPMENT

There are several new drugs for asthma currently in development that may be suited more for patients who do not respond well to corticosteroids.[91] Several cytokines are involved in the pathophysiology of asthma, including Th2 cytokines. Anti–IL-5 antibodies (mepolizumab, reslizumab) are currently in clinical trials for severe eosinophilic asthma that is resistant to corticosteroids, as discussed earlier. IL-13 is increased in severe asthma and causes corticosteroid resistance, so it is a logical target. Currently, anti–IL-13 antibodies, such as lebrikizumab, have been disappointing with little physiologic effect and no effect on symptoms or exacerbations.[121] Blocking antibodies to other cytokines, including IL-9, IL-25, IL-33, and thymus stromal lymphopoietin, are also in development for asthma. Small molecule antagonists of inflammatory mediators have been disappointing in asthma, but there has recently been great interest in blocking prostaglandin (PG) D_2, which is released from mast cells and attracts Th2 cells and eosinophils via the receptor chemoattractant homologous receptor expressed on Th2 cells (CRTH2) (or DP_2 receptors). PGD_2 seems to be increased in patients with severe asthma who are not controlled on inhaled therapy.[122] Several oral CRTH2 antagonists are now in development and have shown some clinical benefit.[123] As discussed earlier, there are several broad-spectrum antiinflammatory treatments that target neutrophilic inflammation, so they may be effective in patients with severe asthma who do not respond well to corticosteroid therapy.[124] Mast-cell

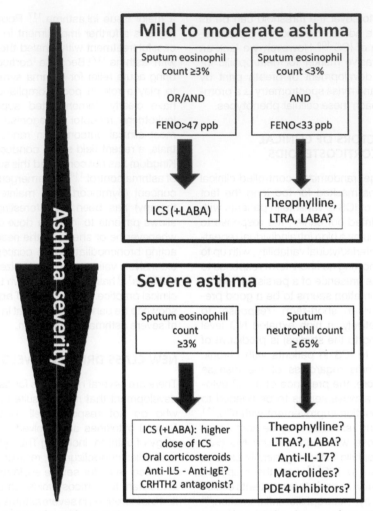

Fig. 1. Proposed strategy for asthma mainstay treatment according to the degree of severity and the sputum inflammatory phenotype. CRTH2, chemoattractant homologous receptor expressed on Th2 cells, also known as DP_2 receptor, a receptor for PGD_2; ICS, inhaled corticosteroids; LABA, long-acting β2-agonists; LTRA, leukotriene receptor antagonist; PDE4, phosphodiesterase 4 inhibitor.

activation is found in patients with severe asthma, suggesting that mast-cell inhibitors may be useful in these patients. As discussed earlier, omalizumab is useful in some patients with severe asthma and reduces exacerbations[66,67] but cannot be used in patients with high circulating IgE concentrations, so antibodies with a higher affinity are now in development. Other drugs that target mast cells include c-kit and Syk inhibitors.

SUMMARY

There is no doubt that ICS have led to considerably improved asthma control and reduced asthma mortality in the Western world over the last 2 decades. ICS are particularly effective in combating Th2-driven inflammation featuring mast-cell and eosinophilic airway infiltration. Their effect on innate immunity-driven neutrophilic inflammation is poor and their ability to prevent airway remodeling and accelerated lung decline is highly controversial. Although ICS remain pivotal drugs in asthma management, research is needed to find drugs complementary to the combination ICS/LABA in refractory asthma and perhaps a new class of drugs as a first-line treatment in mild to moderate noneosinophilic asthma (**Fig. 1**).

ACKNOWLEDGMENTS

The work was supported by federal grant PAI P7/30 Aireway II. We also thank Anne Chevremont for excellent technical assistance.

REFERENCES

1. Barnes PJ. Will It be steroids for ever? Clin Exp Allergy 2005;35:843–5.

2. Global strategy for asthma management and prevention: NHLBI/WHO workshop report March 1993. National Institutes of Health; 2002. Publication number 95–36–59 issued January 1995.

3. Drazen JM, Silverman EK, Lee TH. Heterogeneity of therapeutic responses in asthma. Br Med Bull 2000;56:1054–70.

4. Brown HM, Storey G, George WH. Beclomethasone dipropionate: a new steroid aerosol for the treatment of allergic asthma. Br Med J 1972;1:585–90.

5. Gaddie J, Petrie GR, Reid IW, et al. Aerosol beclomethasone dipropionate: a dose-response study in chronic bronchial asthma. Lancet 1973;2:280–1.

6. Kriz RJ, Chmelik F, doPico G, et al. A short-term double-blind trial of aerosol triamcinolone acetonide in steroid-dependent patients with severe asthma. Chest 1976;69:455–60.

7. Gerdtham UG, Hertzman P, Jonsson B, et al. Impact of inhaled corticosteroids on acute asthma hospitalization in Sweden 1978 to 1991. Med Care 1996;34:1188–98.

8. Blais L, Ernst P, Boivin JF, et al. Inhaled corticosteroids and the prevention of readmission to hospital for asthma. Am J Respir Crit Care Med 1998;158:126–32.

9. Suissa S, Ernst P, Benayoun S, et al. Low-dose inhaled corticosteroids and the prevention of death from asthma. N Engl J Med 2000;343:332–6.

10. Haahtela T, Jarvinen M, Kava T, et al. Comparison of a beta 2-agonist, terbutaline, with an inhaled corticosteroid, budesonide, in newly detected asthma. N Engl J Med 1991;325:388–92.

11. Djukanovic R, Roche WR, Wilson JW, et al. Mucosal inflammation in asthma. Am Rev Respir Dis 1990;142:434–57.

12. Kay AB. Allergy and allergic diseases. First of two parts. N Engl J Med 2001;344:30–7.

13. Corrigan C. The eotaxins in asthma and allergic inflammation: implications for therapy. Curr Opin Investig Drugs 2000;1:321–8.

14. Djukanovic R, Wilson JW, Britten KM, et al. Effect of an inhaled corticosteroid on airway inflammation and symptoms in asthma. Am Rev Respir Dis 1992;145:669–74.

15. Laitinen LA, Laitinen A, Haahtela T. A comparative study of the effects of an inhaled corticosteroid, budesonide, and a beta 2-agonist, terbutaline, on airway inflammation in newly diagnosed asthma: a randomized, double-blind, parallel-group controlled trial. J Allergy Clin Immunol 1992;90:32–42.

16. Aldridge RE, Hancox RJ, Robin TD, et al. Effects of terbutaline and budesonide on sputum cells and bronchial hyperresponsiveness in asthma. Am J Respir Crit Care Med 2000;161:1459–64.

17. Fahy JV, Boushey HA. Effect of low-dose beclomethasone dipropionate on asthma control and airway inflammation. Eur Respir J 1998;11:1240–7.

18. Jatakanon A, Lim S, Chung KF, et al. An inhaled steroid improves markers of airway inflammation in patients with mild asthma. Eur Respir J 1998;12:1084–8.

19. van Rensen EL, Straathof KC, Veselic-Charvat MA, et al. Effect of inhaled steroids on airway hyperresponsiveness, sputum eosinophils, and exhaled nitric oxide levels in patients with asthma. Thorax 1999;54:403–8.

20. Meijer RJ, Kerstjens HA, Arends LR, et al. Effects of inhaled fluticasone and oral prednisolone on clinical and inflammatory parameters in patients with asthma. Thorax 1999;54:894–9.

21. Corrigan CJ, Haczku A, Gemou-Engesaeth V, et al. CD4 T-lymphocyte activation in asthma is accompanied by increased serum concentrations of interleukin-5. Effect of glucocorticoid therapy. Am Rev Respir Dis 1993;147:540–7.

22. Lilly CM, Nakamura H, Kesselman H, et al. Expression of eotaxin by human lung epithelial cells: induction by cytokines and inhibition by glucocorticoids. J Clin Invest 1997;99:1767–73.

23. Maneechotesuwan K, Yao X, Ito K, et al. Suppression of GATA-3 nuclear import and phosphorylation: a novel mechanism of corticosteroid action in allergic disease. PLoS Med 2009;6:e1000076.

24. Pauwels RA, Pedersen S, Busse WW, et al. Early intervention with budesonide in mild persistent asthma: a randomised, double-blind trial. Lancet 2003;361:1071–6.

25. Pauwels RA, Lofdahl CG, Laitinen LA, et al. Long-term treatment with inhaled budesonide in persons with mild chronic obstructive pulmonary disease who continue smoking. European Respiratory Society Study on Chronic Obstructive Pulmonary Disease. N Engl J Med 1999;340:1948–53.

26. James AL, Palmer LJ, Kicic E, et al. Decline in lung function in the Busselton Health Study: the effects of asthma and cigarette smoking. Am J Respir Crit Care Med 2005;171:109–14.

27. Lange P, Parner J, Vestbo J, et al. 15-year follow-up study of ventilatory function in adults with asthma. N Engl J Med 1998;339:1194–200.

28. O'Byrne PM, Pedersen S, Busse WW, et al. Effects of early intervention with inhaled budesonide on lung function in newly diagnosed asthma. Chest 2006;129:1478–85.

29. Sont JK, Willems LN, Bel EH, et al. Clinical control and histopathologic outcome of asthma when using airway hyperresponsiveness as an additional guide to long-term treatment. The AMPUL Study Group. Am J Respir Crit Care Med 1999;159:1043–51.

30. Ward C, Pais M, Bish R, et al. Airway inflammation, basement membrane thickening and bronchial hyperresponsiveness in asthma. Thorax 2002;57:309–16.

31. Cokugras H, Akcakaya N, Seckin I, et al. Ultrastructural examination of bronchial biopsy

specimens from children with moderate asthma. Thorax 2001;56:25–9.

32. Jenkins HA, Cool C, Szefler SJ, et al. Histopathology of severe childhood asthma: a case series. Chest 2003;124:32–41.

33. Davies DE, Wicks J, Powell RM, et al. Airway remodeling in asthma: new insights. J Allergy Clin Immunol 2003;111:215–25.

34. Grainge CL, Lau LC, Ward JA, et al. Effect of bronchoconstriction on airway remodeling in asthma. N Engl J Med 2011;364:2006–15.

35. Bateman ED, Boushey HA, Bousquet J, et al. Can guideline-defined asthma control be achieved? The Gaining Optimal Asthma Control study. Am J Respir Crit Care Med 2004;170:836–44.

36. Antonicelli L, Bucca C, Neri M, et al. Asthma severity and medical resource utilisation. Eur Respir J 2004;23:723–9.

37. Barnes PJ, Jonsson B, Klim JB. The costs of asthma. Eur Respir J 1996;9:636–42.

38. Godard P, Chanez P, Siraudin L, et al. Costs of asthma are correlated with severity: a 1-yr prospective study. Eur Respir J 2002;19:61–7.

39. Serra-Batlles J, Plaza V, Morejon E, et al. Costs of asthma according to the degree of severity. Eur Respir J 1998;12:1322–6.

40. Proceedings of the ATS workshop on refractory asthma: current understanding, recommendations, and unanswered questions. American Thoracic Society. Am J Respir Crit Care Med 2000;162:2341–51.

41. Chanez P, Wenzel SE, Anderson GP, et al. Severe asthma in adults: what are the important questions? J Allergy Clin Immunol 2007;119:1337–48.

42. Jatakanon A, Uasuf C, Maziak W, et al. Neutrophilic inflammation in severe persistent asthma. Am J Respir Crit Care Med 1999;160:1532–9.

43. Louis R, Lau LC, Bron AO, et al. The relationship between airways inflammation and asthma severity. Am J Respir Crit Care Med 2000;161:9–16.

44. Wenzel SE, Schwartz LB, Langmack EL, et al. Evidence that severe asthma can be divided pathologically into two inflammatory subtypes with distinct physiologic and clinical characteristics. Am J Respir Crit Care Med 1999;160:1001–8.

45. ten Brinke A, Grootendorst DC, Schmidt JT, et al. Chronic sinusitis in severe asthma is related to sputum eosinophilia. J Allergy Clin Immunol 2002;109:621–6.

46. The ENFUMOSA cross-sectional European multicentre study of the clinical phenotype of chronic severe asthma. European Network for Understanding Mechanisms of Severe Asthma. Eur Respir J 2003;22:470–7.

47. ten Brinke A, Zwinderman AH, Sterk PJ, et al. "Refractory" eosinophilic airway inflammation in severe asthma: effect of parenteral corticosteroids. Am J Respir Crit Care Med 2004;170:601–5.

48. Green RH, Brightling CE, McKenna S, et al. Asthma exacerbations and sputum eosinophil counts: a randomised controlled trial. Lancet 2002;360:1715–21.

49. Jayaram L, Pizzichini MM, Cook RJ, et al. Determining asthma treatment by monitoring sputum cell counts: effect on exacerbations. Eur Respir J 2006;27:483–94.

50. Duncan CJ, Lawrie A, Blaylock MG, et al. Reduced eosinophil apoptosis in induced sputum correlates with asthma severity. Eur Respir J 2003;22:484–90.

51. Barnes PJ, Adcock IM. Glucocorticoid resistance in inflammatory diseases. Lancet 2009;373:1905–17.

52. Baraniuk JN, Ali M, Brody D, et al. Glucocorticoids induce beta2-adrenergic receptor function in human nasal mucosa. Am J Respir Crit Care Med 1997;155:704–10.

53. Mak JC, Nishikawa M, Barnes PJ. Glucocorticosteroids increase beta 2-adrenergic receptor transcription in human lung. Am J Physiol 1995;268:L41–6.

54. Roth M, Johnson PR, Rudiger JJ, et al. Interaction between glucocorticoids and beta2 agonists on bronchial airway smooth muscle cells through synchronised cellular signalling. Lancet 2002;360:1293–9.

55. Thomson NC, Spears M. The influence of smoking on the treatment response in patients with asthma. Curr Opin Allergy Clin Immunol 2005;5:57–63.

56. Barnes PJ. Reduced histone deacetylase in COPD: clinical implications. Chest 2006;129:151–5.

57. Hew M, Bhavsar P, Torrego A, et al. Relative corticosteroid insensitivity of peripheral blood mononuclear cells in severe asthma. Am J Respir Crit Care Med 2006;174:134–41.

58. Ito K, Ito M, Elliott WM, et al. Decreased histone deacetylase activity in chronic obstructive pulmonary disease. N Engl J Med 2005;352:1967–76.

59. Irusen E, Matthews JG, Takahashi A, et al. p38 mitogen-activated protein kinase-induced glucocorticoid receptor phosphorylation reduces its activity: role in steroid-insensitive asthma. J Allergy Clin Immunol 2002;109:649–57.

60. Matthews JG, Ito K, Barnes PJ, et al. Defective glucocorticoid receptor nuclear translocation and altered histone acetylation patterns in glucocorticoid-resistant patients. J Allergy Clin Immunol 2004;113:1100–8.

61. Goleva E, Li LB, Eves PT, et al. Increased glucocorticoid receptor beta alters steroid response in glucocorticoid-insensitive asthma. Am J Respir Crit Care Med 2006;173:607–16.

62. Pujols L, Mullol J, Picado C. Alpha and beta glucocorticoid receptors: relevance in airway diseases. Curr Allergy Asthma Rep 2007;7:93–9.

63. Alcorn JF, Crowe CR, Kolls JK. TH17 cells in asthma and COPD. Annu Rev Physiol 2010;72: 495–516.

64. McKinley L, Alcorn JF, Peterson A, et al. TH17 cells mediate steroid-resistant airway inflammation and airway hyperresponsiveness in mice. J Immunol 2008;181:4089–97.

65. Peters SP, Kunselman SJ, Icitovic N, et al. Tiotropium bromide step-up therapy for adults with uncontrolled asthma. N Engl J Med 2010;363: 1715–26.

66. Hanania NA, Alpan O, Hamilos DL, et al. Omalizumab in severe allergic asthma inadequately controlled with standard therapy: a randomized trial. Ann Intern Med 2011;154:573–82.

67. Humbert M, Beasley R, Ayres J, et al. Benefits of omalizumab as add-on therapy in patients with severe persistent asthma who are inadequately controlled despite best available therapy (GINA 2002 step 4 treatment): INNOVATE. Allergy 2005; 60:309–16.

68. Louis R. Anti-IgE: a significant breakthrough in the treatment of airway allergic diseases. Allergy 2004; 59:698–700.

69. Djukanovic R, Wilson SJ, Kraft M, et al. Effects of treatment with anti-immunoglobulin E antibody omalizumab on airway inflammation in allergic asthma. Am J Respir Crit Care Med 2004;170: 583–93.

70. van Rensen EL, Evertse CE, van Schadewijk WA, et al. Eosinophils in bronchial mucosa of asthmatics after allergen challenge: effect of anti-IgE treatment. Allergy 2009;64:72–80.

71. Wu AC, Paltiel AD, Kuntz KM, et al. Cost-effectiveness of omalizumab in adults with severe asthma: results from the Asthma Policy Model. J Allergy Clin Immunol 2007;120:1146–52.

72. Manise M, Schleich F, Gusbin N, et al. Cytokine production from sputum cells and blood leukocytes in asthmatics according to disease severity. Allergy 2010;65:889–96.

73. Cho SH, Stanciu LA, Holgate ST, et al. Increased interleukin-4, interleukin-5, and interferon-gamma in airway CD4+ and CD8+ T cells in atopic asthma. Am J Respir Crit Care Med 2005;171:224–30.

74. Haldar P, Brightling CE, Hargadon B, et al. Mepolizumab and exacerbations of refractory eosinophilic asthma. N Engl J Med 2009;360:973–84.

75. Nair P, Pizzichini MM, Kjarsgaard M, et al. Mepolizumab for prednisone-dependent asthma with sputum eosinophilia. N Engl J Med 2009;360:985–93.

76. Kips JC, O'Connor BJ, Langley SJ, et al. Effect of SCH55700, a humanized anti-human interleukin-5 antibody, in severe persistent asthma: a pilot study. Am J Respir Crit Care Med 2003;167:1655–9.

77. Leckie MJ, ten Brinke A, Khan J, et al. Effects of an interleukin-5 blocking monoclonal antibody on eosinophils, airway hyper-responsiveness, and the late asthmatic response. Lancet 2000;356:2144–8.

78. Castro M, Mathur S, Hargreave F, et al. Reslizumab for poorly controlled, eosinophilic asthma: a randomized, placebo-controlled study. Am J Respir Crit Care Med 2011;184:1125–32.

79. Berry MA, Hargadon B, Shelley M, et al. Evidence of a role of tumor necrosis factor alpha in refractory asthma. N Engl J Med 2006;354:697–708.

80. Howarth PH, Babu KS, Arshad HS, et al. Tumour necrosis factor (TNF alpha) as a novel therapeutic target in symptomatic corticosteroid dependent asthma. Thorax 2005;60:1012–8.

81. Morjaria JB, Chauhan AJ, Babu KS, et al. The role of a soluble TNF alpha receptor fusion protein (etanercept) in corticosteroid refractory asthma: a double blind, randomised, placebo controlled trial. Thorax 2008;63:584–91.

82. Erin EM, Leaker BR, Nicholson GC, et al. The effects of a monoclonal antibody directed against tumor necrosis factor-alpha in asthma. Am J Respir Crit Care Med 2006;174:753–62.

83. Wenzel SE, Barnes PJ, Bleecker ER, et al. A randomized, double-blind, placebo-controlled study of tumor necrosis factor-alpha blockade in severe persistent asthma. Am J Respir Crit Care Med 2009;179:549–58.

84. Holgate ST, Noonan M, Chanez P, et al. Efficacy and safety of etanercept in moderate-to-severe asthma: a randomised, controlled trial. Eur Respir J 2011;37:1352–9.

85. Simpson JL, Powell H, Boyle MJ, et al. Clarithromycin targets neutrophilic airway inflammation in refractory asthma. Am J Respir Crit Care Med 2008;177:148–55.

86. Louis R, Djukanovic R. Is the neutrophil a worthy target in severe asthma and chronic obstructive pulmonary disease? Clin Exp Allergy 2006;36: 563–7.

87. Keatings VM, Barnes PJ. Granulocyte activation markers in induced sputum: comparison between chronic obstructive pulmonary disease, asthma, and normal subjects. Am J Respir Crit Care Med 1997;155:449–53.

88. Moermans C, Heinen V, Nguyen M, et al. Local and systemic cellular inflammation and cytokine release in chronic obstructive pulmonary disease. Cytokine 2011;56:298–304.

89. Albert RK, Connett J, Bailey WC, et al. Azithromycin for prevention of exacerbations of COPD. N Engl J Med 2011;365:689–98.

90. Martinez FJ, Curtis JL, Albert R. Role of macrolide therapy in chronic obstructive pulmonary disease. Int J Chron Obstruct Pulmon Dis 2008;3:331–50.

91. Barnes PJ. New therapies for asthma: is there any progress? Trends Pharmacol Sci 2010;31: 335–43.

92. Cox G, Thomson NC, Rubin AS, et al. Asthma control during the year after bronchial thermoplasty. N Engl J Med 2007;356:1327–37.

93. Cox G. Bronchial thermoplasty for severe asthma. Curr Opin Pulm Med 2011;17:34–8.

94. Pavord ID, Cox G, Thomson NC, et al. Safety and efficacy of bronchial thermoplasty in symptomatic, severe asthma. Am J Respir Crit Care Med 2007; 176:1185–91.

95. Castro M, Rubin AS, Laviolette M, et al. Effectiveness and safety of bronchial thermoplasty in the treatment of severe asthma: a multicenter, randomized, double-blind, sham-controlled clinical trial. Am J Respir Crit Care Med 2010;181:116–24.

96. Louis R, Sele J, Henket M, et al. Sputum eosinophil count in a large population of patients with mild to moderate steroid-naive asthma: distribution and relationship with methacholine bronchial hyperresponsiveness. Allergy 2002;57:907–12.

97. Gibson PG, Simpson JL, Saltos N. Heterogeneity of airway inflammation in persistent asthma: evidence of neutrophilic inflammation and increased sputum interleukin-8. Chest 2001;119: 1329–36.

98. Simpson JL, Scott R, Boyle MJ, et al. Inflammatory subtypes in asthma: assessment and identification using induced sputum. Respirology 2006;11: 54–61.

99. Green RH, Brightling CE, Woltmann G, et al. Analysis of induced sputum in adults with asthma: identification of subgroup with isolated sputum neutrophilia and poor response to inhaled corticosteroids. Thorax 2002;57:875–9.

100. Anderson GP. Endotyping asthma: new insights into key pathogenic mechanisms in a complex, heterogeneous disease. Lancet 2008;372:1107–19.

101. Douwes J, Gibson P, Pekkanen J, et al. Non-eosinophilic asthma: importance and possible mechanisms. Thorax 2002;57:643–8.

102. Kharitonov SA, Yates D, Robbins RA, et al. Increased nitric oxide in exhaled air of asthmatic patients. Lancet 1994;343:133–5.

103. Berry MA, Shaw DE, Green RH, et al. The use of exhaled nitric oxide concentration to identify eosinophilic airway inflammation: an observational study in adults with asthma. Clin Exp Allergy 2005;35: 1175–9.

104. Schleich FN, Seidel L, Sele J, et al. Exhaled nitric oxide thresholds associated with a sputum eosinophil count ≥3% in a cohort of unselected patients with asthma. Thorax 2010;65:1039–44.

105. Szefler SJ, Martin RJ, King TS, et al. Significant variability in response to inhaled corticosteroids for persistent asthma. J Allergy Clin Immunol 2002;109:410–8.

106. Berry M, Morgan A, Shaw DE, et al. Pathological features and inhaled corticosteroid response of eosinophilic and non-eosinophilic asthma. Thorax 2007;62:1043–9.

107. Cowan DC, Cowan JO, Palmay R, et al. Effects of steroid therapy on inflammatory cell subtypes in asthma. Thorax 2010;65:384–90.

108. Meijer RJ, Postma DS, Kauffman HF, et al. Accuracy of eosinophils and eosinophil cationic protein to predict steroid improvement in asthma. Clin Exp Allergy 2002;32:1096–103.

109. Pavord ID, Brightling CE, Woltmann G, et al. Non-eosinophilic corticosteroid unresponsive asthma. Lancet 1999;353:2213–4.

110. Smith AD, Cowan JO, Brassett KP, et al. Exhaled nitric oxide: a predictor of steroid response. Am J Respir Crit Care Med 2005;172:453–9.

111. Woodruff PG, Modrek B, Choy DF, et al. T-helper type 2-driven inflammation defines major subphenotypes of asthma. Am J Respir Crit Care Med 2009;180:388–95.

112. Godon P, Boulet LP, Malo JL, et al. Assessment and evaluation of symptomatic steroid-naive asthmatics without sputum eosinophilia and their response to inhaled corticosteroids. Eur Respir J 2002;20: 1364–9.

113. Bacci E, Cianchetti S, Bartoli M, et al. Low sputum eosinophils predict the lack of response to beclomethasone in symptomatic asthmatic patients. Chest 2006;129:565–72.

114. Culpitt SV, Maziak W, Loukidis S, et al. Effect of high dose inhaled steroid on cells, cytokines, and proteases in induced sputum in chronic obstructive pulmonary disease. Am J Respir Crit Care Med 1999;160:1635–9.

115. Keatings VM, Jatakanon A, Worsdell YM, et al. Effects of inhaled and oral glucocorticoids on inflammatory indices in asthma and COPD. Am J Respir Crit Care Med 1997;155:542–8.

116. Tantisira KG, Lasky-Su J, Harada M, et al. Genome-wide association between GLCCI1 and response to glucocorticoid therapy in asthma. N Engl J Med 2011;365:1173–83.

117. Cochrane MG, Bala MV, Downs KE, et al. Inhaled corticosteroids for asthma therapy: patient compliance, devices, and inhalation technique. Chest 2000;117:542–50.

118. Price D, Musgrave SD, Shepstone L, et al. Leukotriene antagonists as first-line or add-on asthma-controller therapy. N Engl J Med 2011;364: 1695–707.

119. Barnes PJ. Scientific rationale for using a single inhaler for asthma control. Eur Respir J 2007;29: 587–95.

120. Louis R, Joos G, Michils A, et al. A comparison of budesonide/formoterol maintenance and reliever therapy vs. conventional best practice in asthma management. Int J Clin Pract 2009; 63:1479–88.

121. Corren J, Lemanske RF, Hanania NA, et al. Lebrikizumab treatment in adults with asthma. N Engl J Med 2011;365:1088–98.

122. Balzar S, Fajt ML, Comhair SA, et al. Mast cell phenotype, location, and activation in severe asthma. Data from the Severe Asthma Research Program. Am J Respir Crit Care Med 2011;183:299–309.

123. Pettipher R, Hansel TT, Armer R. Antagonism of the prostaglandin D2 receptors DP1 and CRTH2 as an approach to treat allergic diseases. Nat Rev Drug Discov 2007;6:313–25.

124. Barnes PJ. New molecular targets for the treatment of neutrophilic diseases. J Allergy Clin Immunol 2007;119:1055–62.

Airway Smooth Muscle in Asthma
Just a Target for Bronchodilation?

Judith L. Black, MD, PhD[a], Reynold A. Panettieri Jr, MD[b],
Audreesh Banerjee, MD[b], Patrick Berger, MD, PhD[c,d,e,*]

KEYWORDS

- Bronchodilators • Hyperresponsiveness • Inflammation • Remodeling • Smooth muscle

KEY POINTS

- A better knowledge of the various roles of airway smooth muscle (ASM) in the pathophysiology of asthma is necessary to understand that ASM is not just a target for bronchodilation.
- Changes in ASM contractile properties or impaired function of relaxant receptors play an important role in the development of bronchial hyperresponsiveness in asthma.
- The roles of ASM in the pathophysiology of asthma are complex and need further specific pharmaceutical developments.

INTRODUCTION

Asthma is a chronic disease, characterized by the association of bronchial hyperresponsiveness (BHR), inflammation, and remodeling.[1] Airway smooth muscle (ASM) has long been recognized as the main cell type responsible for bronchial contraction and BHR.[2] It has, thus, been logically considered as the key target for bronchodilation. Regarding asthmatic inflammation, a high number of eosinophils infiltrate bronchial epithelium and submucosa,[3] but there is apparently no eosinophil infiltration of the ASM layer.[4] However, other inflammatory cells, such as mast cells[4] or T lymphocytes,[5] have been shown to infiltrate the ASM, suggesting a complex relationship between ASM cells and inflammatory cells and even a possible role for ASM to organize inflammation. Asthmatic bronchial remodeling is characterized by various structural changes, including abnormal epithelium, subepithelial membrane thickening, alteration of the extracellular matrix (ECM) deposition, neoangiogenesis, mucus gland hypertrophy, and increased ASM mass.[6] Recent evidence

All authors contributed equally to this article.
Financial disclosures and conflicts of interest: Grant support for R.A.P. is from NIEHS ES013508 and NIH HL097796; Grant support for P.B. is from ANR N 2010 CESA 001 01 (2010-0145). P.B. has received fees for speaking or consulting from Novartis, Glaxo-Smith Kline, Astra-Zeneca, Nycomed, Boehringer, and Chiesi and has received funds for research from Novartis, Glaxo-Smith Kline, and Nycomed. Travel to the European Respiratory Society and American Thoracic Society Congress was funded by Novartis, Glaxo-Smith Kline, and Astra-Zeneca.
[a] University of Sydney, Discipline of Pharmacology and Woolcock Institute of Medical Research, University of Sydney, Sydney, New South Wales, 2006, Australia; [b] Pulmonary, Allergy and Critical Care Division, Department of Medicine, Perelman School of Medicine, University of Pennsylvania, Airways Biology Initiative, Philadelphia, PA 19104-3403, USA; [c] Univ Bordeaux, Centre de Recherche Cardio-thoracique de Bordeaux, F-33000 Bordeaux, France; [d] INSERM, U1045, CIC 0005, F-33000 Bordeaux, France; [e] CHU de Bordeaux, Service d'Exploration Fonctionnelle Respiratoire, CIC0005, F-33604 Pessac, France
* Corresponding author. Centre de Recherche Cardio-thoracique de Bordeaux, INSERM U1045, Equipe: Remodelage bronchique, Université Bordeaux Segalen, 146 rue Léo Saignat, F33076 Bordeaux Cedex, France.
E-mail address: patrick.berger@u-bordeaux2.fr

chestmed.theclinics.com

suggests that the increased ASM mass is the key feature of bronchial remodeling in asthma because, on the one hand, it is associated with severe asthma phenotype[7] and, on the other hand, it is correlated with a decrease in lung function.[5,8]

This article reviews the main concepts about the 3 possible roles of ASM in asthma: (1) contractile tone, (2) inflammatory response, and (3) remodeling.

ASM SHORTENING AND RELAXATION

In normal airways, ASM cell contraction regulates airway caliber and bronchomotor tone. Using isolated bronchial preparations, studies have compared the isotonic length or force generation of tissues derived from patients with asthma and those without asthma. Not all studies demonstrated an increased force generation in asthmatic tissues when compared with control tissues.[9] These conflicting data likely can be attributed to differences in the experimental and methodological approaches used.[10] Several parameters, such as the degree of tissue elastance, smooth muscle mass, and knowledge of the optimal length, were found to be important factors when evaluating the force-generating capacity of ASM preparations derived from patients with asthma.[9,10]

Although conflicting data exist in studies comparing smooth muscle responsiveness between normal subjects and patients with asthma, several studies report that passive sensitization of human ASM with asthmatic serum induces a nonspecific increase in smooth muscle responsiveness,[11–14] demonstrating the existence of mediators in the serum of patients with asthma that promote airway responsiveness. Although the precise nature of these mediators remains incompletely defined, evidence suggests that tumor necrosis factor (TNF)-α, interleukin (IL)-13, or IL-1β can induce BHR in both humans and animals. Cytokines also can prime ASM to become hyperresponsive to contractile agonists in vitro, supporting the concept that cytokines modulate agonist-induced ASM contractile function. Other proinflammatory mediators, such as lysophosphatidic acid, a bioactive lipid released from activated platelets, phospholipase A_2 and leukotriene C4, also enhance ASM responsiveness in vitro to contractile agonists, such as acetylcholine, methacholine, and serotonin. Together, these studies suggest that proinflammatory mediators induce BHR by enhancing ASM contraction or altering ASM relaxation (Fig. 1). Understanding the mechanisms by which inflammatory mediators modulate ASM contractile reactivity may offer new insight into the molecular mechanisms that modulate BHR in asthma.[15]

The level of intracellular calcium regulates, in part, ASM shortening. The activation of an ASM cell by an agonist induces a rapid increase in intracellular calcium concentration ($[Ca^{2+}]_i$), associated with the release of intracellular calcium stores, to a peak level roughly tenfold higher than the resting level (100 nM to greater than 1 μM with maximum agonist stimulation). Following this peak, calcium levels decrease but remain elevated provided that the excitatory stimulus remains present. The elevation in $[Ca^{2+}]_i$ activates the calcium/calmodulin-sensitive myosin light chain kinase, leading to phosphorylation of the regulatory myosin light chain (MLC_{20}) at Serine 19. Phosphorylation of this residue by myosin ATPase activity initiates cross-bridge cycling between myosin and actin. ATP binding, hydrolysis, and ADP release continue as long as MLC_{20} is phosphorylated; dephosphorylation by the MLC phosphatase terminates cross-bridge cycling and relaxes smooth muscle.[16]

Considering the central role of Ca^{2+} in regulating ASM contractile function, investigators postulate that alterations in Ca^{2+} regulatory mechanisms likely impair ASM contractility. Studies using cultured human tracheal or bronchial smooth muscle cells, as in vitro models of ASM responsiveness, convincingly demonstrated that G protein–coupled receptors (GPCR)–associated signaling in ASM can be modulated by a variety of inflammatory stimuli. Cytokines, such as TNF-α, augment agonist-induced ASM contractility by enhancing, in a nonspecific manner, agonist-evoked Ca^{2+} transients (to bradykinin, carbachol).[15] The hypothesis that changes in GPCR-associated Ca^{2+} signaling represent an important mechanism underlying the development of BHR has also been supported by other studies. Tao and colleagues[17] showed that ASM cells derived from hyperresponsive inbred rats have an augmented bradykinin-induced Ca^{2+} response when compared with ASM cells derived from normoresponsive rats. Deshpande and colleagues[18] demonstrated that in addition to TNF-α, other cytokines, including IL-1β and, to a lesser degree, interferon (IFN)γ, augment Ca^{2+} responses induced by carbachol, bradykinin, and thrombin. In a similar manner, IL-13, a T-helper type 2 (Th2) important mediator in allergic asthma,[19] also nonspecifically increased Ca^{2+} responses to agonists.[20–23] Microarray technology used to study the modulation of gene expression of ASM by IL-13 revealed a diversity of potential molecular mechanisms influencing ASM responsiveness, including changes in cytoskeletal proteins, receptors, or calcium regulators.[24] Together, these data show that proasthmatic cytokines, in a nonspecific manner, enhance GPCR-associated Ca^{2+} responses in ASM, a mechanism likely to affect ASM contractility.

Reports in C3H/HeJ, Balb/C, and A/J mice revealed that differences in ASM contractility among species may not require changes in GPCR

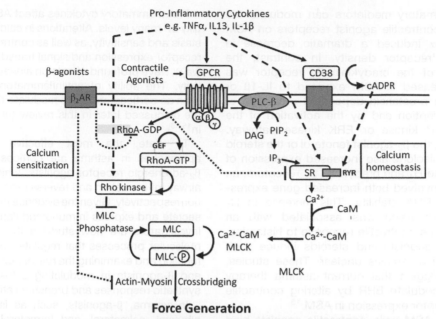

Force Generation

Fig. 1. Excitation-contraction coupling in ASM. Effects of proinflammatory cytokines and β_2-adrenergic receptor agonists on excitation-contraction coupling in ASM cells. Contractile agonists activate receptors that influence intracellular signaling, affecting calcium homeostasis and sensitization as well as the function and expression of GPCRs and CD38. Inflammatory cytokines bind to receptors and modulate calcium homeostasis by increasing expression of CD38 and increasing Ca^{2+} release from the sarcoplasmic reticulum. Inflammatory cytokines, such as IL-13, IL-1β, and TNF-α, also increase Rho kinase activity to modulate the calcium sensitization pathways. β_2-adrenergic receptor agonists regulate calcium homeostasis and calcium sensitization by inhibiting RhoA activation, Ca^{2+} release from the sarcoplasmic reticulum, and actin-myosin cross bridging. β_2AR, β_2-adrenergic receptor; cADPR, cyclic ADP ribose; CaM, calmodulin; DAG, diacylglycerol; GEF, guanine exchange factor; GPCR, G protein–coupled receptor; IP$_3$, inositol triphosphate; MLC, myosin light chain; MLCK, myosin light chain kinase; PIP$_2$, phosphatidylinositol 4,5 biphosphate; PLC, phospholipase C; RyR, ryanodine receptor; SR, sarcoplasmic reticulum.

agonist–induced Ca^{2+} responses but rather involve changes in the Ca^{2+} sensitivity of the contractile apparatus.[25] A possible mechanism involves the small monomeric G protein Rho that can augment ASM contractility by increasing levels of MLC phosphorylation via the Rho-activated kinase (ROCK)–dependent suppression of MLC phosphatase.[26,27] Both RhoA and ROCK are activated by a variety of stimuli associated with the development of BHR, including cytokines,[28–31] sphingolipids,[32–34] mechanical stress,[35] and isoprostane.[36] The RhoA/Rho kinase pathway regulates the expression of serum response factor–dependent smooth muscle–specific genes in canine ASM cells,[37] a mechanism that identifies the importance of the Rho kinase pathway in maintaining a contractile phenotype recently described in bovine ASM tissues.[38] Rho pathways modulate diverse cellular responses in ASM cells, including the regulation of Ca^{2+} influx[39] and cell proliferation.[40] Possibly, abnormal RhoA activity or expression will dramatically alter ASM contractility not only via the Ca^{2+} sensitization but also through the increased

expression of Rho-dependent contractile proteins. A report using the Y-27632 inhibitor confirmed that the nonspecific BHR and the specific allergen responsiveness induced by passive sensitization requires the activation of Rho kinase.[41]

Changes in ASM contractile properties play an important role in the development of BHR associated with chronic airway diseases, such as asthma. In vitro studies support the concept that a variety of proasthmatic signals, such as physical (repeated stretch) or chemical exposures (cytokines), drastically augment ASM contractile force by altering multiple key pathways: (1) via the aberrant activation of contractile or impaired function of relaxant receptors (desensitization), (2) the alteration of Ca^{2+} regulatory signaling molecules (CD38, sarco/endoplasmic reticulum Ca^{2+}-ATPase, Ca^{2+} channels), and (3) the activity of elements of the contractile apparatus through Rho-dependent pathways. Defining the inflammatory signals (factors and associated mechanisms) involved in the regulation of ASM responsiveness may represent a potential new target for the treatment of BHR.

Proinflammatory mediators can modulate the density of contractile agonist receptors on ASM cells. TNF-α induced a dramatic decrease in muscarinic receptor density. In contrast, the expression of the bradykinin B_2 receptor was rapidly increased in ASM exposed to IL-1β or TNF-α by a prostanoid-dependent regulation of gene transcription and by the activation of the Ras/Raf/MAP kinase or ERK kinase pathway. Surprisingly, the β_2-agonist fenoterol or the steroid methylprednisolone also increased expression of the histamine H_1 and bradykinin B_2 receptors, an effect that involved both increased gene expression and mRNA stability. This increase in H_1 receptor expression was associated with an increase in the contractile response to histamine. Whether β_2-agonists and steroids induce such effects in vivo remains unclear. These studies, however, suggest that current asthma therapy may also modulate BHR by altering contractile agonist receptor expression in ASM.[15]

In human ASM cells, contractile agonists bind GPCR and activate phospholipase C. The subsequent hydrolysis of phosphatidylinositol 4,5 bisphosphate into inositol triphosphate and diacylglycerol ultimately results in an increase in $[Ca^{2+}]_i$.[16] Because most of the inflammatory agents do not evoke either a calcium response or phosphoinositide hydrolysis in human ASM, the modulation of agonist-induced increases in $[Ca^{2+}]_i$ by extracellular stimuli may be caused by the modulation of downstream GPCR signaling. TNF-α increased the amount, as well as the activity, of G-proteins in several cell types, including ASM.[42,43] The finding that TNF-α potentiated calcium mobilization in response to sodium fluoride,[44] an agent that bypasses membrane receptors and directly activates G proteins,[45,46] supports the notion that TNF-α may act directly at the level of G proteins.

Studies now show that bradykinin-evoked phosphoinositide accumulation in human ASM is significantly enhanced by various cytokines, such as TNF-α and IL-1β.[44,47–49] The effect of cytokines on agonist-evoked calcium responses seems to be stimulus specific, however, because the pretreatment of ASM cells with IL-1β diminished phosphoinositide metabolism induced by histamine.[50] In addition to their effect on calcium signaling, cytokines may also modulate β_2-adrenergic function. TNF-α and IL-1β also suppress isoproterenol-stimulated activation of adenylyl cyclase.[51–53] A recent report showed that IL-13 is also able to impair ASM responsiveness to β_2-adrenergic stimuli,[54] showing that cytokines may promote BHR by impairing β_2-adrenergic responsiveness in ASM cells.

Proinflammatory cytokines affect ASM contractility on many levels. Alterations in calcium homeostasis and sensitivity, as well as contractile agonist receptor expression and signal transduction pathways, have profound effects on airway hyperreactivity. The ability of antiinflammatory therapies, such as corticosteroids, to modulate these effects are discussed later in this review (also reviewed in[15,55]).

To date, the most effective therapeutic approaches in asthma are corticosteroids and β_2-adrenergic receptor agonists, which abrogate airway inflammation and reverse bronchoconstriction respectively. Given the evidence that ASM cells secrete and express immunomodulatory proteins, investigators are now studying the cellular and molecular processes that regulate ASM synthetic function and examining the role of dexamethasone and β-agonists in modulating cytokine-induced synthetic responses and bronchodilation.

In asthma, β-agonists, such as isoproterenol, albuterol, salmeterol, and formoterol, are therapeutic agents that promote bronchodilation by stimulating receptors coupled to Gs and that, in turn, activate adenylyl cyclase, increase intracellular cyclic AMP concentration ($[cAMP]_i$), and stimulate cAMP-dependent protein kinase (A kinase) in ASM. In a similar manner, prostaglandin E2 (PGE$_2$), which is produced in large quantities at sites of inflammation, also increases $[cAMP]_i$ in human ASM cells and is a potent and effective bronchodilator.[56] Evidence suggests that $[cAMP]_i$ mobilizing agents in ASM cells also modulate cytokine-induced synthetic function. In TNF-α–stimulated ASM cells, both eotaxin and regulated upon activation, normal T-cell expressed, and secreted (RANTES) expression are effectively inhibited by isoproterenol, PGE$_2$, dibutyl-$[cAMP]_i$, or the phosphodiesterase inhibitors, rolipram and cilomast.[57–59] TNF-α–induced IL-8 secretion was also inhibited by the combination of $[cAMP]_i$ mobilizing agents and corticosteroids.[60] Similarly, sphingosine-1-phosphate, which activates a Gs protein coupled receptor and increases $[cAMP]_i$, abrogated TNF-α–induced RANTES secretion in ASM cells.[61]

In contrast to the effects of $[cAMP]_i$ on chemokine secretion, pharmacologic agents that increase $[cAMP]_i$ also markedly stimulate the secretion of IL-6 in human ASM cells.[57] This stimulation seems to be caused by the effects on basal IL-6 promoter activity.[62] Whether the secreted IL-6 modulates ASM cell function in an autocrine manner or alters leukocyte function in the submucosa remains unknown. Because studies show that overexpression of IL-6 decreases acetylcholine responsiveness in transgenic mice,[63] the role of IL-6 in asthma may be that of an antiinflammatory signal.

More recently, investigators reported that cAMP limits the secretion of granulocyte-macrophage colony-stimulating factor (GM-CSF) by ASM cells. Cyclooxygenase inhibitors reduce PGE_2 and enhance cytokine-induced secretion of GM-CSF,[64,65] whereas PDE type IV inhibitors reduce GM-CSF secretion in vitro and antigen-induced BHR in an animal model.[64,66] Taken together, current evidence suggests that some but not all proinflammatory functions in ASM cells are inhibited by $[cAMP]_i$ mobilizing agents.

Conflicting reports exist, however, concerning the effects of increased $[cAMP]_i$ on lymphocyte adhesion and migration through cytokine-activated endothelial cells.[67,68] The controversy regarding the role of $[cAMP]_i$ in modulating cell adhesion likely reflects differences in the cytokines used to stimulate endothelial cells or the temporal differences in the addition of the agonists used to increase $[cAMP]_i$. Far less is known concerning the effects of $[cAMP]_i$ on smooth muscle–leukocyte adhesion. In human ASM cells, the activation of $[cAMP]_i$-dependent pathways inhibited, in part, both the TNF-α–mediated induction of intercellular adhesion molecule 1 (ICAM-1) and vascular cell adhesion molecule 1 (VCAM-1) expression and the adhesion of activated T cells to ASM cells. The basal expression of ICAM-1 and VCAM-1, as well as the binding of activated T cells to unstimulated ASM, was resistant to increases in $[cAMP]_i$.[69] Together these studies suggest that cytokine-induced expression of cell adhesion molecules and T cell adhesion to ASM cells are modulated by changes in $[cAMP]_i$.

ASM CAN ALSO ORGANIZE INFLAMMATION

There is plenty of evidence that, in asthma, a complex relationship involves ASM and inflammatory cells. Indeed, ASM produces a variety of chemotactic mediators and expresses different adhesion molecules (**Table 1**), which can participate to both the recruitment and the microlocalization of inflammatory cells within the ASM. Asthmatic ASM is infiltrated by both mast cells[4] and T lymphocytes[5] but apparently not eosinophil.[4]

The mast cell infiltration of the ASM layer, also called mast cell myositis,[70] seemed to be a specific feature of asthma, compared with that of patients suffering from eosinophilic bronchitis and healthy subjects.[4,71] The ASM mast cell infiltration is observed in various asthma phenotypes, including eosinophilic and noneosinophilic asthma[72]; severe and nonsevere asthma[71,73–75]; and also atopic and nonatopic asthma, even if the number of mast cells were significantly higher in the ASM of patients with atopic asthma.[76] Moreover, asthma treatments,

including inhaled corticosteroids, did not change mast cell myositis.[71,73] The mechanism of such a myositis has been firstly related with the production of mast cell chemotactic factors by the ASM itself, through an auto-activation loop.[77] Indeed, on activation, mast cells release tryptase and proinflammatory cytokines, such as TNF-α, which stimulate the production of transforming growth factor (TGF)-β_1 and, to a lesser extent, stem cell factor (SCF) by ASM cells, which induce mast cell chemotaxis.[77] Moreover, ASM promotes mast cell chemotaxis through the secretion of a wide array of chemotactic factors, on stimulation by Th1,[78] Th2,[78,79] or proinflammatory cytokines.[77,80] ASM also produces functionally active CXCL10[78]; CXCL8[79]; CCL11[79]; and CX_3CL1,[80] even if for CX_3CL1, the additional presence of vasoactive intestinal peptide is necessary.[80] Taken together, mast cell migration is induced by the production of various mediators secreted by the ASM itself, which is closely related to the ASM inflammatory microenvironment.

Once present within the ASM bundle, mast cells can adhere to ASM. This adhesion has been initially reported to be a cell-cell direct interaction involving an immunoglobulin (Ig) superfamily member (ie, cell adhesion molecule 1 [CADM1]), previously known as tumor suppressor in lung cancer (TLSC-1) (**Fig. 2**).[81,82] However, blocking CADM1 partially reduced the adhesion of mast cells to ASM, suggesting an alternative mechanism.[81] Indeed, mast cell–ASM adherence also involved cell-ECM-cell interaction through type I collagen, CD44, and CD51 (see **Fig. 2**).[83] This adhesion was improved under inflammatory conditions or using asthmatic ASM cells.[83] These latter in vitro findings are in agreement with ex vivo ultrastructural analysis of asthmatic ASM using electron microscopy.[84] Indeed, such analysis did not demonstrate any direct cell-cell contact between ASM and mast cells but only close contacts without tight junction.[84] Most mast cells infiltrating the asthmatic ASM bundles are typically of the MC_{TC} phenotype, containing both tryptase and chymase.[4,85,86] These mast cells infiltrate the ASM of both large and small airways and exhibit marked features of chronic ongoing activation.[74,76] Such findings were also confirmed by ultrastructural analysis of asthmatic ASM using electron microscopy.[84] However, little is known about the mechanisms by which mast cell activation may occur within the ASM layer.[87] Mast cell degranulation may result from IgE-dependent activation, especially in atopic patients.[76] However, IgE-independent mechanisms have also been evoked, following mast cell–ASM interaction through the complement C3a or SCF,[82,88–90] for instance, or following bacterial or viral infection through Toll-like receptors.[87]

Table 1
ASM production of chemotactic mediators and adhesion molecules

Factors	Spontaneous	After Stimulation	References
Chemokines			
CCL2 (MCP-1)	-	+ (IL-1β, TNF-α)	Watson et al[146], Pype et al[147]
CCL5 (RANTES)	-	+ (IL-1β, TNF-α)	Pype et al[147], John et al[148], Amrani et al[149]
CCL11 (eotaxin)	+	+ (IL-1β, TNF-α)	Brightling et al[78], Chung et al[150], Ghaffar et al[151]
CCL19 (MIP-3β)	+	...	Kaur et al[95]
CXCL8 (IL-8)		+ (IL-1α, IL-1β, TNF-α)	Brightling et al[78], Watson et al[146], John et al[152]
CXCL9 (Mig)	-	+ (IFN-γ, IL-1β, TNF-α)	Brightling et al[78]
CXCL10 (IP-10)	-	+ (IFN-γ, IL-1β, TNF-α)	Brightling et al[78]
CXCL12 (SDF-1α)	-	+ (IFN-γ, IL-1β, TNF-α)	Brightling et al[78]
CX₃CL1 (fractalkine)	-	+ (TNF-α)	El-Shazly et al[80]
Cytokines			
SCF	+	...	Kassel et al[153]
TGF-β1	+	+ (Angiotensin II)	McKay et al[154]
IFN-γ	+	+ (AS)	Hakonarson et al[155]
GM-CSF	+	+ (AS, IL-1β, TNF-α)	Hakonarson et al[155], Hallsworth et al[156], Saunders et al[157]
IL-2	+	+ (AS)	Hakonarson et al[155]
IL-5	+	+ (AS)	Hakonarson et al[155]
IL-6	-	+ (IL-1, TGF-β, TNF-α)	Amrani et al[149], Elias et al[158]
IL-11	-	+ (IL-1, TGF-β, virus)	Elias et al[158]
IL-12	+	+ (AS)	Hakonarson et al[155]
IL-33	+	+ (IFN-γ, TNF-α)	Prefontaine et al[159]
Adhesion and costimulatory molecules			
CD11a	+	...	Hakonarson et al[100]
CD40	+	+ (TNF-α, IFN-γ)	Lazaar et al[103]
CD40L	+	...	Lazaar et al[103]
CD44	+	...	Lazaar et al[99]
CD80, CD86	+	...	Hakonarson et al[100]
ICAM-1	+	+ (TNF-α, IL-1β, IL-5, AS)	Lazaar et al[99], Amrani et al[160], Grunstein et al[161]
VCAM-1	+	+ (TNF-α, IL-1β)	Lazaar et al[99], Amrani et al[160]

Abbreviations: AS, asthmatic serum; IP-10, interferon gamma-induced protein 10; MCP, membrane cofactor protein; MIP, macrophage inflammatory protein; SCF, stem cell factor; SDF, stromal cell-derived factor; TGF, transforming growth factor.

Taking into account the microlocalization of mast cells within the asthmatic ASM layer, the adherence of mast cells to the ASM, and the features of mast cell activation within the ASM, it may be suggested that a close functional relationship exists between these two cell types. On the one hand, mast cells are likely to alter functional and phenotypic properties of ASM cells. Indeed, mast cell–derived mediators may contribute to BHR (see earlier discussion) and ASM remodeling

(see earlier discussion).[6] For instance, the major mast cell product tryptase induces ASM calcium increase[91] and nonspecific BHR to histamine in vitro[92] and in vivo.[93] Tryptase also increases the production TGF-β1 by ASM cells,[77] which promotes the differentiation of ASM cells toward a more contractile phenotype, characterized by both an increased expression of α–smooth muscle actin and an enhanced ASM contractility.[88] The number of mast cells within the ASM layer is

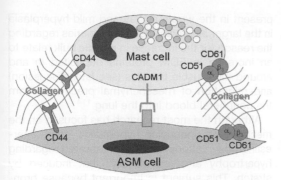

Fig. 2. ASM: mast cell interaction. ASM can adhere to mast cells through cell-cell direct interaction involving CADM1 and through cell-extracellular matrix interaction involving type I collagen and both CD44 and CD51.

positively correlated with the degree of BHR[4,71] and with the intensity of α–smooth muscle actin staining.[88] Furthermore, mast cell myositis may also promote ASM remodeling. Indeed, mast cell–derived tryptase has been shown to stimulate ASM proliferation.[94] Moreover, mast cell–derived CCL19 mediates ASM migration through the activation of ASM CCR7.[95] However, neither ASM proliferation[89,96] nor ASM survival seemed to be modulated by cocultured mast cells.[89] In addition, CCL11/CCR3-mediated ASM cell migration was inhibited by mast cells.[97] Furthermore, no correlation was found between the number of mast cells within the ASM and ASM mass, supporting the modest role of mast cells in ASM remodeling.[76] On the other hand, ASM cells can alter mast cell functional and phenotypic properties. Indeed, ASM cells can promote mast cell survival and proliferation through a mechanism involving a cooperative interaction between ASM membrane-bound SCF, soluble IL-6, and mast cell–CADM1.[82] ASM cell-derived ECM proteins may also promote mast cells differentiation toward a fibroblastoid phenotype, characterized by the expression of fibroblast markers and fibroblastlike morphology. This feature seems to be specific of mast cells within the ASM layer, since fibroblast markers were not expressed by mast cells within the submucosa.[75]

Regarding T-cell infiltration within the asthmatic ASM layer, only a few studies have been performed. CD4+ T-cell microlocalization was initially reported in an experimental asthma model within the ASM layer of ovalbumine-sensitized rats compared with nonsensitized animals.[98] These findings have been further confirmed in human patients with asthma[5,84] and are related to asthma severity.[5] As compared with mast cell infiltration, the number of T cells seems to be lower within

the ASM layer.[4,84] ASM cells are able to produce appropriate chemotactic factors for T cells, including CCL5 (RANTES) or CXCL10 interferon gamma-induced protein 10 (IP-10).[78] However, direct chemotactic properties of ASM to T cells remain to be demonstrated.

Close contacts between ASM and T cells have been shown in asthma,[5,84] suggesting cell-cell adherence between these two cell types. Lazaar and coworkers[99] first demonstrated that activated T cells can adhere in vitro to resting ASM cells from nonasthmatic patients and that such an adhesion was enhanced when ASM cells were primed with proinflammatory cytokines, such as TNF-α. These findings were further confirmed independently.[100] This adhesion involves, on the one hand, CD44, ICAM-1, and VCAM-1 expressed by ASM cells and, on the other hand, CD44, lymphocyte function-associated antigen 1, and very late antigen 4 expressed by T cells.[99] More recently, nonasthmatic ASM cells, pulsed to the superantigen staphylococcal enterotoxin A (SEA), have been shown to adhere to T cells by presenting the SEA via their major histocompatibility complex (MHC) class II.[101] Although ASM cells express MHC class II constitutively and under stimulation,[100,102] these cells are not classically considered to be an antigen-presenting cell. Consequently, these findings support an emerging role of ASM cells as an immunomodulatory cells. However, except for VCAM1, which forms clusters in the asthmatic ASM ex vivo suggesting VCAM1-mediated intercellular signaling, the role of the previously mentioned molecules in adherence between T cell and ASM cell from patients with asthma has not yet been considered. Two other ASM cell-surface molecules, CD40[100,103–105] and OX40 ligand,[105–107] both expressed in asthmatic and nonasthmatic ASM cells, have also been suggested in promoting ASM cell–T-cell adherence. These costimulatory cell-surface molecules, members of the TNF superfamily, respectively bind to CD154 and OX40 on activated T cells.[108,109] However, their role in the adherence of T cells to asthmatic ASM remains to be investigated. By contrast, a possible role for mast cell chymase has been suggested because this mast cell protease is able to inhibit T-cell adhesion to nonasthmatic ASM cells in vitro.[110]

Close interaction between T cells and ASM cells can stimulate a crosstalk between these two cell types but little is known about the functional consequences of such interaction. On the one hand, T cells may alter functional properties of ASM cells. Firstly, T cells may alter ASM contractile phenotype, enhancing ASM contractility to acetylcholine and reducing its relaxation to isoproterenol in isolated rabbit bronchi.[100] Moreover, T cells may also induce ASM remodeling and, more precisely, ASM hyperplasia.[5,98,99] Indeed, in an experimental rat asthma model, adoptively transferred CD4[+] T cells from ovalbumine-sensitized rats induced an increase in ASM mass, which was both related to an increased ASM proliferation and decreased apoptosis ex vivo.[98] Such findings were confirmed in vitro only on direct CD4[+] T-cells–ASM cells contact, highlighting the need for close cellular interaction between these two cell types.[98] These observations are in agreement with a previous study demonstrating in vitro a role for T cell in ASM DNA synthesis and proliferation in ASM cells from nonasthmatic patients.[99] The role of T cells in driving ASM remodeling was later confirmed in human patients with asthma.[5] Moreover, the number of T cells infiltrating the asthmatic ASM correlated with ASM mass.[5] Collectively, these findings suggest an emerging role of T cells in both ASM hyperresponsiveness and remodeling. On the other hand, ASM cells may also alter functional properties of T cells. Indeed, direct contact between CD4[+] T cells and ASM cells also enhances T-cell survival, thus possibly contributing to the perpetuation of bronchial inflammation.[98] Cultured, human, nonasthmatic ASM cells are able to present superantigens via their MHC class II molecules to resting CD4[+] T cells,[101] which induces CD4[+] T-cell activation, adherence between these cells, and finally the release of IL-13, which, in turns, allow increasing the contractile response to acetylcholine of isolated rabbit bronchi.[101]

ASM REMODELING

It is well recognized that the increased ASM mass in the asthmatic airway is one of the key features of the structural changes that constitute airway remodeling.[111] Moreover, this increase has been attributed with a pivotal role in determining one of the key functional characteristics of the asthmatic airway, namely airway hyperresponsiveness.[112] The increased muscle mass is likely to be the most important abnormality responsible for the exaggerated response to bronchoconstricting stimuli in asthma, resulting in the development of greater narrowing of the lumen. More recently, there has been much investigation into the mechanisms underlying this increase. Whether the major contributing process is hyperplasia, hypertrophy, or their combination remains unclear, and it is possible that the changes in the muscle are not homogeneous throughout the airway. Ebina and colleagues[113] described 2 patterns in lungs harvested postmortem: type I in which hyperplasia was present in the walls of large bronchi with no hypertrophy and type II in which hypertrophy was

present in the whole airway and mild hyperplasia in the larger airways. Additional theories regarding the reason for the increase in muscle bulk relate to an increase in ECM proteins deposited in and around the muscle bundles (see later discussion) and migration of mesenchymal precursors from the peripheral blood into the lung.[114]

Although the most research has focused on the mechanisms underlying hyperplasia, some interesting observations have been reported regarding hypertrophy and, specifically, that induced by stretch. This subject is important because bronchoconstriction itself constitutes a form of stretch or strain[115] and this is highly relevant to the asthmatic airway. The effect of mechanical stretch is to induce hypertrophy of human ASM and this seems to be mediated by the action of a miRNA, specifically miR-26a.[116] Stretch or overexpression of miR-26a induces human ASM hypertrophy via an effect on glycogen synthase kinase-3β. In these experiments, stretch also induced hyperplasia but the predominant effect was hypertrophy and miR26a did not affect proliferation.

A lot more attention has been focused on the underlying causes of hyperplasia, which, in some studies, has been reported to be the sole pathologic condition underlying the increase in muscle mass.[117] This finding has been attributed to an upregulation of proproliferative pathways or, alternatively, a lack of endogenous braking mechanisms (**Table 2**). In 2001,[118] it was noted that ASM cells obtained from patients with asthma proliferated at a greater rate than those obtained from people without asthma and this finding was confirmed and extended by Trian and colleagues,[119] although this has not always been a consistent finding.[89,120] In the study by Trian and colleagues,[119] the increased growth was attributed to mitochondrial biogenesis and to dysfunctional calcium regulation. Further studies on calcium homeostasis have demonstrated that the expression and function of sarco-endoplasmic reticulum calcium ATPases, which play a role in the extrusion of calcium from the ASM cell, are downregulated.[121,122] With respect to hyperproliferative pathways, almost every signal transduction protein has been associated with exaggerated proliferation, including, but not limited to, the mitogen-activated protein kinases extracellular signal-regulated kinase[123] and p38,[124] as well as phosphatidylinositol 3 kinases.[125] Studies conducted using intact tissue, as opposed to cells from patients with asthma, have revealed an increased immunohistochemical detection of a marker of proliferation-proliferative cell nuclear antigen, indicating that evidence for increased proliferation of ASM is not merely a phenomenon of cell culture.[5,126]

Table 2
Modulation of human ASM proliferation

Proproliferative	Antiproliferative
Growth factors	
EGF[162]	PGE$_2$[127,163]
IGF[164]	Heparin[163]
PDGF[165]	IL-13[166]
FGF-2[167]	VIP[168]
Plasma/Inflammatory cell mediators	
β-hexosaminidases[169]	Glucocorticoids[a,128]
Elastase[170]	IL-4[167]
α-thrombin[171]	beta agonists[127]
Tryptase[94]	
Sphingosine-1 phosphate[61]	
Contractile agents	
Endothelin-1[b,162]	
Leukotriene D4[b,172]	
Cysteinyl leukotriene[173]	
Histamine[168]	
Extracellular matrix proteins	
Fibronectin[174]	
Collagen-1[174]	

Abbreviations: EGF, epidermal growth factor; FGF-2, fibroblast growth factor-2; IGF, insulinlike growth factor; PDGF, platelet-derived growth factor; VIP, vasoactive intestinal peptide.
[a] Nonasthmatic cells only.
[b] A comitogen.
Reviewed in Hirst SJ, Martin JG, Bonacci JV, et al. Proliferative aspects of airway smooth muscle. J Allergy Clin Immunol 2004;114:S2–17.

It is possible that internal mechanisms for limiting proliferation could be dysfunctional (see **Table 2**). Levels of endogenous PGE$_2$, which is an inhibitor of mitogenesis,[127] are decreased in cultures of asthma-derived ASM and this was also found to be the case for protein levels of the transcription factor CCAAT/enhancer binding protein α-, an inhibitor of proliferation.[128] In addition, evidence that vitamin D inhibits ASM cell proliferation may suggest that low levels in vivo could contribute to unopposed growth.[129]

It was originally thought that the structural changes in asthmatic airways that constitute airway remodeling developed as a result of a persistent inflammatory stimulus. This idea has been challenged by some recent reports regarding the mechanisms underlying remodeling. Bronchoconstriction induced by a noninflammatory stimulus, such as methacholine, resulted in significant increases in parameters of remodeling to approximately the same extent as an allergen challenge.[130] These changes were assessed by means of biopsies; although there was no actual measurement of ASM, the number of proliferating cells in the lamina propria was increased in each challenge. The exact nature of these cells was not explored but they could have been myocytes that had dedifferentiated into myofibroblasts and migrated into the submucosa in response to allergen challenge.[131] Increases in sub-basement membrane collagen and alterations in epithelial cell morphology, both hallmarks of airway remodeling, were a consistent feature observed in the study by Grainge[130] in response to inflammatory (allergen) and noninflammatory (methacholine) challenges. Thus, it may be that the structural changes that constitute remodeling are not a consequence of chronic persistent inflammation, as was previously thought, but rather the two processes develop along separate parallel pathways, which is a hypothesis put forward by Martinez in 2007.[132]

Not only ASM cells per se but also their products (eg, ECM proteins) contribute to the area of the muscle bundle.[133] The fractional area of the matrix is increased in the smooth muscle in cases of fatal asthma.[134] The ECM provides a scaffold for support of the cells embedded in it. In addition, ECM proteins have profound biologic effects on the smooth muscle, influencing the proliferation, formation, and release of growth factors and matrix metalloproteinases (MMPs), which may cleave factors embedded in the matrix and release them to alter function. There is now accumulating evidence that remodeling in the asthmatic airway is associated with changes in the ECM proteins. When ASM cells are exposed to serum from patients with asthma, increases in many ECM proteins are observed.[135] Alterations in the ECM are a well-recognized component of remodeling in the asthmatic airway, including enhanced deposition of collagens I, III, and V; fibronectin; tenascin; hyaluronan; versican; laminin α2/β2; and perlecan,[136–139] whereas decorin, collagen IV, and elastin are decreased.[140] ASM cells derived from patients with asthma produce a different profile of matrix proteins,[141] including increased amounts of fibulin 1-C.[142] The importance of these alterations in the matrix proteins lies in the fact that they can profoundly alter the properties of the ASM. Fibulin 1-C, for example, plays a role in vitro in the enhanced proliferation of asthmatic ASM. The components of the matrix may also modulate response to pharmacotherapy, conferring resistance to corticosteroids and β2 adrenoceptor agonists.[143,144] In intensive studies of tissue from patients with asthma who have suffered a fatal attack, elastic fibers and fibronectin are increased and in this same cohort, changes in the MMPs were also noted, with increases in both MMP-9 and -12 detected immunohistochemically in the ASM of large airways.[145] Whether these changes are consistent throughout the airways is unclear.

SUMMARY

A better knowledge of the various roles of ASM in the pathophysiology of asthma is necessary to understand that ASM is not just a target for bronchodilation. Of course, changes in ASM contractile properties or impaired function of relaxant receptors play an important role in the development of BHR in asthma. Bronchodilators can also inhibit some but not all proinflammatory functions of ASM in vitro. Moreover, steroids are not able to reduce both mast cell myositis and increased proliferation of asthmatic ASM. This latter seems to be an important mechanism of ASM remodeling. Moreover, T cells may induce ASM hyperplasia and have been involved in BHR. All of these findings confirm that the roles of ASM in the pathophysiology of asthma are complex and need further specific pharmaceutical developments.

REFERENCES

1. Busse WW, Lemanske RF Jr. Asthma. N Engl J Med 2001;344:350–62.
2. Huber HL, Koessler KK. The pathology of bronchial asthma. Arch Intern Med 1922;30:689–760.
3. Bousquet J, Chanez P, Lacoste JY, et al. Eosinophilic inflammation in asthma. N Engl J Med 1990;323:1033–9.
4. Brightling CE, Bradding P, Symon FA, et al. Mast-cell infiltration of airway smooth muscle in asthma. N Engl J Med 2002;346:1699–705.
5. Ramos-Barbon D, Fraga-Iriso R, Brienza NS, et al. T Cells localize with proliferating smooth muscle alpha-actin+ cell compartments in asthma. Am J Respir Crit Care Med 2010;182:317–24.
6. Bara I, Ozier A, Tunon de Lara JM, et al. Pathophysiology of bronchial smooth muscle remodelling in asthma. Eur Respir J 2010;36:1174–84.
7. Pepe C, Foley S, Shannon J, et al. Differences in airway remodeling between subjects with severe and moderate asthma. J Allergy Clin Immunol 2005;116:544–9.
8. Kaminska M, Foley S, Maghni K, et al. Airway remodeling in subjects with severe asthma with or without chronic persistent airflow obstruction. J Allergy Clin Immunol 2009;124:45–51

9. Seow CY, Schellenberg RR, Pare PD. Structural and functional changes in the airway smooth muscle of asthmatic subjects. Am J Respir Crit Care Med 1998;158:S179–86.
10. James A, Carroll N. Airway smooth muscle in health and disease; methods of measurement and relation to function. Eur Respir J 2000;15:782–9.
11. Schmidt D, Ruehlmann E, Branscheid D, et al. Passive sensitization of human airways increases responsiveness to leukotriene C4. Eur Respir J 1999;14:315–9.
12. Black J, Marthan R, Armour CL, et al. Sensitization alters contractile responses and calcium influx in human airway smooth muscle. J Allergy Clin Immunol 1989;84:440–7.
13. Marthan R, Crevel H, Guénard H, et al. Responsiveness to histamine in human sensitized airway smooth muscle. Respir Physiol 1992;90:239–50.
14. Roux E, Hyvelin JM, Savineau JP, et al. Calcium signaling in airway smooth muscle cells is altered by in vitro exposure to the aldehyde acrolein. Am J Respir Cell Mol Biol 1998;19:437–44.
15. Amrani Y, Panettieri RA Jr. Modulation of calcium homeostasis as a mechanism for altering smooth muscle responsiveness in asthma. Curr Opin Allergy Clin Immunol 2002;2:39–45.
16. Amrani Y, Panettieri RA Jr. Cytokines induce airway smooth muscle cell hyperresponsiveness to contractile agonists. Thorax 1998;53:713–6.
17. Tao FC, Shah S, Pradhan AA, et al. Enhanced calcium signaling to bradykinin in airway smooth muscle from hyperresponsive inbred rats. Am J Physiol Lung Cell Mol Physiol 2003;284:L90–9.
18. Deshpande DA, Walseth TF, Panettieri RA, et al. CD38/cyclic ADP-ribose-mediated Ca2+ signaling contributes to airway smooth muscle hyper-responsiveness. FASEB J 2003;17:452–4.
19. Wills-Karp M. IL-12/IL-13 axis in allergic asthma. J Allergy Clin Immunol 2001;107:9–18.
20. Deshpande DA, Dogan S, Walseth TF, et al. Modulation of calcium signaling by interleukin-13 in human airway smooth muscle: role of CD38/cyclic adenosine diphosphate ribose pathway. Am J Respir Cell Mol Biol 2004;31:36–42.
21. Deshpande DA, White TA, Dogan S, et al. CD38/cyclic ADP-ribose signaling: role in the regulation of calcium homeostasis in airway smooth muscle. Am J Physiol Lung Cell Mol Physiol 2005;288:L773–88.
22. Kellner J, Gamarra F, Welsch U, et al. IL-13Ralpha2 reverses the effects of IL-13 and IL-4 on bronchial reactivity and acetylcholine-induced Ca+ signaling. Int Arch Allergy Immunol 2007;142:199–210.
23. Tliba O, Deshpande D, Chen H, et al. IL-13 enhances agonist-evoked calcium signals and contractile responses in airway smooth muscle. Br J Pharmacol 2003;140:1159–62.

24. Syed F, Panettieri RA Jr, Tliba O, et al. The effect of IL-13 and IL-13R130Q, a naturally occurring IL-13 polymorphism, on the gene expression of human airway smooth muscle cells. Respir Res 2005;6:9.

25. Bergner A, Sanderson MJ. Airway contractility and smooth muscle Ca(2+) signaling in lung slices from different mouse strains. J Appl Physiol 2003; 95:1325–32.

26. Amrani Y, Chen H, Panettieri RA Jr. Activation of tumor necrosis factor receptor 1 in airway smooth muscle: a potential pathway that modulates bronchial hyper-responsiveness in asthma? Respir Res 2000;1:49–53.

27. Ito S, Kume H, Honjo H, et al. Possible involvement of Rho kinase in Ca2+ sensitization and mobilization by MCh in tracheal smooth muscle. Am J Physiol Lung Cell Mol Physiol 2001;280:L1218–24.

28. Hunter I, Cobban HJ, Vandenabeele P, et al. Tumor necrosis factor-alpha-induced activation of RhoA in airway smooth muscle cells: role in the Ca2+ sensitization of myosin light chain20 phosphorylation. Mol Pharmacol 2003;63:714–21.

29. Parris JR, Cobban HJ, Littlejohn AF, et al. Tumour necrosis factor-alpha activates a calcium sensitization pathway in guinea-pig bronchial smooth muscle. J Physiol 1999;518(Pt 2):561–9.

30. Sakai H, Otogoto S, Chiba Y, et al. Involvement of p42/44 MAPK and RhoA protein in augmentation of ACh-induced bronchial smooth muscle contraction by TNF-alpha in rats. J Appl Physiol 2004;97:2154–9.

31. Sakai H, Otogoto S, Chiba Y, et al. TNF-alpha augments the expression of RhoA in the rat bronchus. J Smooth Muscle Res 2004;40:25–34.

32. Kume H, Takeda N, Oguma T, et al. Sphingosine 1-phosphate causes airway hyper-reactivity by rho-mediated myosin phosphatase inactivation. J Pharmacol Exp Ther 2007;320:766–73.

33. Rosenfeldt HM, Amrani Y, Watterson KR, et al. Sphingosine-1-phosphate stimulates contraction of human airway smooth muscle cells. FASEB J 2003;17:1789–99.

34. Sakai J, Oike M, Hirakawa M, et al. Theophylline and cAMP inhibit lysophosphatidic acid-induced hyperresponsiveness of bovine tracheal smooth muscle cells. J Physiol 2003;549:171–80.

35. Smith PG, Roy C, Zhang YN, et al. Mechanical stress increases RhoA activation in airway smooth muscle cells. Am J Respir Cell Mol Biol 2003;28:436–42.

36. Liu C, Tazzeo T, Janssen LJ. Isoprostane-induced airway hyperresponsiveness is dependent on internal Ca2+ handling and Rho/ROCK signaling. Am J Physiol Lung Cell Mol Physiol 2006;291:L1177–84.

37. Liu HW, Halayko AJ, Fernandes DJ, et al. The RhoA/Rho kinase pathway regulates nuclear localization of serum response factor. Am J Respir Cell Mol Biol 2003;29:39–47.

38. Gosens R, Schaafsma D, Meurs H, et al. Role of Rho-kinase in maintaining airway smooth muscle contractile phenotype. Eur J Pharmacol 2004;483:71–8.

39. Ito S, Kume H, Oguma T, et al. Roles of stretch-activated cation channel and Rho-kinase in the spontaneous contraction of airway smooth muscle. Eur J Pharmacol 2006;552:135–42.

40. Takeda N, Kondo M, Ito S, et al. Role of RhoA inactivation in reduced cell proliferation of human airway smooth muscle by simvastatin. Am J Respir Cell Mol Biol 2006;35:722–9.

41. Schaafsma D, Zuidhof AB, Nelemans SA, et al. Inhibition of Rho-kinase normalizes nonspecific hyperresponsiveness in passively sensitized airway smooth muscle preparations. Eur J Pharmacol 2006;531:145–50.

42. Reithmann C, Gierschik P, Werdan K, et al. Tumor necrosis factor alpha up-regulates Gi alpha and G beta proteins and adenylyl cyclase responsiveness in rat cardiomyocytes. Eur J Pharmacol 1991;206:53–60.

43. Hakonarson H, Herrick DJ, Grunstein MM. Mechanism of impaired beta-adrenoceptor responsiveness in atopic sensitized airway smooth muscle. Am J Physiol 1995;269:L645–52.

44. Amrani Y, Krymskaya V, Maki C, et al. Am J Physiol 1997;273:L1020–8.

45. Hall IP, Donaldson J, Hill SJ. Modulation of fluoroaluminate-induced inositol phosphate formation by increases in tissue cyclic AMP content in bovine tracheal smooth muscle. Br J Pharmacol 1990;100:646–50.

46. Hardy E, Farahani M, Hall IP. Regulation of histamine H1 receptor coupling by dexamethasone in human cultured airway smooth muscle. Br J Pharmacol 1996;118:1079–84.

47. Hsu YM, Chiu CT, Wang CC, et al. Tumour necrosis factor-alpha enhances bradykinin-induced signal transduction via activation of Ras/Raf/MEK/MAPK in canine tracheal smooth muscle cells. Cell Signal 2001;13:633–43.

48. Yang CM, Chien CS, Wang CC, et al. Interleukin-1beta enhances bradykinin-induced phosphoinositide hydrolysis and Ca2+ mobilization in canine tracheal smooth-muscle cells: involvement of the Ras/Raf/mitogen-activated protein kinase (MAPK) kinase (MEK)/MAPK pathway. Biochem J 2001;354:439–46.

49. Schmidlin F, Scherrer D, Daeffler L, et al. Interleukin-1beta induces bradykinin B2 receptor gene expression through a prostanoid cyclic AMP-dependent pathway in human bronchial smooth muscle cells. Mol Pharmacol 1998;53:1009–15.

50. Pype JL, Xu H, Schuermans M, et al. Mechanisms of interleukin 1beta-induced human airway smooth

muscle hyporesponsiveness to histamine. Involvement of p38 MAPK NF-kappaB. Am J Respir Crit Care Med 2001;163:1010–7.

51. Emala CW, Kuhl J, Hungerford CL, et al. TNF-alpha inhibits isoproterenol-stimulated adenylyl cyclase activity in cultured airway smooth muscle cells. Am J Physiol 1997;272:L644–50.

52. Shore SA, Laporte J, Hall IP, et al. Effect of IL-1 beta on responses of cultured human airway smooth muscle cells to bronchodilator agonists. Am J Respir Cell Mol Biol 1997;16:702–12.

53. Moore PE, Lahiri T, Laporte JD, et al. Selected contribution: synergism between TNF-alpha and IL-1 beta in airway smooth muscle cells: implications for beta-adrenergic responsiveness. J Appl Physiol 2001;91:1467–74.

54. Laporte JC, Moore PE, Baraldo S, et al. Direct effects of interleukin-13 on signaling pathways for physiological responses in cultured human airway smooth muscle cells. Am J Respir Crit Care Med 2001;164:141–8.

55. Amrani Y, Tliba O, Deshpande DA, et al. Bronchial hyperresponsiveness: insights into new signaling molecules. Curr Opin Pharmacol 2004;4:230–4.

56. Hall IP, Widdop S, Townsend P, et al. Control of cyclic AMP levels in primary cultures of human tracheal smooth muscle cells. Br J Pharmacol 1992;107:422–8.

57. Ammit AJ, Hoffman RK, Amrani Y, et al. Tumor necrosis factor-alpha-induced secretion of RANTES and interleukin-6 from human airway smooth-muscle cells. Modulation by cyclic adenosine monophosphate. Am J Respir Cell Mol Biol 2000;23:794–802.

58. Pang L, Knox AJ. Regulation of TNF-alpha-induced eotaxin release from cultured human airway smooth muscle cells by beta2-agonists and corticosteroids. FASEB J 2001;15:261–9.

59. Hallsworth MP, Twort CH, Lee TH, et al. beta(2)-adrenoceptor agonists inhibit release of eosinophil-activating cytokines from human airway smooth muscle cells. Br J Pharmacol 2001;132:729–41.

60. Pang L, Knox AJ. Synergistic inhibition by beta(2)-agonists and corticosteroids on tumor necrosis factor-alpha-induced interleukin-8 release from cultured human airway smooth-muscle cells. Am J Respir Cell Mol Biol 2000;23:79–85.

61. Ammit AJ, Hastie AT, Edsall LC, et al. Sphingosine 1-phosphate modulates human airway smooth muscle cell functions that promote inflammation and airway remodeling in asthma. FASEB J 2001;15:1212–4.

62. Ammit AJ, Lazaar AL, Irani C, et al. Tumor necrosis factor-alpha-induced secretion of RANTES and interleukin-6 from human airway smooth muscle cells: modulation by glucocorticoids and

beta-agonists. Am J Respir Cell Mol Biol 2002;26:465–74.

63. DiCosmo BF, Geba GP, Picarella D, et al. Airway epithelial cell expression of interleukin-6 in transgenic mice. Uncoupling of airway inflammation and bronchial hyperreactivity. J Clin Invest 1994;94:2028–35.

64. Lazzeri N, Belvisi MG, Patel HJ, et al. Effects of prostaglandin E2 and cAMP elevating drugs on GM-CSF release by cultured human airway smooth muscle cells. Relevance to asthma therapy. Am J Respir Cell Mol Biol 2001;24:44–8.

65. Bonazzi A, Bolla M, Buccellati C, et al. Effect of endogenous and exogenous prostaglandin E(2) on interleukin-1 beta-induced cyclooxygenase-2 expression in human airway smooth-muscle cells. Am J Respir Crit Care Med 2000;162:2272–7.

66. Kanehiro A, Ikemura T, Makela MJ, et al. Inhibition of phosphodiesterase 4 attenuates airway hyperresponsiveness and airway inflammation in a model of secondary allergen challenge. Am J Respir Crit Care Med 2001;163:173–84.

67. Oppenheimer-Marks N, Kavanaugh AF, Lipsky PE. Inhibition of the transendothelial migration of human T lymphocytes by prostaglandin E2. J Immunol 1994;152:5703–13.

68. To SS, Schrieber L. Effect of leukotriene B4 and prostaglandin E2 on the adhesion of lymphocytes to endothelial cells. Clin Exp Immunol 1990;81:160–5.

69. Panettieri RA Jr, Lazaar AL, Pure E, et al. Activation of cAMP-dependent pathways in human airway smooth muscle cells inhibits TNF-alpha-induced ICAM-1 and VCAM-1 expression and T lymphocyte adhesion. J Immunol 1995;154:2358–65.

70. Berger P, Girodet PO, Tunon De Lara JM. Mast cell myositis: a new feature of allergic asthma? Allergy 2005;60:1238–40.

71. Siddiqui S, Mistry V, Doe C, et al. Airway hyperresponsiveness is dissociated from airway wall structural remodeling. J Allergy Clin Immunol 2008;122:335–41.

72. Berry M, Morgan A, Shaw DE, et al. Pathological features and inhaled corticosteroid response of eosinophilic and non-eosinophilic asthma. Thorax 2007;62:1043–9.

73. Saha SK, Berry MA, Parker D, et al. Increased sputum and bronchial biopsy IL-13 expression in severe asthma. J Allergy Clin Immunol 2008;121:685–91.

74. Carroll NG, Mutavdzic S, James AL. Distribution and degranulation of airway mast cells in normal and asthmatic subjects. Eur Respir J 2002;19:879–85.

75. Kaur D, Saunders R, Hollins F, et al. Mast cell fibroblastoid differentiation mediated by airway smooth muscle in asthma. J Immunol 2010;185:6105–14.

76. Amin K, Janson C, Boman G, et al. The extracellular deposition of mast cell products is increased

in hypertrophic airways smooth muscles in allergic asthma but not in non-allergic asthma. Allergy 2005;60(10):1241–7.

77. Berger P, Girodet PO, Begueret H, et al. Tryptase-stimulated human airway smooth muscle cells induce cytokine synthesis and mast cell chemotaxis. FASEB J 2003;17:2139–41.

78. Brightling CE, Ammit AJ, Kaur D, et al. The CXCL10/CXCR3 axis mediates human lung mast cell migration to asthmatic airway smooth muscle. Am J Respir Crit Care Med 2005;171:1103–8.

79. Sutcliffe A, Kaur D, Page S, et al. Mast cell migration to Th2 stimulated airway smooth muscle from asthmatics. Thorax 2006;61:657–62.

80. El-Shazly A, Berger P, Girodet PO, et al. Fraktalkine produced by airway smooth muscle cells contributes to mast cell recruitment in asthma. J Immunol 2006;176:1860–8.

81. Yang W, Kaur D, Okayama Y, et al. Human lung mast cells adhere to human airway smooth muscle, in part, via tumor suppressor in lung cancer-1. J Immunol 2006;176:1238–43.

82. Hollins F, Kaur D, Yang W, et al. Human airway smooth muscle promotes human lung mast cell survival, proliferation, and constitutive activation: cooperative roles for CADM1, stem cell factor, and IL-6. J Immunol 2008;181:2772–80.

83. Girodet PO, Ozier A, Trian T, et al. Mast cell adhesion to bronchial smooth muscle in asthma specifically depends on CD51 and CD44 variant 6. Allergy 2010;65:1004–12.

84. Begueret H, Berger P, Vernejoux JM, et al. Inflammation of bronchial smooth muscle in allergic asthma. Thorax 2007;62:8–15.

85. Carter RJ, Bradding P. The role of mast cells in the structural alterations of the airways as a potential mechanism in the pathogenesis of severe asthma. Curr Pharm Des 2011;17:685–98.

86. Brightling CE, Symon FA, Holgate ST, et al. Interleukin-4 and -13 expression is co-localized to mast cells within the airway smooth muscle in asthma. Clin Exp Allergy 2003;33:1711–6.

87. Bradding P, Walls AF, Holgate ST. The role of the mast cell in the pathophysiology of asthma. J Allergy Clin Immunol 2006;117:1277–84.

88. Woodman L, Siddiqui S, Cruse G, et al. Mast cells promote airway smooth muscle cell differentiation via autocrine up-regulation of TGF-beta 1. J Immunol 2008;181:5001–7.

89. Kaur D, Hollins F, Saunders R, et al. Airway smooth muscle proliferation and survival is not modulated by mast cells. Clin Exp Allergy 2010; 40:279–88.

90. Thangam EB, Venkatesha RT, Zaidi AK, et al. Airway smooth muscle cells enhance C3a-induced mast cell degranulation following cell-cell contact. FASEB J 2005;19:798–800.

91. Berger P, Tunon-de-Lara JM, Savineau JP, et al. Tryptase-induced PAR-2-mediated Ca(2+) signaling in human airway smooth muscle cells. J Appl Physiol 2001;91:995–1003.

92. Berger P, Compton SJ, Molimard M, et al. Mast cell tryptase as a mediator of hyperresponsiveness in human isolated bronchi. Clin Exp Allergy 1999;29:804–12.

93. Molinari JF, Scuri M, Moore WR, et al. Inhaled tryptase causes bronchoconstriction in sheep via histamine release. Am J Respir Crit Care Med 1996;154:649–53.

94. Berger P, Perng DW, Thabrew H, et al. Tryptase and agonists of PAR-2 induce the proliferation of human airway smooth muscle cells. J Appl Physiol 2001;91:1372–9.

95. Kaur D, Saunders R, Berger P, et al. Airway smooth muscle and mast cell-derived CC chemokine ligand 19 mediate airway smooth muscle migration in asthma. Am J Respir Crit Care Med 2006;174:1179–88.

96. Alkhouri H, Hollins F, Moir LM, et al. Human lung mast cells modulate the functions of airway smooth muscle cells in asthma. Allergy 2011;66:1231–41.

97. Saunders R, Sutcliffe A, Woodman L, et al. The airway smooth muscle CCR3/CCL11 axis is inhibited by mast cells. Allergy 2008;63:1148–55.

98. Ramos-Barbon D, Presley JF, Hamid QA, et al. Antigen-specific CD4+ T cells drive airway smooth muscle remodeling in experimental asthma. J Clin Invest 2005;115:1580–9.

99. Lazaar AL, Albelda SM, Pilewski JM, et al. T lymphocytes adhere to airway smooth muscle cells via integrins and CD44 and induce smooth muscle cell DNA synthesis. J Exp Med 1994;180:807–16.

100. Hakonarson H, Kim C, Whelan R, et al. Bi-directional activation between human airway smooth muscle cells and T lymphocytes: role in induction of altered airway responsiveness. J Immunol 2001;166:293–303.

101. Veler H, Hu A, Fatma S, et al. Superantigen presentation by airway smooth muscle to CD4+ T lymphocytes elicits reciprocal proasthmatic changes in airway function. J Immunol 2007;178:3627–36.

102. Lazaar AL, Reitz HE, Panettieri RA Jr, et al. Antigen receptor-stimulated peripheral blood and bronchoalveolar lavage- derived T cells induce MHC class II and ICAM-1 expression on human airway smooth muscle. Am J Respir Cell Mol Biol 1997;16:38–45.

103. Lazaar AL, Amrani Y, Hsu J, et al. CD40-mediated signal transduction in human airway smooth muscle. J Immunol 1998;161:3120–7.

104. Burgess JK, Blake AE, Boustany S, et al. CD40 and OX40 ligand are increased on stimulated asthmatic

airway smooth muscle. J Allergy Clin Immunol 2005;115:302–8.

105. Krimmer DI, Loseli M, Hughes JM, et al. CD40 and OX40 ligand are differentially regulated on asthmatic airway smooth muscle. Allergy 2009;64:1074–82.

106. Burgess JK, Carlin S, Pack RA, et al. Detection and characterization of OX40 ligand expression in human airway smooth muscle cells: a possible role in asthma? J Allergy Clin Immunol 2004;113:683–9.

107. Siddiqui S, Mistry V, Doe C, et al. Airway wall expression of OX40/OX40L and interleukin-4 in asthma. Chest 2010;137:797–804.

108. Xu Y, Song G. The role of CD40-CD154 interaction in cell immunoregulation. J Biomed Sci 2004;11:426–38.

109. Fujita T, Ukyo N, Hori T, et al. Functional characterization of OX40 expressed on human CD8+ T cells. Immunol Lett 2006;106:27–33.

110. Lazaar AL, Plotnick MI, Kucich U, et al. Mast cell chymase modifies cell-matrix interactions and inhibits mitogen-induced proliferation of human airway smooth muscle cells. J Immunol 2002;169:1014–20.

111. Durrani SR, Viswanathan RK, Busse WW. What effect does asthma treatment have on airway remodeling? Current perspectives. J Allergy Clin Immunol 2011;128:439–48.

112. Lambert RK, Wiggs BR, Kuwano K, et al. Functional significance of increased airway smooth muscle in asthma and COPD. J Appl Physiol 1993;74:2771–81.

113. Ebina M, Takahashi T, Chiba T, et al. Cellular hypertrophy and hyperplasia of airway smooth muscles underlying bronchial asthma. A 3-D morphometric study. Am Rev Respir Dis 1993;148:720–6.

114. Bai TR. Evidence for airway remodeling in chronic asthma. Curr Opin Allergy Clin Immunol 2010;10:82–6.

115. Tschumperlin DJ, Drazen JM. Mechanical stimuli to airway remodeling. Am J Respir Crit Care Med 2001;164:S90–4.

116. Mohamed JS, Lopez MA, Boriek AM. Mechanical stretch up-regulates microRNA-26a and induces human airway smooth muscle hypertrophy by suppressing glycogen synthase kinase-3beta. J Biol Chem 2010;285:29336–47.

117. Woodruff PG, Dolganov GM, Ferrando RE, et al. Hyperplasia of smooth muscle in mild to moderate asthma without changes in cell size or gene expression. Am J Respir Crit Care Med 2004;169:1001–6.

118. Johnson PR, Roth M, Tamm M, et al. Airway smooth muscle cell proliferation is increased in asthma. Am J Respir Crit Care Med 2001;164:474–7.

119. Trian T, Benard G, Begueret H, et al. Bronchial smooth muscle remodeling involves calcium-dependent enhanced mitochondrial biogenesis in asthma. J Exp Med 2007;204:3173–81.

120. Ward JE, Harris T, Bamford T, et al. Proliferation is not increased in airway myofibroblasts isolated from asthmatics. Eur Respir J 2008;32:362–71.

121. Mahn K, Hirst SJ, Ying S, et al. Diminished sarco/endoplasmic reticulum Ca2+ ATPase (SERCA) expression contributes to airway remodelling in bronchial asthma. Proc Natl Acad Sci U S A 2009;106:10775–80.

122. Mahn K, Ojo OO, Chadwick G, et al. Ca(2+) homeostasis and structural and functional remodelling of airway smooth muscle in asthma. Thorax 2010;65:547–52.

123. Lee JH, Johnson PR, Roth M, et al. ERK activation and mitogenesis in human airway smooth muscle cells. Am J Physiol Lung Cell Mol Physiol 2001;280:L1019–29.

124. Chung KF. p38 mitogen-activated protein kinase pathways in asthma and COPD. Chest 2011;139:1470–9.

125. Burgess JK, Lee JH, Ge Q, et al. Dual ERK and phosphatidylinositol 3-kinase pathways control airway smooth muscle proliferation: differences in asthma. J Cell Physiol 2008;216:673–9.

126. Hassan M, Jo T, Risse PA, et al. Airway smooth muscle remodeling is a dynamic process in severe long-standing asthma. J Allergy Clin Immunol 2010;125:1037–45.

127. Yan H, Deshpande DA, Misior AM, et al. Anti-mitogenic effects of beta-agonists and PGE2 on airway smooth muscle are PKA dependent. FASEB J 2011;25:389–97.

128. Roth M, Johnson PR, Borger P, et al. Dysfunctional interaction of C/EBPalpha and the glucocorticoid receptor in asthmatic bronchial smooth-muscle cells. N Engl J Med 2004;351:560–74.

129. Damera G, Fogle HW, Lim P, et al. Vitamin D inhibits growth of human airway smooth muscle cells through growth factor-induced phosphorylation of retinoblastoma protein and checkpoint kinase 1. Br J Pharmacol 2009;158:1429–41.

130. Grainge CL, Lau LC, Ward JA, et al. Effect of bronchoconstriction on airway remodeling in asthma. N Engl J Med 2011;364:2006–15.

131. Kelly MM, O'Connor TM, Leigh R, et al. Effects of budesonide and formoterol on allergen-induced airway responses, inflammation, and airway remodeling in asthma. J Allergy Clin Immunol 2010;125:349–356.e13.

132. Martinez FD. Asthma treatment and asthma prevention: a tale of 2 parallel pathways. J Allergy Clin Immunol 2007;119:30–3.

133. An SS, Bai TR, Bates JH, et al. Airway smooth muscle dynamics: a common pathway of airway obstruction in asthma. Eur Respir J 2007;29:834–60.

134. Bai TR, Cooper J, Koelmeyer T, et al. The effect of age and duration of disease on airway structure in

fatal asthma. Am J Respir Crit Care Med 2000;162: 663–9.

135. Johnson PR, Black JL, Carlin S, et al. The production of extracellular matrix proteins by human passively sensitized airway smooth-muscle cells in culture: the effect of beclomethasone. Am J Respir Crit Care Med 2000;162:2145–51.

136. Laitinen LA, Laitinen A, Altraja A, et al. Bronchial biopsy findings in intermittent or "early" asthma. J Allergy Clin Immunol 1996;98:S3–6 [discussion: S33–40].

137. Laitinen A, Altraja A, Kampe M, et al. Tenascin is increased in airway basement membrane of asthmatics and decreased by an inhaled steroid. Am J Respir Crit Care Med 1997;156:951–8.

138. Roberts CR, Burke AK. Remodelling of the extracellular matrix in asthma: proteoglycan synthesis and degradation. Can Respir J 1998;5:48–50.

139. Roche WR, Beasley R, Williams JH, et al. Subepithelial fibrosis in the bronchi of asthmatics. Lancet 1989;1:520–4.

140. Bousquet J, Chanez P, Lacoste JY, et al. Asthma: a disease remodeling the airways. Allergy 1992; 47:3–11.

141. Johnson PR, Burgess JK, Underwood PA, et al. Extracellular matrix proteins modulate asthmatic airway smooth muscle cell proliferation via an autocrine mechanism. J Allergy Clin Immunol 2004;113: 690–6.

142. Lau JY, Oliver BG, Baraket M, et al. Fibulin-1 is increased in asthma–a novel mediator of airway remodeling? PLoS One 2010;5:e13360.

143. Schuliga M, Ong SC, Soon L, et al. Airway smooth muscle remodels pericellular collagen fibrils: implications for proliferation. Am J Physiol Lung Cell Mol Physiol 2010;298:L584–92.

144. Bourke JE, Li X, Foster SR, et al. Collagen remodelling by airway smooth muscle is resistant to steroids and beta-agonists. Eur Respir J 2011;37: 173–82.

145. Araujo BB, Dolhnikoff M, Silva LF, et al. Extracellular matrix components and regulators in the airway smooth muscle in asthma. Eur Respir J 2008;32:61–9.

146. Watson ML, Grix SP, Jordan NJ, et al. Interleukin 8 and monocyte chemoattractant protein 1 production by cultured human airway smooth muscle cells. Cytokine 1998;10:346–52.

147. Pype JL, Dupont LJ, Menten P, et al. Expression of monocyte chemotactic protein (MCP)-1, MCP-2, and MCP-3 by human airway smooth-muscle cells. Modulation by corticosteroids and T-helper 2 cytokines. Am J Respir Cell Mol Biol 1999;21:528–36.

148. John M, Hirst SJ, Jose PJ, et al. Human airway smooth muscle cells express and release RANTES in response to T helper 1 cytokines: regulation by T helper 2 cytokines and corticosteroids. J Immunol 1997;158:1841–7.

149. Amrani Y, Ammit AJ, Panettieri RA Jr. Tumor necrosis factor receptor (TNFR) 1, but not TNFR2, mediates tumor necrosis factor-alpha-induced interleukin-6 and RANTES in human airway smooth muscle cells: role of p38 and p42/44 mitogen-activated protein kinases. Mol Pharmacol 2001; 60:646–55.

150. Chung KF, Patel HJ, Fadlon EJ, et al. Induction of eotaxin expression and release from human airway smooth muscle cells by IL-1beta and TNFalpha: effects of IL-10 and corticosteroids. Br J Pharmacol 1999;127:1145–50.

151. Ghaffar O, Hamid Q, Renzi PM, et al. Constitutive and cytokine-stimulated expression of eotaxin by human airway smooth muscle cells. Am J Respir Crit Care Med 1999;159:1933–42.

152. John M, Au BT, Jose PJ, et al. Expression and release of interleukin-8 by human airway smooth muscle cells: inhibition by Th-2 cytokines and corticosteroids. Am J Respir Cell Mol Biol 1998;18:84–90.

153. Kassel O, Schmidlin F, Duvernelle C, et al. Human bronchial smooth muscle cells in culture produce stem cell factor. Eur Respir J 1999;13:951–4.

154. McKay S, de Jongste JC, Saxena PR, et al. Angiotensin II induces hypertrophy of human airway smooth muscle cells: expression of transcription factors and transforming growth factor-beta1. Am J Respir Cell Mol Biol 1998;18:823–33.

155. Hakonarson H, Maskeri N, Carter C, et al. Regulation of TH1- and TH2-type cytokine expression and action in atopic asthmatic sensitized airway smooth muscle. J Clin Invest 1999;103:1077–87.

156. Hallsworth MP, Soh CP, Twort CH, et al. Cultured human airway smooth muscle cells stimulated by interleukin-1beta enhance eosinophil survival. Am J Respir Cell Mol Biol 1998;19:910–9.

157. Saunders MA, Mitchell JA, Seldon PM, et al. Release of granulocyte-macrophage colony stimulating factor by human cultured airway smooth muscle cells: suppression by dexamethasone. Br J Pharmacol 1997;120:545–6.

158. Elias JA, Wu Y, Zheng T, et al. Cytokine- and virus-stimulated airway smooth muscle cells produce IL-11 and other IL-6-type cytokines. Am J Physiol 1997;273:L648–55.

159. Prefontaine D, Lajoie-Kadoch S, Foley S, et al. Increased expression of IL-33 in severe asthma: evidence of expression by airway smooth muscle cells. J Immunol 2009;183:5094–103.

160. Amrani Y, Lazaar AL, Panettieri RA Jr. Up-regulation of ICAM-1 by cytokines in human tracheal smooth muscle cells involves an NF-kappa B-dependent signaling pathway that is only partially sensitive to dexamethasone. J Immunol 1999;163: 2128–34.

161. Grunstein MM, Hakonarson H, Maskeri N, et al. Intrinsic ICAM-1/LFA-1 activation mediates altered

responsiveness of atopic asthmatic airway smooth muscle. Am J Physiol Lung Cell Mol Physiol 2000; 278:L1154–63.

162. Panettieri RA Jr, Goldie RG, Rigby PJ, et al. Endothelin-1-induced potentiation of human airway smooth muscle proliferation: an ETA receptor-mediated phenomenon. Br J Pharmacol 1996; 118:191–7.

163. Johnson PR, Armour CL, Carey D, et al. Heparin and PGE2 inhibit DNA synthesis in human airway smooth muscle cells in culture. Am J Physiol 1995;269:L514–9.

164. Kelleher MD, Abe MK, Chao TS, et al. Role of MAP kinase activation in bovine tracheal smooth muscle mitogenesis. Am J Physiol 1995;268:L894–901.

165. Hirst SJ, Barnes PJ, Twort CH. PDGF isoform-induced proliferation and receptor expression in human cultured airway smooth muscle cells. Am J Physiol 1996;270:L415–28.

166. Risse PA, Jo T, Suarez F, et al. Interleukin-13 inhibits proliferation and enhances contractility of human airway smooth muscle cells without change in contractile phenotype. Am J Physiol Lung Cell Mol Physiol 2011;300:L958–66.

167. Hawker KM, Johnson PR, Hughes JM, et al. Interleukin-4 inhibits mitogen-induced proliferation of human airway smooth muscle cells in culture. Am J Physiol 1998;275:L469–77.

168. Maruno K, Absood A, Said SI. VIP inhibits basal and histamine-stimulated proliferation of human airway smooth muscle cells. Am J Physiol 1995; 268:L1047–51.

169. Lew DB, Dempsey BK, Zhao Y, et al. beta-hexosaminidase-induced activation of p44/42 mitogen-activated protein kinase is dependent on p21Ras and protein kinase C and mediates bovine airway smooth-muscle proliferation. Am J Respir Cell Mol Biol 1999;21:111–8.

170. Huang CD, Chen HH, Wang CH, et al. Human neutrophil-derived elastase induces airway smooth muscle cell proliferation. Life Sci 2004;74:2479–92.

171. Panettieri RA Jr, Hall IP, Maki CS, et al. alpha-thrombin increases cytosolic calcium and induces human airway smooth muscle cell proliferation. Am J Respir Cell Mol Biol 1995;13:205–16.

172. Panettieri RA, Tan EM, Ciocca V, et al. Effects of LTD4 on human airway smooth muscle cell proliferation, matrix expression, and contraction in vitro: differential sensitivity to cysteinyl leukotriene receptor antagonists. Am J Respir Cell Mol Biol 1998;19:453–61.

173. Ravasi S, Citro S, Viviani B, et al. CysLT1 receptor-induced human airway smooth muscle cells proliferation requires ROS generation, EGF receptor transactivation and ERK1/2 phosphorylation. Respir Res 2006;7:42.

174. Nguyen TT, Ward JP, Hirst SJ. beta1-integrins mediate enhancement of airway smooth muscle proliferation by collagen and fibronectin. Am J Respir Crit Care Med 2005;171:217–23.

Resolution of Inflammation in Asthma

Bruce D. Levy, MD[a,b,*], Isabelle Vachier, PhD[c],
Charles N. Serhan, PhD[d]

KEYWORDS

- Inflammation • Resolution • Lipoxins • Mediators • Asthma

KEY POINTS

- Resolution of inflammation is an active process with specific cellular and molecular events.
- Specialized proresolving mediators are enzymatically derived from polyunsaturated fatty acids, including the ω-3 fatty acids eicosapentaenoic acid and docosahexaenoic acid.
- Proresolving mediators interact with specific receptors to regulate allergic airway responses and asthma.
- Uncontrolled asthma is associated with a defect in proresolving mediator signaling.

INTRODUCTION

Asthma is characterized by increased and chronic airway inflammation.[1] Airway sampling by bronchoscopy or sputum analysis most often reveals abundant eosinophils and activated T cells, and lung histology demonstrates airway remodeling with disordered mucosal epithelium.[2,3] Whereas noxious stimuli, including potential allergens, can initiate an acute inflammatory response that is self-limited, nonresolving inflammation is linked to asthma and other chronic inflammatory diseases (reviewed in Ref.[4]). The overall magnitude and duration of inflammation depends on competing physiologic processes, namely prophlogistic mechanisms that amplify inflammation and endogenous braking programs that control the resolution of inflammation (reviewed in Ref.[5]). In health, the resolution of inflammation is an active coordinated

Funding sources: Dr Levy: National Institutes of Health. Dr Vachier: Med Bio Med. Dr Serhan: National Institutes of Health.
This research was supported in part by the US National Institutes of Health grants AI068084, P01-GM095467, U10-HL109172 and P50-HL107166.
Conflicts of interest: Dr Levy: Consultant for Resolvyx Pharmaceuticals; patents licensed to Bayer Healthcare and Resolvyx; Equity in Resolvyx Pharmaceuticals. Dr Levy's interests were reviewed and are managed by the Brigham and Women's Hospital and Partners HealthCare in accordance with their conflict of interest policies. Dr Vachier: No conflict of Interest. Dr Serhan is an inventor of patents (resolvins) and proresolving mediators and related compounds assigned to Brigham and Women's Hospital and licensed to Resolvyx Pharmaceuticals. Dr Serhan is a scientific founder of Resolvyx Pharmaceuticals and owns equity in the company. His interests were reviewed and are managed by the Brigham and Women's Hospital and Partners HealthCare in accordance with their conflict of interest policies.
a Harvard Medical School, Department of Internal Medicine, Brigham and Women's Hospital, Boston, MA 02115, USA; b Center for Experimental Therapeutics and Reperfusion Injury, Department of Anesthesiology, Perioperative and Pain Medicine, Brigham and Women's Hospital, Boston, MA 02115, USA; c Respiratory Disease Department, Arnaud de Villeneuve Hospital, CHRU Montpellier, 34295 Montpellier, France; d Center for Experimental Therapeutics and Reperfusion Injury, Department of Anesthesiology, Perioperative and Pain Medicine, Brigham and Women's Hospital, HIM829, 77 Avenue Louis Pasteur, Boston, MA 02115, USA
* Corresponding author. Brigham and Women's Hospital, Harvard Institutes of Medicine, HIM855, 77 Avenue Louis Pasteur, Boston, MA 02115.
E-mail address: blevy@partners.org

0272-5231/12/$ – see front matter © 2012 Elsevier Inc. All rights reserved.

process that is spatiotemporally controlled by endogenously generated autacoids at sites of inflammation.[6] While several classes of mediators participate in resolution, the enzymatic transformations of polyunsaturated fatty acids (PUFAs) to specific proresolving agonists are of particular interest. The discovery that PUFAs are essential dietary constituents[7] led to the recognition of their immunoregulatory actions.[8] These PUFA-derived mediators display cell type–selective anti-inflammatory, proresolving, antifibrotic, antiangiogenic, and anti-infective actions (reviewed in Ref.[5]).

This article reviews recent findings on new mechanisms and mediators for resolution of airway inflammation, with a focus on their relevance to asthma.

RESOLUTION OF ACUTE INFLAMMATION

The acute inflammatory response to inhaled pathogens, particles, and toxins is inherently protective and essential to ultimately restoring the injured airway to its normal physiologic functioning. Acute inflammation is initiated within minutes of recognition of a danger signal, and is generally self-limited, resolving within hours or days. In several conditions that are clinically recognized as lung disease, including asthma, chronic inflammation persists. Somehow, a naturally protective response becomes unrestrained and leads to chronic changes to airway structure and function. In most individuals with asthma, it is this chronic inflammation that causes the clinical expression of symptoms, namely cough, mucus, chest tightness, wheeze, and shortness of breath. There is a rapidly expanding exploration of the natural mechanisms and mediators of resolution that limit acute inflammation in healthy tissues, and this information has turned conventional thinking on its head regarding the pathophysiology of asthma and other chronic inflammatory diseases.

Resolution is now appreciated to be an active process that terminates acute inflammation.[6,9,10] At present, it is known that efficient restoration of inflamed tissues to their basal state requires that inflammatory cells are effectively cleared and further neutrophil recruitment is abrogated. During this process, tissue neutrophils undergo apoptosis, and are recognized and subsequently engulfed by phagocytic macrophages in a noninflammatory manner.[11,12] Clearance of apoptotic neutrophils also leads to the production of additional mediators that suppress the progression of inflammation and promote repair of damaged tissues.[13–15] Dysregulation of this process leads to unresolved inflammation, which underlies the pathology of several chronic inflammatory disease processes.[5,16] Hence,

resolution of inflammation requires cellular interactions in the affected tissues to reestablish a homeostatic state after a limited period of inflammation. This sequence of events is also referred to as catabasis: the reversion from a pathologic to a noninflammatory state of tissue homeostasis.[17,18]

In health, the acute inflammatory response is self-limited. Early tissue edema (minutes to hours) and neutrophil accumulation (hours to days) will decrease with time, and lymphocytes, macrophages, and other monocytoid cells will traffic to the inflamed tissue to restore homeostasis.[19] While antileukocyte actions are commonly considered anti-inflammatory, it is important to view the role of each cell type in this dynamic process of inflammation resolution (ie, catabasis). Inhibition of neutrophil transmigration and activation is anti-inflammatory, whereas restitution of barrier integrity (endothelial, epithelial, or both), recruitment of monocytoid cells, and promotion of macrophage clearance of apoptotic cells, microbes, and tissue debris are all proresolving. In the lung, restitution of barrier integrity is of heightened importance, secondary to concern for alveolar edema leading to hypoxemia. Thus, lung-specific proresolving events include clearance of edema and transitional matrix, repopulation of the airway epithelia, and restoration of pulmonary surfactants.

For resolution of adaptive immune responses, allergen-specific or pathogen-specific effector T cells and inflammatory macrophages need to be cleared from the lung. Direct and indirect mechanisms for T-cell clearance include natural killer (NK) cell direct cytotoxicity, macrophage engulfment of apoptotic T cells, and decrements in proinflammatory mediators.

Most individuals with asthma have chronic inflammation of the airways that does not resolve. Perhaps as many as 50% of adult asthmatics and an even higher proportion of pediatric asthmatic individuals have an expansion of allergy airway inflammation that is characterized by an abundance of CD4[+] TH2 cells with increased interleukin (IL)-5 and IL-13 production.[20,21] IL-5 is a potent chemoattractant and activator of eosinophils, which are also present in large numbers in most asthmatic subjects.[1] Eosinophils and mast cells release significant amounts of the cysteinyl leukotrienes (CysLTs; LTC_4, LTD_4, and LTE_4), of which LTD_4 is the most potent constrictor of airway smooth muscle identified to date.[22] These mediators also induce changes in vascular permeability and edema in tissue. IL-13 leads to mucous metaplasia of the bronchial epithelium, with increased airway mucus.[23,24] Together, the increased numbers of airway leukocytes (T cells, eosinophils), proinflammatory (IL-5, IL-13), and prophlogistic (CysLTs) mediators, smooth muscle constriction, and mucus production by epithelial cells lead to airway narrowing and hyperactivity.

Although chronic eosinophilic bronchitis is common in asthma, the condition is syndromic, and airway pathobiology is more complex in many individuals with asthma. Some experience a predominately neutrophilic infiltration and others are pauci-immune, likely reflecting a primary disorder of airway smooth muscle.[25] Environmental factors, such as cigarette smoke, microbial pathogens, and air pollution, can lead to mixed and more complex airway inflammation.[1] Despite the presence of airway inflammation in the vast majority of individuals with asthma, there is still limited understanding of why the asthmatic airway inflammation fails to resolve. In addition, potent anti-inflammatory agents such as glucocorticoids are available, yet their use does not cure asthma. Once adults are diagnosed with asthma, it most often remains a life-long illness. Thus important questions remain to be answered in determining why asthmatic inflammation fails to resolve, so that proresolving therapeutics can be developed.

Anti-inflammation and proresolution are distinct physiologic processes.[26] The identification of proresolving mediators that facilitate the clearance of inflammatory cells and debris from inflamed tissue has improved our understanding of the distinction between proresolving and purely anti-inflammatory mediators (reviewed in Ref.[5]). While anti-inflammatory mediators block granulocyte tissue entry and activation, endogenous proresolving mediators accelerate the restitution of tissue homeostasis and clearance of inflammatory cells without concomitant immunosuppression. To this end, proresolving mediators decrease allergic edema,[27] recruit monocytes in a nonphlogistic fashion,[28] increase phagocytosis and efferocytosis by macrophages,[29] increase chemokine scavenging by apoptotic neutrophils (via C-C chemokine receptor type 5 [CCR5] expression),[30] enhance luminal clearance of tissue neutrophils by CD55 expression,[31] and augment mucosal host defense via expression of antimicrobial proteins.[32,33] These proresolution mediators can also stimulate the secretion of transforming growth factor (TGF)-β1 and IL-10, which can also dampen inflammation.[17,34]

To combat asthma, currently available anti-inflammatory agents (eg, glucocorticoids and the biological therapeutic agents anti–immunoglobulin E, IL-5, and IL-13) target proinflammatory mediator pathways.[1] In addition, asthmatic individuals may use nonsteroidal anti-inflammatory drugs that inhibit cyclooxygenases (COX), and zileuton, which inhibits arachidonate 5-lipoxygenase (ALOX5).

These agents can interfere with resolution of inflammation, because these enzymes are also involved in the endogenous formation of proresolving mediators.[35–37] Thus, new disease-modifying therapeutic agents are needed that are specifically designed to prevent further inflammation and promote resolution.

POLYUNSATURATED FATTY ACID METABOLISM TO PRORESOLVING MEDIATORS

PUFAs are essential nutrients. The ω-6 PUFA, arachidonic acid (AA; 20:4n-6) is incorporated into cellular phospholipids, and on cell activation, specific phospholipase A_2 enzymes release AA from the sn-2 fatty acyl bond of phospholipids. AA can then be converted enzymatically by COX to prostaglandins (PGs), by ALOX5 to leukotrienes (LTs) or, by ALOX5 in collaboration with ALOX12 or ALOX15 to lipoxins (LXs).[5,38] The ω-3 PUFAs eicosapentaenoic acid (EPA; 20:5n-3) and docosahexaenoic acid (DHA; 22:6n-3) are enriched in neural and mucosal tissues.[39,40] In whole blood from healthy subjects, the total fatty acid pool contains both EPA (~0.5%–2.8% of total fatty acids) and DHA (~1.3%–5.0%).[41–46] These ω-3 PUFAs are also available at sites of inflammation for enzymatic transformation to resolvins, protectins, maresins, and other new families of proresolving mediators.[9,10,47–49] These new specialized mediators display receptor-mediated cell type–specific actions (**Table 1**). Because information on these mediators in airway health and asthma is limited at present, this review focuses on lipoxin A_4 (LXA$_4$), the E-series resolvin termed resolvin E1 (RvE1), and protectin D1 (PD1), and highlight their formation, sites of action, and potential anti-inflammatory and proresolving actions, with particular reference to available information on allergic airway inflammation and asthma.

Lipoxin A_4

LXs are trihydroxytetraene-containing mediators derived from the sequential actions of lipoxygenases (LOXs) (reviewed in Ref.[5]). Because LX biosynthetic enzymes (ie, LOXs) are predominately compartmentalized in distinct cell types, LXs are principally generated during heterotypic cell-cell interactions in multicellular host responses, such as inflammation. LXs are structurally and functionally distinct from PGs and LTs. Tissue levels of these prophlogistic eicosanoids (PGs and LTs) are prominent during the onset of inflammation, whereas LXs are increased during resolution. LXs have cell type–specific actions (see **Table 1**), including inhibition of neutrophil (PMN) and

Table 1
Cellular actions of proresolving mediators

Proresolving Mediator	Cell Type	Action	Ref.
Lipoxin A$_4$	Eosinophils	Inhibits eosinophil migration	107
	T cells	Inhibits TNF release	108
	Neutrophils	Inhibits PMN chemotaxis	62
		Inhibits transendothelial migration	109,110
		Inhibits transepithelial migration	109
		Inhibits superoxide anion generation	69
		Inhibits azurophilic granule release	111
	NK cells	Inhibits NK cell cytotoxicity	112
	Monocytes	Increases adhesion and transmigration	28
		Inhibits IL-8 release induced by TNF	113
	Macrophages	Increases engulfment of apoptotic PMN	29
	Smooth muscle	Inhibits LTC$_4$-initiated migration	114
	Endothelium	Stimulates prostacyclin release	115
	Epithelial cells	Increases proliferation after acid injury	116
		Inhibits cytokine release	116
		Increases intracellular Ca^{2+}	117
Resolvin E1	T cells	Increases CCR5 expression	30
	Neutrophils	Inhibits transendothelial migration	32
Protectin D1	T cells	Increases CCR5 expression	30
	Neutrophils	Inhibits TNF-α and IFN-γ release	118
		Inhibits PMN transmigration	17

Abbreviations: CCR5, C-C chemokine receptor type 5; IFN, interferon; IL, interleukin; LTC$_4$, leukotriene C$_4$; NK, natural killer; PMN, polymorphonuclear neutrophil; TNF, tumor necrosis factor.

eosinophil transendothelial and transepithelial migration, PMN reactive oxygen species generation, and stimulation of monocyte chemotaxis and macrophage engulfment of apoptotic PMNs. LXs also display neuromodulatory actions at capsaicin-sensitive sensory nerves in the guinea pig[50] and can dampen inflammatory pain processing in mice.[51] In the lung, ALOX15 is a key enzyme for LX generation and is expressed by many cells in the inflamed lung, including bronchial epithelial cells, macrophages, and eosinophils.[52–55] ALOX15 converts C20:4 to 15S-hydroperoxyeicosatetraenoic acid (15S-H(p)ETE) that can be further converted to LXs by ALOX5.[53] Thus, LX biosynthesis can occur when infiltrating PMNs or eosinophils interact with epithelia in inflamed airways.[6,56] LXs can also be generated in the vasculature during collaborations between leukocyte ALOX5 and platelet ALOX12. Human platelet ALOX12 is an LX synthase that can generate LXs from ALOX5-derived leukotriene A$_4$ (LTA$_4$).

LX epimers are also generated during inflammation and can be increased in the presence of aspirin (acetylsalicylic acid [ASA]).[57] Acetylation of COX-2 by ASA blocks PG synthesis; however, the enzyme remains catalytically active, converting AA to 15R-hydroxyeicosapentaenoic acid (15R-HETE) rather than PG. 15R-HETE can serve as a substrate for leukocyte ALOX5 for subsequent transformation to 15-epimer LXs (15-epi-LX).[57] 15R-HETE can also be generated by cytochrome P450 metabolism of C20:4 in epithelial cells.[58] Of interest, statins can also increase 15-epi-LX production,[59] including in the airway.[60]

At sites of inflammation, LXs are rapidly formed and rapidly inactivated. The enzyme 15-hydroxyprostaglandin dehydrogenase (15-PGDH) metabolizes LXs by dehydration to convert LXA$_4$ to 15-oxo-LXA$_4$.[61] This conversion inactivates the LXs, as the oxo-LXs no longer display counterregulatory bioactions. 15-oxo-LXA$_4$ can be further metabolized by eicosanoid oxidoreductase, which specifically reduces the double bond adjacent to the ketone, and then again by 15-PGDH to a 13,14-dihydro-LXA$_4$. LX metabolism is stereospecific, so 15-epi-LXs are metabolized less efficiently than LXs, increasing their biological half-life approximately 2-fold and thereby enhancing their ability to evoke bioactions.[62] Thus, ASA's unique pharmacologic properties arise from both its ability to inhibit proinflammatory PG formation and its capacity to generate anti-inflammatory lipid mediators, including the 15-epi-LXs.[63] This biosynthetic paradigm for ASA-triggered counterregulatory lipid mediators from AA is also observed for the ω-3 PUFAs C20:5 (eicosapentaenoic acid) and C22:6 (docosahexaenoic acid).[63]

Lipoxin A₄ Receptors

LXA$_4$ is an agonist, interacting with specific receptors (termed ALX/FPR2). ALX/FPR2 receptors are 7-transmembrane, G-protein–coupled receptors that are expressed on several cell types, including human PMNs, eosinophils, monocytes/macrophages, enterocytes, synovial fibroblasts, and airway epithelium.[64] LXs bind to ALX/FPR2 with high affinity (K_d = 1.7 nM).[65] Asthma biologists will recognize that the DP2 receptor can bind both peptide and lipid ligands,[66] but ALX/FPR2 was the first receptor described with these properties.[67] This dual recognition of structurally distinct ligands is now appreciated to be a more generalized phenomenon.[64,68] In PMNs, ALX/FPR2 transduces stop signals in part via polyisoprenyl phosphate remodeling[69] and inhibition of leukocyte-specific protein (LSP-1) phosphorylation, a downstream regulator of the p38-MAPK cascade.[70]

Cytokines, including IL-13 and interferon (IFN)-γ, can induce ALX/FPR2 expression in airway epithelial cells and enterocytes,[71] and the ALX/FPR2 promoter was recently characterized.[72] Lung ALX/FPR2 expression is also induced in vivo in a murine model of allergic airway inflammation.[56] Transgenic mice that express human ALX/FPR2 receptors have demonstrated the importance of these receptors in regulating experimental inflammation,[73] including allergic airway responses.[56]

In addition to ALX/FPR2, additional receptors have been identified for LXA$_4$, including the intracellular aryl hydrocarbon receptor (AhR)[74] and CysLT1 receptor.[75,76] LX signaling via AhR can attenuate IL-12 release from dendritic cells.[77] LXA$_4$ interaction with CysLT1 receptors antagonizes CysLT binding.[76] Together, these findings indicate that LXs can serve as agonists (via ALX and AhR) to transduce cell type–specific anti-inflammatory and proresolving actions, and as antagonists (at CysLT1) to block prophlogistic signaling.

Lipoxin A₄ in Allergic Airway Responses and Asthma

Lipoxins are present in bronchoalveolar lavage fluids (BALFs) and sputum in asthma.[78–80] Because LXs can block LTD$_4$-mediated constriction of isolated lung strips in vitro,[81] LXA$_4$ was given via nebulizer to asthmatic subjects before airway provocation challenges with inhaled LTC$_4$, and LXA$_4$ displayed protective actions in human asthmatic airways.[82]

Translational research has uncovered a decreased ability to generate LXs in ASA-exacerbated respiratory disease[83] and other forms of severe asthma (**Table 2**).[79,84] Relative to milder asthma, blood from severe asthmatics has a reduced capacity to convert AA to ALOX15 catalyzed products, including 15-HETE and LXA$_4$,[84,85] and levels of LXA$_4$ in BALFs

Table 2
Uncontrolled asthma: a defect in proresolving mediators

Proresolving Mediator	Evidence	Age	Country	Ref.
Lipoxin A$_4$	Aspirin-tolerant asthmatics generate more lipoxins than aspirin-intolerant asthmatics	Adults	Poland	83
	Diminished lipoxin biosynthesis in severe asthma	Adults	USA	84
	Severe asthma is associated with a loss of LXA$_4$, an endogenous anti-inflammatory compound	Adults	France	80
	Lipoxin A$_4$ levels in asthma: relation with disease severity and aspirin sensitivity	Adults	Turkey	85
	Airway lipoxin A$_4$ generation and lipoxin A$_4$ receptor expression are decreased in severe asthma	Adults	USA	79
	The role of lipoxin A$_4$ in exercise-induced bronchoconstriction in asthma	Adults	Turkey	86
	Corticosteroid suppression of lipoxin A$_4$ and leukotriene B$_4$ from alveolar macrophages in severe asthma	Adults	UK	119
	Reversed changes of lipoxin A$_4$ and leukotrienes in children with asthma in different degrees of severity	Children	China	120
Protectin D1	Generated in asthma, and dampens airway inflammation and hyperresponsiveness	Adults	USA	106

are markedly decreased in severe asthma in comparison with nonsevere asthma.[79] LXA$_4$ levels are also lower in supernatants of induced sputum in severe asthma compared with those in mild asthma.[80] In addition, lower levels of LXA$_4$ are associated with exercise-induced asthma.[86] Decreased formation of LXs in uncontrolled asthma has now been identified in culturally distinct populations of adults and children from several countries, including the United States, Poland, France, Turkey, and China (see **Table 2**). Decreased LX generation in uncontrolled asthma is partially explained by dysregulated expression of LX biosynthetic genes that vary by both disease severity and anatomic compartment.[79] By contrast, generation of the ALOX5-derived products 5-HETE, LTB$_4$, and CysLTs are all increased in asthma, particularly severe asthma.[84] Peripheral blood LXA$_4$ and the individualized ratio of LXA$_4$/CysLTs correlate with lung function (predicted percentage values of forced expiratory volume in 1 second),[84,85] suggesting a link between AA metabolism and these bioactive lipids and airflow obstruction in asthma. Lower LX levels have also been described in the airways of patients suffering from cystic fibrosis and interstitial lung disease, and appear to play important roles in the pathobiology of these inflammatory lung diseases as well.[87,88] Together, these results indicate that LXs are generated during airway inflammation and that decrements in their generation can contribute to the pathogenesis of asthma.

NOVEL ω-3 FATTY ACID–DERIVED LIPID MEDIATORS

Population surveys report that diets rich in ω-3 fatty acids are associated with lower asthma prevalence.[89] However, the underlying mechanisms behind this observation remain unclear. Recently, specialized proresolving mediators derived from ω-3 fatty acids were identified in self-limited models of acute inflammation, and were termed resolvins (resolution-phase interaction products).[9,10] Similar to LXs, resolvins can be generated via ALOX5-catalyzed reactions during transcellular biosynthesis (reviewed in Ref.[5]). Based on the ω-3 fatty acid of origin, resolvins are divided into the D-series (docosahexaenoic acid; DHA, C22:6) or E-series (eicosapentaenoic acid; EPA, C20:5). Dietary modification or transgenic expansion of the *fat-1* gene (GeneID: 178291 [NC_003282.5]), which encodes a prokaryote ω-3 fatty acid desaturase, can increase resolvin production.[90,91]

Resolvin E1

Resolvin E1 (RvE1) is present in resolving exudates[9] and lung.[92] RvE1 transcellular biosynthesis occurs

in human vasculature in the presence of ASA with transformation of EPA to 18R-hydroxyeicosapentaenoic acid (18R-HEPE) by ASA-acetylated COX-2 in endothelial cells.[68] 18R-HEPE is subsequently converted by leukocyte ALOX5 to RvE1 via a 5(6) epoxide-containing intermediate.[9,68] RvE1 biosynthesis in humans can be increased by ingestion of ASA (100 g) and/or following dietary EPA supplementation (1 g).[68] The stereochemical assignment for RvE1 is 5S,12R,18R-trihydroxyeicosa-6Z,8E,10E,14Z,16E-pentaenoic acid,[9,68] and structure-activity relationships have established that RvE1's actions are highly stereoselective.[5]

Resolvin E1 Receptors

Receptors RvE1 have been recently identified.[68,93] RvE1 interacts with the G-protein–coupled receptor CMKLR1 as an agonist. CMKLR1 (aka ChemR23) was first identified as a receptor for the peptide chemerin. Thus, like ALX/FPR2, this receptor also recognizes both lipid and peptide ligands. CMKLR1 is expressed on monocytes/macrophages and plasmacytoid dendritic cells.[94–96] Human CMKLR1 binds RvE1 with high affinity (K_d = 11.3 ± 5.4 nM).[68] RvE1 also interacts with a second G-protein–coupled receptor, leukotriene B$_4$ receptor 1 (BLT1).[93] In humans, BLT1 receptors are expressed by neutrophils, eosinophils, monocytes/macrophages, mast cells, dendritic cells, and effector T cells.[97] RvE1 effectively competes with LTB$_4$ for BLT1 binding to functionally antagonize LTB$_4$-mediated responses.[93] RvE1's affinity for BLT1 (K_d = 45 nM) is relatively lower than for CMKLR1 and in addition to LTB$_4$ antagonism, RvE1 can serve as a partial agonist for BLT1 signaling.

Resolvin E1 in Allergic Airway Responses and Asthma

Resolvin E1 has potent anti-inflammatory and proresolving actions in several murine models of inflammation, and is bioactive in very low concentrations (nanomolar to picomolar) in vivo and in vitro.[9] RvE1 dampens the development and promotes the resolution of allergic airway responses in a murine experimental model of asthma.[98–100] In nanogram quantities, intravenous administration of RvE1 decreases eosinophil and lymphocyte accumulation and airway mucous metaplasia and improves airway hyperresponsiveness to inhaled methacholine.[100] To promote resolution of inflammation, RvE1 decreases IL-6, IL-17, and IL-23 in the lung while increasing IFN-γ and LXA$_4$ formation.[100] RvE1's actions were additive with those of LXs, as these proresolving mediators both regulate IL-17. Of interest, only RvE1, and not

LXA_4, regulated IL-23 and IFN-γ levels.[100] Together, these findings support the presence of independent proresolving signaling circuits for RvE1 and LXA_4 that converge on the regulation of IL-17 to hasten catabasis in this model of allergic asthma exacerbations. RvE1 is also bioactive when given intraperitoneally before and during the sensitization and aeroallergen challenge phases of this asthma model.[98] Administration with RvE1 concurrent with allergen challenge can prevent the development of bronchial hyperresponsiveness, mucous metaplasia, eosinophil accumulation, and T-helper type 2 (Th2) cytokine mediator release (eg, IL-13).[98] Because immune responses are pathologically sustained in asthma, models of self-limited allergic airway responses have been used to determine mechanisms for downregulating adaptive immune responses in health with the goal of establishing the critical checkpoints for maintaining lung tissue homeostasis. In a murine model of asthma exacerbation with self-limited allergic airway inflammation, NK cell phenotype and trafficking to draining mediastinal lymph nodes is temporally regulated during resolution in a CXCL9-CXCR3 (ligand-receptor) dependent manner.[99] Depletion of NK cells disrupts the endogenous resolution program, leading to delayed resolution of airway eosinophils and antigen-specific $CD4^+$ T cells, increased LTB_4 and IL-23, and decreased LXA_4.[99] In addition, NK cells express CMKLR1, and RvE1-mediated resolution is markedly inhibited in this setting by NK-cell depletion. These findings indicate new functions for NK cells in promoting resolution of adaptive immune responses, and suggest that NK cells are targets for specialized proresolving mediators for clearance of activated T cells from inflamed lung. No published reports are currently available on resolvin E1 in human asthma.

Protectin D1

DHA is also present in resolving exudates, and DHA is converted into D-series resolvins.[10] Of interest, the DHA metabolome includes several additional classes of proresolving mediators, including protectins and maresins.[47,48] Mucosal surfaces, including the airway, are enriched with DHA,[40] and airway mucosal epithelial cells from individuals with asthma or cystic fibrosis have depleted stores of DHA compared with healthy control subjects.[40] This section focuses on protectin D1 (PD1). Roles for D-series resolvins, maresins, and other DHA-derived mediators in asthma are the subject of ongoing research; however, there is currently only limited information on these compounds in asthma.

At sites of inflammation, DHA is rapidly converted by LOX activity to a 17S-hydroperoxy–containing intermediate and via an epoxide-containing intermediate to protectins, such as PD1 (10R,17S-dihydroxy-docosa-4Z,7Z,11E,13E,15Z,19Z-hexaenoic acid).[101] When produced in neural systems, this bioactive mediator is termed neuroprotectin D1 (NPD1/PD1) (for detailed reviews, see Refs.[5,102,103]). NPD1/PD1 is distinguished from D-series resolvins by the presence of a conjugated triene and 2 alcohol groups in a specific chirality required for potent bioactions. Structure-activity relationships suggest that PD1's actions are receptor mediated in human leukocytes[104]; however, the PD1 receptor has yet to be molecularly characterized.

Protectin D1 in Allergic Airway Responses and Asthma

DHA can be delivered during the early stages of an acute inflammatory response in albumin-rich edema fluid.[105] It is noteworthy that the cellular components of the airway mucosa are enriched with DHA,[40] and both 17S-HDHA (17S-hydroxy-docosa-4Z,7Z,11E,13E,15Z,19Z-hexaenoic acid) and PD1 are generated in human airways.[106] Of interest, PD1 levels decrease during acute exacerbations of asthma (see **Table 2**) and PD1 mediates bronchoprotective actions in a murine experimental model of allergic asthma in vivo.[106] Using ovalbumin-sensitized mice, PD1 (2–200 ng) given by the intravenous route before aeroallergen challenge markedly suppressed bronchial hyperresponsiveness, mucous metaplasia, pulmonary eosinophil accumulation, and release of proinflammatory cytokines and lipid mediators. PD1 also mediates proresolving actions on established pulmonary inflammation when given after allergen challenge, leading to significantly expedited resolution of allergic airway inflammation.[106] In a head-to-head comparison with a lipoxin stable analogue and RvE1 in acute, self-limited murine peritonitis, PD1 displayed the lowest ψ_{max} (maximum number of infiltrating leukocytes) and T_{max} (time to resolve), and the shortest R_l (resolution interval, time taken from maximal leukocyte infiltration to 50% of maximum), indicating PD1's potent bioactons.[17]

SUMMARY

The resolution of inflammation is an integral and natural part of the physiologic response to tissue injury, infection, and allergen or other noxious stimuli. Resolution is an active process with highly regulated cellular and biochemical events. Several discrete families of natural small molecules have recently been uncovered using a lipidomics approach. Select members are proresolving and stimulate tissue catabasis. These agents include resolvins, protectins and, most recently, maresins. Insights into these chemical mediators and their signaling pathways provide an opportunity to develop agonists of resolution as a potential novel class of therapeutics. The chronic and uncontrolled airway inflammation that characterizes asthma, especially severe variants of the disease, appears to result in part from a defect in resolution. It is notable that in uncontrolled asthma there is also a defect in the generation of specialized pro-resolving mediators, including LXA_4 and PD1. Thus, bioactive stable analogue mimetics of these mediators that can harness endogenous resolution mechanisms for inflammation may offer new therapeutic strategies for asthma and associated diseases of airway inflammation.

REFERENCES

1. Fanta CH. Asthma. N Engl J Med 2009;360:1002.
2. Bousquet J, Jeffery PK, Busse WW, et al. Asthma. From bronchoconstriction to airways inflammation and remodeling. Am J Respir Crit Care Med 2000;161:1720.
3. Busse WW, Lemanske RF Jr. Asthma. N Engl J Med 2001;344:350.
4. Nathan C, Ding A. Nonresolving inflammation. Cell 2010;140:871.
5. Serhan CN. Resolution phase of inflammation: novel endogenous anti-inflammatory and proresolving lipid mediators and pathways. Annu Rev Immunol 2007;25:101.
6. Levy BD, Clish CB, Schmidt B, et al. Lipid mediator class switching during acute inflammation: signals in resolution. Nat Immunol 2001;2:612.
7. Burr GO, Burr MM. A new deficiency disease produced by the rigid exclusion of fat from the diet. J Biol Chem 1929;82:345.
8. Serhan CN. The resolution of inflammation: the devil in the flask and in the details. FASEB J 2011;25:1441.
9. Serhan CN, Clish CB, Brannon J, et al. Novel functional sets of lipid-derived mediators with antiinflammatory actions generated from omega-3 fatty acids via cyclooxygenase 2-nonsteroidal antiinflammatory drugs and transcellular processing. J Exp Med 2000;192:1197.
10. Serhan CN, Hong S, Gronert K, et al. Resolvins: a family of bioactive products of omega-3 fatty acid transformation circuits initiated by aspirin treatment that counter proinflammation signals. J Exp Med 2002;196:1025.
11. Savill J, Apoptosis. Phagocytic docking without shocking. Nature 1998;392:442.
12. Savill JS, Wyllie AH, Henson JE, et al. Macrophage phagocytosis of aging neutrophils in inflammation. Programmed cell death in the neutrophil leads to its recognition by macrophages. J Clin Invest 1989; 83:865.
13. Fadok VA, Bratton DL, Konowal A, et al. Macrophages that have ingested apoptotic cells in vitro inhibit proinflammatory cytokine production through autocrine/paracrine mechanisms involving TGF-beta, PGE2, and PAF. J Clin Invest 1998;101:890.
14. Freire-de-Lima CG, Xiao YQ, Gardai SJ, et al. Apoptotic cells, through transforming growth factor-beta, coordinately induce anti-inflammatory and suppress pro-inflammatory eicosanoid and NO synthesis in murine macrophages. J Biol Chem 2006;281:38376.
15. Savill J, Fadok V. Corpse clearance defines the meaning of cell death. Nature 2000;407:784.
16. Gilroy DW, Lawrence T, Perretti M, et al. Inflammatory resolution: new opportunities for drug discovery. Nat Rev Drug Discov 2004;3:401.
17. Bannenberg GL, Chiang N, Ariel A, et al. Molecular circuits of resolution: formation and actions of resolvins and protectins [Erratum appears in J Immunol. 2005 May 1;174(9):5884]. J Immunol 2005; 174:4345.
18. Serhan CN, Savill J. Resolution of inflammation: the beginning programs the end. Nat Immunol 2005;6: 1191.
19. Majno G. Cells, tissues and disease: principles of general pathology. Cambridge (MA): Blackwell; 1996.
20. Woodruff PG, Boushey HA, Dolganov GM, et al. Genome-wide profiling identifies epithelial cell genes associated with asthma and with treatment response to corticosteroids. Proc Natl Acad Sci U S A 2007;104:15858.
21. Woodruff PG, Modrek B, Choy DF, et al. T-helper type 2-driven inflammation defines major subphenotypes of asthma. Am J Respir Crit Care Med 2009;180:388.
22. Samuelsson B. From studies of biochemical mechanisms to novel biological mediators: prostaglandin endoperoxides, thromboxanes and leukotrienes. In: Les prix Nobel: Nobel prizes, presentations, biographies and lectures. Stockholm (Sweden): Almqvist & Wiksell; 1982. p. 153.
23. Wills-Karp M, Luyimbazi J, Xu X, et al. Interleukin-13: central mediator of allergic asthma. Science 1998;282:2258.
24. Zhen G, Park SW, Nguyenvu LT, et al. IL-13 and epidermal growth factor receptor have critical but distinct roles in epithelial cell mucin production. Am J Respir Cell Mol Biol 2007;36:244.
25. Moore WC, Bleecker ER, Curran-Everett D, et al. Characterization of the severe asthma phenotype by the National Heart, Lung, and Blood Institute's

Severe Asthma Research Program. J Allergy Clin Immunol 2007;119:405.

26. Serhan CN, Brain SD, Buckley CD, et al. Resolution of inflammation: state of the art, definitions and terms. FASEB J 2007;21:325.

27. Bandeira-Melo C, Serra MF, Diaz BL, et al. Cyclooxygenase-2-derived prostaglandin E2 and lipoxin A4 accelerate resolution of allergic edema in Angiostrongylus costaricensis-infected rats: relationship with concurrent eosinophilia. J Immunol 2000;164:1029.

28. Maddox JF, Serhan CN. Lipoxin A4 and B4 are potent stimuli for human monocyte migration and adhesion: selective inactivation by dehydrogenation and reduction. J Exp Med 1996;183:137.

29. Godson C, Mitchell S, Harvey K, et al. Cutting edge: lipoxins rapidly stimulate nonphlogistic phagocytosis of apoptotic neutrophils by monocyte-derived macrophages. J Immunol 2000;164:1663.

30. Ariel A, Fredman G, Sun YP, et al. Apoptotic neutrophils and T cells sequester chemokines during immune response resolution through modulation of CCR5 expression. Nat Immunol 2006;7:1209.

31. Lawrence DW, Bruyninckx WJ, Louis NA, et al. Anti-adhesive role of apical decay-accelerating factor (CD55) in human neutrophil transmigration across mucosal epithelia. J Exp Med 2003;198:999.

32. Campbell EL, Louis NA, Tomassetti SE, et al. Resolvin E1 promotes mucosal surface clearance of neutrophils: a new paradigm for inflammatory resolution. FASEB J 2007;21:3162.

33. Canny G, Levy O, Furuta GT, et al. Lipid mediator-induced expression of bactericidal/permeability-increasing protein (BPI) in human mucosal epithelia. Proc Natl Acad Sci U S A 2002;99:3902.

34. Souza DG, Fagundes CT, Amaral FA, et al. The required role of endogenously produced lipoxin A4 and annexin-1 for the production of IL-10 and inflammatory hyporesponsiveness in mice. J Immunol 2007;179:8533.

35. Fukunaga K, Kohli P, Bonnans C, et al. Cyclooxygenase 2 plays a pivotal role in the resolution of acute lung injury. J Immunol 2005;174:5033.

36. Gilroy DW, Colville-Nash PR, Willis D, et al. Inducible cyclooxygenase may have anti-inflammatory properties [see comments]. Nat Med 1999;5:698.

37. Schwab JM, Chiang N, Arita M, et al. Resolvin E1 and protectin D1 activate inflammation-resolution programmes. Nature 2007;447:869.

38. Samuelsson B, Dahlen SE, Lindgren JA, et al. Leukotrienes and lipoxins: structures, biosynthesis, and biological effects. Science 1987;237:1171.

39. Bazan NG. Synaptic lipid signaling: significance of polyunsaturated fatty acids and platelet-activating factor. J Lipid Res 2003;44:2221.

40. Freedman SD, Blanco PG, Zaman MM, et al. Association of cystic fibrosis with abnormalities in fatty acid metabolism. N Engl J Med 2004;350:560.

41. Albert CM, Campos H, Stampfer MJ, et al. Blood levels of long-chain n-3 fatty acids and the risk of sudden death. N Engl J Med 2002;346:1113.

42. Gong J, Rosner B, Rees DG, et al. Plasma docosahexaenoic acid levels in various genetic forms of retinitis pigmentosa. Invest Ophthalmol Vis Sci 1992;33:2596.

43. Kew S, Mesa MD, Tricon S, et al. Effects of oils rich in eicosapentaenoic and docosahexaenoic acids on immune cell composition and function in healthy humans. Am J Clin Nutr 2004;79:674.

44. Miles EA, Noakes PS, Kremmyda LS, et al. The Salmon in Pregnancy Study: study design, subject characteristics, maternal fish and marine n-3 fatty acid intake, and marine n-3 fatty acid status in maternal and umbilical cord blood. Am J Clin Nutr 2011;94:1986S.

45. Newcomer LM, King IB, Wicklund KG, et al. The association of fatty acids with prostate cancer risk. Prostate 2001;47:262.

46. Wakai K, Ito Y, Kojima M, et al. Intake frequency of fish and serum levels of long-chain n-3 fatty acids: a cross-sectional study within the Japan Collaborative Cohort Study. J Epidemiol 2005;15:211.

47. Serhan CN, Fredman G, Yang R, et al. Novel proresolving aspirin-triggered DHA pathway. Chem Biol 2011;18:976.

48. Serhan CN, Yang R, Martinod K, et al. Maresins: novel macrophage mediators with potent antiinflammatory and proresolving actions. J Exp Med 2009;206:15.

49. Yang R, Fredman G, Krishnamoorthy S, et al. Decoding functional metabolomics with docosahexaenoyl ethanolamide (DHEA) identifies novel bioactive signals. J Biol Chem 2011;286:31532.

50. Meini S, Evangelista S, Geppetti P, et al. Pharmacologic and neurochemical evidence for the activation of capsaicin-sensitive sensory nerves by lipoxin A4 in guinea pig bronchus. Am Rev Respir Dis 1992;146:930.

51. Svensson CI, Zattoni M, Serhan CN. Lipoxins and aspirin-triggered lipoxin inhibit inflammatory pain processing. J Exp Med 2007;204:245.

52. Hunter JA, Finkbeiner WE, Nadel JA, et al. Predominant generation of 15-lipoxygenase metabolites of arachidonic acid by epithelial cells from human trachea. Proc Natl Acad Sci U S A 1985;82:4633.

53. Levy BD, Romano M, Chapman HA, et al. Human alveolar macrophages have 15-lipoxygenase and generate 15(S)-hydroxy-5,8,11-cis-13-trans-eicosatetraenoic acid and lipoxins. J Clin Invest 1993;92:1572.

54. Serhan CN, Hirsch U, Palmblad J, et al. Formation of lipoxin A by granulocytes from eosinophilic donors. FEBS Lett 1987;217:242.

55. Shannon VR, Chanez P, Bousquet J, et al. Histochemical evidence for induction of arachidonate 15-lipoxygenase in airway disease. Am Rev Respir Dis 1993;147:1024.

56. Levy BD, De Sanctis GT, Devchand PR, et al. Multipronged inhibition of airway hyperresponsiveness and inflammation by lipoxin A(4) [see comment]. Nat Med 2002;8:1018.

57. Claria J, Serhan CN. Aspirin triggers previously undescribed bioactive eicosanoids by human endothelial cell-leukocyte interactions. Proc Natl Acad Sci U S A 1995;92:9475.

58. Claria J, Lee MH, Serhan CN. Aspirin-triggered lipoxins (15-epi-LX) are generated by the human lung adenocarcinoma cell line (A549)-neutrophil interactions and are potent inhibitors of cell proliferation. Mol Med 1996;2:583.

59. Birnbaum Y, Ye Y, Lin Y, et al. Augmentation of myocardial production of 15-epi-lipoxin-a4 by pioglitazone and atorvastatin in the rat. Circulation 2006;114:929.

60. Planaguma A, Pfeffer MA, Rubin G, et al. Lovastatin decreases acute mucosal inflammation via 15-epi-lipoxin A4. Mucosal Immunol 2010;3:270.

61. Serhan CN, Fiore S, Brezinski DA, et al. Lipoxin A4 metabolism by differentiated HL-60 cells and human monocytes: conversion to novel 15-oxo and dihydro products. Biochemistry 1993;32:6313.

62. Serhan CN, Maddox JF, Petasis NA, et al. Design of lipoxin A4 stable analogs that block transmigration and adhesion of human neutrophils. Biochemistry 1995;34:14609.

63. Spite M, Serhan CN. Novel lipid mediators promote resolution of acute inflammation: impact of aspirin and statins. Circ Res 2010;107:1170.

64. Chiang N, Serhan CN, Dahlen SE, et al. The lipoxin receptor ALX: potent ligand-specific and stereoselective actions in vivo. Pharmacol Rev 2006;58:463.

65. Chiang N, Fierro IM, Gronert K, et al. Activation of lipoxin A(4) receptors by aspirin-triggered lipoxins and select peptides evokes ligand-specific responses in inflammation. J Exp Med 2000;191:1197.

66. Hirai H, Tanaka K, Yoshie O, et al. Prostaglandin D2 selectively induces chemotaxis in T helper type 2 cells, eosinophils, and basophils via seven-transmembrane receptor CRTH2. J Exp Med 2001;193:255.

67. Serhan CN, Fiore S, Levy BD. Cell-cell interactions in lipoxin generation and characterization of lipoxin A4 receptors. Ann N Y Acad Sci 1994;744:166.

68. Arita M, Bianchini F, Aliberti J, et al. Stereochemical assignment, antiinflammatory properties, and receptor for the omega-3 lipid mediator resolvin E1. J Exp Med 2005;201:713.

69. Levy BD, Fokin VV, Clark JM, et al. Polyisoprenyl phosphate (PIPP) signaling regulates phospholipase D activity: a 'stop' signaling switch for aspirin-triggered lipoxin A4. FASEB J 1999;13:903.

70. Ohira T, Bannenberg G, Arita M, et al. A stable aspirin-triggered lipoxin A4 analog blocks phosphorylation of leukocyte-specific protein 1 in human neutrophils. J Immunol 2004;173:2091.

71. Gronert K, Gewirtz A, Madara JL, et al. Identification of a human enterocyte lipoxin A4 receptor that is regulated by interleukin (IL)-13 and interferon gamma and inhibits tumor necrosis factor alpha-induced IL-8 release. J Exp Med 1998;187:1285.

72. Simiele F, Recchiuti A, Mattoscio D, et al. Transcriptional regulation of the human FPR2/ALX gene: evidence of a heritable genetic variant that impairs promoter activity. FASEB J 2012;26(3):1323–33.

73. Devchand PR, Arita M, Hong S, et al. Human ALX receptor regulates neutrophil recruitment in transgenic mice: roles in inflammation and host defense [Erratum appears in FASEB J. 2003 Jun;17(9):4]. FASEB J 2003;17:652.

74. Schaldach CM, Riby J, Bjeldanes LF. Lipoxin A4: a new class of ligand for the Ah receptor. Biochemistry 1999;38:7594.

75. Badr KF, DeBoer DK, Schwartzberg M, et al. Lipoxin A4 antagonizes cellular and in vivo actions of leukotriene D4 in rat glomerular mesangial cells: evidence for competition at a common receptor. Proc Natl Acad Sci U S A 1989;86:3438.

76. Gronert K, Martinsson-Niskanen T, Ravasi S, et al. Selectivity of recombinant human leukotriene D(4), leukotriene B(4), and lipoxin A(4) receptors with aspirin-triggered 15-epi-LXA(4) and regulation of vascular and inflammatory responses. Am J Pathol 2001;158:3.

77. Aliberti J, Hieny S, Reis e Sousa C, et al. Lipoxin-mediated inhibition of IL-12 production by DCs: a mechanism for regulation of microbial immunity. Nat Immunol 2002;3:76.

78. Lee TH, Crea AE, Gant V, et al. Identification of lipoxin A4 and its relationship to the sulfidopeptide leukotrienes C4, D4, and E4 in the bronchoalveolar lavage fluids obtained from patients with selected pulmonary diseases. Am Rev Respir Dis 1990;141:1453.

79. Planaguma A, Kazani S, Marigowda G, et al. Airway lipoxin A4 generation and lipoxin A4 receptor expression are decreased in severe asthma. Am J Respir Crit Care Med 2008;178:574.

80. Vachier I, Bonnans C, Chavis C, et al. Severe asthma is associated with a loss of LX4, an endogenous anti-inflammatory compound. J Allergy Clin Immunol 2005;115:55.

81. Dahlen SE, Franzen L, Raud J, et al. Actions of lipoxin A4 and related compounds in smooth muscle preparations and on the microcirculation in vivo. Adv Exp Med Biol 1988;229:107.

82. Christie PE, Spur BW, Lee TH. The effects of lipoxin A4 on airway responses in asthmatic subjects. Am Rev Respir Dis 1992;145:1281.

83. Sanak M, Levy BD, Clish CB, et al. Aspirin-tolerant asthmatics generate more lipoxins than aspirin-intolerant asthmatics. Eur Respir J 2000;16:44.

84. Levy BD, Bonnans C, Silverman ES, et al. Diminished lipoxin biosynthesis in severe asthma. Am J Respir Crit Care Med 2005;172:824.

85. Celik GE, Erkekol FO, Misirligil Z, et al. Lipoxin A4 levels in asthma: relation with disease severity and aspirin sensitivity. Clin Exp Allergy 2007;37:1494.

86. Tahan F, Saraymen R, Gumus H. The role of lipoxin A4 in exercise-induced bronchoconstriction in asthma. J Asthma 2008;45:161.

87. Karp CL, Flick LM, Park KW, et al. Defective lipoxin-mediated anti-inflammatory activity in the cystic fibrosis airway. Nat Immunol 2004;5:388.

88. Kowal-Bielecka O, Kowal K, Distler O, et al. Cyclooxygenase- and lipoxygenase-derived eicosanoids in bronchoalveolar lavage fluid from patients with scleroderma lung disease: an imbalance between proinflammatory and antiinflammatory lipid mediators. Arthritis Rheum 2005;52:3783.

89. Schwartz J, Weiss ST. The relationship of dietary fish intake to level of pulmonary function in the first National Health and Nutrition Survey (NHANES I). Eur Respir J 1994;7:1821.

90. Connor KM, SanGiovanni JP, Lofqvist C, et al. Increased dietary intake of omega-3-polyunsaturated fatty acids reduces pathological retinal angiogenesis. Nat Med 2007;13:868.

91. Hudert CA, Weylandt KH, Lu Y, et al. Transgenic mice rich in endogenous omega-3 fatty acids are protected from colitis. Proc Natl Acad Sci U S A 2006;103:11276.

92. Bilal S, Haworth O, Wu L, et al. Fat-1 transgenic mice with elevated omega-3 fatty acids are protected from allergic airway responses. Biochim Biophys Acta 2011;1812:1164.

93. Arita M, Ohira T, Sun YP, et al. Resolvin E1 selectively interacts with leukotriene B4 receptor BLT1 and ChemR23 to regulate inflammation. J Immunol 2007;178:3912.

94. Cash JL, Hart R, Russ A, et al. Synthetic chemerin-derived peptides suppress inflammation through ChemR23. J Exp Med 2008;205:767.

95. Samson M, Edinger AL, Stordeur P, et al. ChemR23, a putative chemoattractant receptor, is expressed in monocyte-derived dendritic cells and macrophages and is a coreceptor for SIV and some primary HIV-1 strains. Eur J Immunol 1998;28:1689.

96. Wittamer V, Franssen JD, Vulcano M, et al. Specific recruitment of antigen-presenting cells by chemerin, a novel processed ligand from human inflammatory fluids. J Exp Med 2003;198:977.

97. Yokomizo T, Izumi T, Chang K, et al. A G-protein-coupled receptor for leukotriene B4 that mediates chemotaxis. Nature 1997;387:620.

98. Aoki H, Hisada T, Ishizuka T, et al. Resolvin E1 dampens airway inflammation and hyperresponsiveness in a murine model of asthma. Biochem Biophys Res Commun 2008;367:509.

99. Haworth O, Cernadas M, Levy BD. NK cells are effectors for resolvin E1 in the timely resolution of allergic airway inflammation. J Immunol 2011;186:6129.

100. Haworth O, Cernadas M, Yang R, et al. Resolvin E1 regulates interleukin 23, interferon-gamma and lipoxin A4 to promote the resolution of allergic airway inflammation. Nat Immunol 2008;9:873.

101. Serhan CN, Gotlinger K, Hong S, et al. Anti-inflammatory actions of neuroprotectin D1/protectin D1 and its natural stereoisomers: assignments of dihydroxy-containing docosatrienes. J Immunol 2006;176:1848.

102. Bazan NG. Neuroprotectin D1-mediated anti-inflammatory and survival signaling in stroke, retinal degenerations, and Alzheimer's disease. J Lipid Res 2009;50:S400.

103. Serhan CN, Chiang N, Van Dyke TE. Resolving inflammation: dual anti-inflammatory and pro-resolution lipid mediators. Nat Rev Immunol 2008;8:349.

104. Marcheselli VL, Mukherjee PK, Arita M, et al. Neuroprotectin D1/protectin D1 stereoselective and specific binding with human retinal pigment epithelial cells and neutrophils. Prostaglandins Leukot Essent Fatty Acids 2010;82:27.

105. Kasuga K, Yang R, Porter TF, et al. Rapid appearance of resolvin precursors in inflammatory exudates: novel mechanisms in resolution. J Immunol 2008;181:8677.

106. Levy BD, Kohli P, Gotlinger K, et al. Protectin D1 is generated in asthma and dampens airway inflammation and hyperresponsiveness. J Immunol 2007;178:496.

107. Bandeira-Melo C, Bozza PT, Diaz BL, et al. Cutting edge: lipoxin (LX) A4 and aspirin-triggered 15-epi-LXA4 block allergen-induced eosinophil trafficking. J Immunol 2000;164:2267.

108. Ariel A, Chiang N, Arita M, et al. Aspirin-triggered lipoxin A4 and B4 analogs block extracellular signal-regulated kinase-dependent TNF-alpha secretion from human T cells. J Immunol 2003;170:6266.

109. Colgan SP, Serhan CN, Parkos CA, et al. Lipoxin A4 modulates transmigration of human neutrophils across intestinal epithelial monolayers. J Clin Invest 1993;92:75.

110. Papayianni A, Serhan CN, Brady HR. Lipoxin A4 and B4 inhibit leukotriene-stimulated interactions of human neutrophils and endothelial cells. J Immunol 1996;156:2264.

111. Soyombo O, Spur BW, Lee TH. Effects of lipoxin A4 on chemotaxis and degranulation of human

eosinophils stimulated by platelet-activating factor and N-formyl-L-methionyl-L-leucyl-L-phenylalanine. Allergy 1994;49:230.

112. Ramstedt U, Serhan CN, Nicolaou KC, et al. Lipoxin A-induced inhibition of human natural killer cell cytotoxicity: studies on stereospecificity of inhibition and mode of action. J Immunol 1987;138:266.

113. Bonnans C, Vachier I, Chavis C, et al. Lipoxins are potential endogenous antiinflammatory mediators in asthma. Am J Respir Crit Care Med 2002;165:1531.

114. Parameswaran K, Radford K, Fanat A, et al. Modulation of human airway smooth muscle migration by lipid mediators and Th-2 cytokines. Am J Respir Cell Mol Biol 2007;37:240.

115. Brezinski ME, Gimbrone MA Jr, Nicolaou KC, et al. Lipoxins stimulate prostacyclin generation by human endothelial cells. FEBS Lett 1989;245:167.

116. Bonnans C, Fukunaga K, Levy MA, et al. Lipoxin A(4) regulates bronchial epithelial cell responses to acid injury. Am J Pathol 2006;168:1064.

117. Bonnans C, Mainprice B, Chanez P, et al. Lipoxin A4 stimulates a cytosolic Ca^{2+} increase in human bronchial epithelium. J Biol Chem 2003;278:10879.

118. Ariel A, Li PL, Wang W, et al. The docosatriene protectin D1 is produced by TH2 skewing and promotes human T cell apoptosis via lipid raft clustering. J Biol Chem 2005;280:43079.

119. Bhavsar PK, Levy BD, Hew MJ, et al. Corticosteroid suppression of lipoxin A4 and leukotriene B4 from alveolar macrophages in severe asthma. Respir Res 2010;11:71.

120. Wu SH, Yin PL, Zhang YM, et al. Reversed changes of lipoxin A4 and leukotrienes in children with asthma in different severity degree. Pediatr Pulmonol 2010;45:333.

Severe Asthma in Adults
An Orphan Disease?

Mina Gaga, MD, PhD[a],*, Eleftherios Zervas, MD[a],
Konstantinos Samitas, MD, PhD[a], Elisabeth H. Bel, MD, PhD[b]

KEYWORDS

- Severe asthma • Rare disease • Orphan act • Phenotypes • Treatment-response

KEY POINTS

- Severe asthma is associated with a high risk of death and disability and has a large impact on health, quality of life, and cost to patients and society and large.
- Long-term, multicenter, international studies are needed to enroll a substantial number of well-characterized subjects, examine the evolution of the disease, and evaluate the effect of treatment in specific asthma phenotypes.
- Given the poor response to treatment and side effects associated with medications more efficient, cost-effective, and phenotype-specific medications are needed; considering severe asthma as an orphan disease could encourage the pharmaceutical industry to work towards this end.

INTRODUCTION

Although asthma is a prevalent chronic disease, severe asthma that is refractory to treatment is rare. Epidemiologic data on severe asthma prevalence are missing, but severe asthma probably affects approximately 10% of patients with asthma, whereas severe treatment-resistant/refractory asthma probably affects 1% to 2%.[1,2] Moreover, severe asthma is an extremely heterogeneous disease in terms of clinical presentation and pathophysiologic mechanisms. Studies of severe asthma cohorts, such as the European Network for Understanding Mechanisms of Severe Asthma (ENFUMOSA), Severe Asthma Research Program (SARP), the Epidemiology and Natural History of Asthma: Outcomes and Treatment Regimens study (TENOR), and single-center cohorts (**Table 1**),[3–21] provide important information on severe asthma and introduce the concept of specific phenotypes in terms of clinical, physiologic, pathophysiologic, and treatment response characteristics. Moreover, some patients exhibit concordant disease, such as severe symptoms, inflammation, and impairment, whereas others show discordant disease, with very poor correlation between symptoms, inflammation, bronchial tissue damage, and functional impairment.[22] Although important new information has been gained from these recent severe asthma studies, many questions remain unanswered and the issue of treatment is still unresolved.

Management of severe asthma follows the general principles of overall asthma management, and inhaled steroids and long-acting β-agonists remain the cornerstone of treatment. However, severe asthma requires more classes of medication, including oral steroids and omalizumab, and some newer compounds are currently being tested. Nevertheless, a substantial number of patients have severe asthma that remains uncontrolled. Given the poor response to treatment and the side effects associated with medications for severe asthma, such as oral steroids, new pharmaceutical compounds must be developed

Financial disclosures and/or conflicts of interest: The authors have nothing to disclose.
[a] 7th Respiratory Department and Asthma Centre, Athens Chest Hospital, 152 Mesogion Avenue, Athens 11527, Greece; [b] Department of Pulmonology, Academic Medical Centre, Meibergdreef 9, 1105 AZ, Amsterdam, The Netherlands
* Corresponding author.
E-mail address: minagaga@yahoo.com

Table 1
Important studies on severe asthma

Study Authors	Population	Major Outcomes/Conclusions
European Network for Understanding Mechanisms of Severe Asthma (ENFUMOSA)		
ENFUMOSA Study Group,[3] 2003	• 163 SA • 158 MMA	• Female predominance • Neutrophilic inflammation • Less atopy but ongoing inflammatory mediator release
Gaga et al,[9] 2005	• 155 SA • 148 MMA	• Less atopy and family allergy history • Impaired QoL
Romagnoli et al,[17] 2007	• 67 MMA • 64 SA • 24 NFA	• Patients with NFA less compliant • Lung function, blood gases, and inflammatory markers similar to MMA but not SA
The Epidemiology and Natural History of Asthma: Outcomes and Treatment Regimens study (TENOR)		
Dolan et al,[7] 2004	• 4756 patients with difficult-to-treat asthma	• 48% of patients had severe asthma according to physician evaluation • 17% of patients whose asthma was categorized as severe had a history of intubation • Highest IgE levels in SA • Highest health care use in SA
Miller et al,[14] 2006	• 2821 SA from TENOR cohort	• Health care use in SA was associated with younger age, female sex, non-white race, BMI >35, history of pneumonia, diabetes, cataracts, intubation for asthma, and ≥ three steroid bursts in the prior 3 months
Campell et al,[5] 2008	• 774 SA from TENOR cohort	• Some SA respond better to low-dose ICS-LABA combination therapy • SA on high-dose ICS-LABA combination do not experience significant improvement in many control-related health outcomes
Haselkorn et al,[11] 2009	• 807 SA from TENOR cohort	• Very poorly controlled asthma is a strong predictor of future exacerbations
Severe Asthma Research Program (SARP)		
Busacker et al,[4] 2009	• 60 SA from SARP cohort • 34 MMA • 26 healthy controls	• Air-trapping phenotype associated with asthma duration, history of pneumonia, airway neutrophilia, airflow obstruction, and atopy • Quantitative CT-determined air trapping identifies asthma phenotype at high risk for severe disease

Study	Population	Findings
Moore et al,[15] 2010	• 726 SA from SARP cohort	• Identification of five distinct clinical phenotypes using cluster analysis: Cluster 1: early-onset atopic asthma with normal lung function Cluster 2: early-onset atopic asthma and preserved lung function but increased medication requirements and health care use Cluster 3: mostly older obese women with late-onset nonatopic asthma, moderate reductions in FEV_1, and frequent oral CS use Cluster 4 and 5: patients with severe airflow obstruction, frequent exacerbations, use of oral CS, history of ICU admission, and poor QoL
Hastie et al,[12] 2010	• 242 SA from SARP cohort	• Increased sputum eosinophils and neutrophils associated with SA phenotype characterized by the lowest lung function, worse asthma control, and increased symptoms and health care requirements
Holguin et al,[13] 2011	• 436 SA from SARP cohort • 613 MMA	• Patients with asthma are differentially affected by obesity based on whether they had early- or late-onset asthma • Obese subjects with early-onset asthma had more airway obstruction, AHR, and more oral CS courses or ICU admissions
The Leiden cohort		
ten Brinke et al,[18] 2001	• 132 SA	• Persistent airflow obstruction strongly associated with AHR, late-onset asthma, and sputum eosinophilia
ten Brinke et al,[19] 2004	• 22 SA with sputum eosinophilia	• 2 wk of treatment with CS resolved sputum eosinophilia, decreased rescue medication use, and improved FEV_1
ten Brinke et al,[20] 2005	• 136 patients with difficult-to-treat asthma	• Patients with recurrent exacerbations constitute a distinct phenotype of younger patients with late-onset asthma with frequent common comorbidities
Other studies		
Green et al,[10] 2002	• 34 healthy controls • 259 patients with asthma receiving treatment according to BTS steps 1–3	• Presence of a distinct subgroup of older, predominantly female, nonatopic patients with mainly neutrophilic airway inflammation who respond less well to ICS

(continued on next page)

Table 1
(continued)

Study Authors	Population	Major Outcomes/Conclusions
Fabbri et al,[8] 2003	• 19 patients with asthma with fixed airway obstruction • 27 patients with COPD and fixed airway obstruction	• Patients with asthma with fixed airway obstruction had more eosinophils in blood, sputum, BALF, and airway mucosa; fewer neutrophils in sputum and BALF; higher CD4/CD8 ratio of infiltrating T cells; and thicker RBM
van Veen et al,[21] 2008	• 136 patients with difficult-to-treat asthma	• Obese patients with difficult-to-treat asthma have less sputum eosinophilia and FeNO and are associated with higher presence of comorbid factors and reduced lung volumes
Contoli et al,[6] 2010	• 15 patients with asthma with reversible airflow obstruction • 16 patients with asthma with fixed airway obstruction • 21 patients with COPD with fixed airway obstruction	• The rate of FEV_1 decline was similar in patients with asthma and COPD with fixed airway obstruction, and higher in patients with asthma with reversible obstruction • FEV_1 inversely correlated with sputum eosinophilia and baseline eNO levels in patients with asthma with fixed airway obstruction • Fixed airflow obstruction was associated with increased lung function decline and frequency of exacerbations
Ponte et al,[16] 2011	• 731 SA	• 10% of patients had at least one severe exacerbation that required ICU admission • Patients with near-fatal asthma on admission had worse lung function measurements and were more likely to have asthma exacerbations during the follow-up period and respond poorly to therapy

Abbreviations: AHR, airway hyperresponsiveness; BALF, bronchoalveolar lavage fluid; BMI, body mass index; BTS, British Thoracic Society; COPD, chronic obstructive pulmonary disease; CS, corticosteroids; eNO, endothelial nitric oxide; FeNO, fractional exhaled nitric oxide; FEV_1, forced expiratory volume in the first second of expiration; ICU, intensive care unit; ICS, inhaled corticosteroid; LABA, long-acting β_2-agonist; MMA, patients with mild-to-moderate asthma; NFA, near-fatal asthma; QoL, quality of life; RBM, reticular basement membrane; SA, patients with severe asthma.

and their effects examined. However, patients with severe asthma are few, and pathophysiologic mechanisms and responses to treatment must be examined in each phenotypic group within this small population. Therefore, this severe spectrum of the disease likely fits the definition of a rare or orphan disease.

This article briefly describes severe asthma and its definition, risk factors, phenotypes, and treatment options, and provides a definition of orphan disease. Severe asthma remains a challenge to treat, greatly affects the lives of patients, and represents a huge cost to patients and society. New treatment options are needed and their effectiveness should be examined in long-term studies and meticulously characterized cohorts.

DEFINITION OF SEVERE ASTHMA

The concept of asthma severity has evolved substantially over the years. In the early Global Initiative for Asthma (GINA) and National Asthma Education and Prevention Program (NAEPP) guidelines, overall asthma severity was assessed primarily based on the patient's clinical characteristics before treatment initiation.[23,24] According to the 2009 World Health Organization Consultation,[25] severe asthma comprises three groups: untreated, difficult-to-treat, and treatment-resistant severe.

Untreated severe asthma is, of course, a major issue in areas where asthma drugs are not readily available or reimbursed and deaths from asthma are common—mostly low-income countries. However, in Europe and North America, treatment is widely available and many patients with severe asthma experience response to treatment and lead a normal life. In these areas, the important problems are treatment-resistant asthma and asthma that requires continuous high-dose treatment that is associated with important medication side effects and high long-term risk. This therapy-resistant/refractory/difficult-to-treat asthma has been the subject of several reports published by the European Respiratory Society (ERS), the American Thoracic Society (ATS), and panels of experts, and is currently the issue of a joint ERS/ATS task force.[26–29]

According to these reports, severe difficult-to-treat asthma is defined as disease that requires high-intensity treatment although modifiable factors and comorbidities have been appropriately managed, and includes two categories of patients: (1) those who require continuous high-intensity treatment to maintain control and (2) those with poor asthma control and/or frequent exacerbations despite high-intensity treatment. According to the ongoing ERS/ATS task force on severe asthma, the proposed definition describes severe asthma as asthma that requires treatment with high-dose inhaled corticosteroids (ICS) plus a second controller (and/or systemic corticosteroids) to prevent it from becoming uncontrolled, or that remains uncontrolled despite this therapy. This definition therefore includes treatment-resistant asthma and severe asthma that persists because of inability to effectively treat confounders/comorbidities, such as severe sinus disease or obesity, but does not include untreated asthma.

EVALUATION AND MONITORING

In evaluating the patient, the diagnosis of severe asthma must be confirmed and other diseases excluded, such as vocal cord dysfunction, Churg-Strauss syndrome, panbronchiolitis, chronic obstructive pulmonary disease (COPD), and many others that may be associated with asthma.[28] Once the diagnosis is confirmed, the physician should assess frequency/severity of symptoms and exacerbations. Validated measures to examine symptom severity, such as dyspnea scales, are valuable indicators of a patient's ability to cope at rest and during activity. Lung function testing is clearly paramount and should initially include not only prebronchodilation and postbronchodilation spirometry but also lung volumes.[30] Furthermore, it is clearly important to assess all possible risk factors associated with the disease and suggest avoidance of exposure, when possible. These risk factors include occupational exposure, exposure to pets and other indoor allergens, stress, and sensitivity to medications, such as aspirin.[31] Noninvasive and invasive assessment of inflammation allows better phenotyping of the patient and helps provide more-targeted treatment options.[32] This assessment includes examination of induced sputum and, if possible, tissue samples obtained using fiberoptic bronchoscopy.

Severe asthma is also complicated by significant comorbidities, such as depression and other psychopathologies, rhinosinusitis, recurrent infections, gastroesophageal reflux, osteoporosis, diabetes mellitus, hormonal dysfunction, and obesity, which further incapacitate patients and should be evaluated and managed concurrent with asthma treatment.[33] Compliance is another important issue and always should be evaluated. A good relationship with the patient, continuous discussion of perceptions and fears regarding medications, particularly steroids, and education lead to better compliance and better control.[34]

Evaluation is initially mainly based on history and lung function, but the patient must be reviewed regularly for a period of at least 6 months, preferably longer.[28] This regular long-term follow-up allows physicians to get to know the patients, assess them properly, and adjust treatment. Asthma control questionnaires and quality-of-life questionnaires help doctors understand the patients' problems and perception of disease and are invaluable in the regular follow-up. Many biomarkers have been examined, but those that have been shown to predict response to treatment and/or loss of control are sputum eosinophils and exhaled NO. Nevertheless, more research is needed.

SEVERE ASTHMA PHENOTYPES: A CLUSTER OF RARE DISEASES?

Until a few years ago, severe asthma was usually classified in terms such as *severe occupational*, *aspirin-induced*, *premenstrual*, *intrinsic*, and *brittle*. These classifications still stand; however, it is more important to classify asthma in terms of clinical presentation, pathophysiologic characteristics, and response to treatment (**Box 1**). These features include frequency and severity of exacerbations, age of onset, lung function status, risk factors, and comorbidities, and also the extent, type, and site of inflammation; remodeling changes; and airway smooth muscle dysfunction, all of which could overlap (**Fig. 1**).

Clinical/Physiology Phenotypes

Assessment of inflammation and pathophysiologic changes is not universally performed or available.

In clinical practice, physicians must treat patients with different clinical phenotypes, such as (1) those who, despite high-dose treatment, present with continuous symptoms and/or frequent severe exacerbations but have normal lung function, (2) those with permanent airflow limitation but few symptoms, and (3) those with continuous symptoms, frequent severe exacerbations, and poor lung function. Lung function impairment has been associated with worse outcome,[35] and a history of exacerbations is associated with more severe lung function decline and a higher risk of future exacerbations.[36] Therefore, the last group has the highest risk.[11]

Patients with severe asthma with frequent exacerbations have a specific phenotype of severe asthma that has been addressed in several studies. In the Netherlands,[20] active recruitment in 10 hospitals resulted in the participation of 136 adult patients with difficult-to-treat asthma, showing how small a part of asthma this group represents. Fewer than one-third of these patients exhibited more than three exacerbations during the study. These frequent exacerbators were generally younger and had late-onset asthma with frequent comorbidities. Similar results were observed in the SARP database, in which a small group of patients (59 of 304 with difficult-to-treat asthma) with frequent exacerbations was also found.[15] This exacerbation-prone subgroup represented a difficult-to-manage, late-onset phenotype of mostly older obese women with decreased baseline pulmonary function who required continuous

---

Box 1
Phenotyping severe asthma according to clinical physiology, pathophysiology, and treatment response

1. Clinical/physiology-related phenotypes

   a. Type and number of exacerbations (eg, exacerbation-prone asthma, near-fatal asthma)

   b. Pattern of airflow obstruction (eg, fixed airway obstruction, small airway obstruction)

   c. Presence of comorbidities (eg, obesity-related asthma, asthma with rhinosinusitis)

2. Pathology/pathophysiology-related phenotypes

   a. Type of inflammation (eg, eosinophilic and/ or neutrophilic, paucigranulocytic)

   b. Structural changes (eg, remodeling)

   c. Site of inflammation (eg, large and/or small airways)

   d. Smooth muscle abnormality

3. Treatment-related phenotypes

   a. Corticosteroid responsiveness (eg, corticosteroid-dependent or corticosteroid-resistant asthma)

   b. β-adrenergic responsiveness

   c. Immunomodulated treatment response (eg, anti-IgE, anti–interleukin [IL]-5)

   d. Inflammatory-based treatment (eg, anti–IL-5, CXCR2)

   e. Smooth muscle–targeted therapy (eg, bronchial thermoplasty)

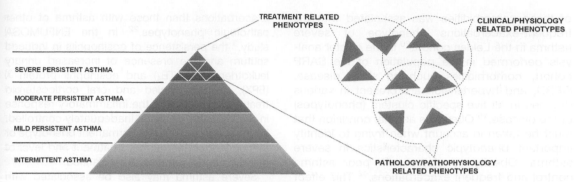

Fig. 1. Schematic representation of asthma severity identifying phenotypes of severe asthma according to clinical, pathologic, and treatment-related features, with potential overlapping of groups.

oral corticosteroid therapy. In the TENOR study, the largest-to-date cohort of patients with severe asthma, a subgroup of patients (n = 244; 8.8%) with frequent exacerbations was also identified.[7] These patients were more likely to be young, black, female, and overweight adults.[14] Furthermore, recent severe asthma exacerbations were strongly associated with future exacerbations, suggesting that this group of patients represents a small specific phenotype of severe asthma.

Patients with near-fatal asthma exacerbations, usually requiring admission to the intensive care unit (ICU) and intubation, have also been recognized in the past as an apparent but rare group of patients with asthma. In the ENFUMOSA cohort, a group of 24 patients was isolated that had a near-fatal episode in the previous 5 years.[17] Surprisingly, these patients' lung function, atopic status, sputum cultures, and blood inflammatory cell counts were similar to those of patients with mild-to-moderate, but not severe, asthma. In the SARP cohort, approximately 12% of the severe asthma population had an ICU stay in the previous year.[15] Contrary to the ENFUMOSA findings, these patients had abnormal lung function despite the use of multiple asthma medications and increased sputum inflammation. In the TENOR study, a significant proportion of patients with severe asthma (17%) reported an ICU admission for asthma, but no further characterization of these patients was performed.[7] Similar percentages of patients with near-fatal exacerbations were reported in a recent prospective 4-year study in Salvador involving 731 patients with severe asthma.[16] As many as 10% of patients had at least one severe exacerbation that required ICU admission. Patients with near-fatal asthma on admission had worse lung function measurements and were more likely to have asthma exacerbations during the follow-up period and to experience a poor response to therapy. Whether near-fatal asthma is a specific phenotype must be elucidated.

Another small subgroup of patients with severe asthma consists of those with reduced lung function and persistent airflow limitation. In the Leiden cohort, approximately half (n = 66; 48.5%) of the nonsmoking patients with severe asthma seemed to have persistent airflow limitation despite treatment.[18] This phenotype was associated with older age, adult-onset asthma, and a longer duration of disease, and with sputum eosinophilia and airway hyperresponsiveness (AHR). Studies from the U.S. National Heart, Lung, and Blood Institute Children's Asthma Management Program (CAMP) suggest that only a fraction of patients with childhood-onset asthma develop progressive loss of lung function over a 5-year period.[37] These children are more likely to be boys, less allergic, and less predisposed to exacerbations than the children with asthma who have no loss of lung function. However, data from the United Kingdom report that children with multiple sensitizations have a worse prognosis, so the data are conflicting.[38] Similar outcomes have been seen in TENOR study,[7] whereas in a study from Italy, eosinophilic inflammation was prominent, with evidence of remodeling changes in bronchial biopsies.[8] In a 5-year prospective study of these subjects, fixed airflow obstruction was associated with accelerated lung function decline and frequency of exacerbations.[6] In clinical practice, this is an important phenotype of severe asthma, often confused with COPD. This phenotype is far less studied, because patients with fixed airway obstruction are usually excluded from clinical trials.

An important issue in severe asthma is the presence of comorbidities, including mainly rhinosinusitis, gastroesophageal reflux disease (GERD), obstructive sleep apnea, hormonal disorders, and psychopathologies.[33] Many of these conditions share common pathophysiologic mechanisms with asthma, influence the response to treatment, and lead to poor asthma control.[39–41] The presence of these comorbidities was associated with the frequent-exacerbations phenotype of severe asthma in the Leiden cohort.[20] In the cluster analysis performed in the population of the SARP cohort, comorbidities such as sinus disease, GERD, and hypertension are present in various degrees in all five specific clusters (phenotypes) of the disease.[15] Obesity is another condition that must be taken in account when trying to identify important phenotypic characteristics in severe asthma. Obesity correlates with poor asthma control and frequent exacerbations.[42] This effect is modified by age of asthma onset, as illustrated in the SARP cohort, in which a phenotype of obese subjects with early-onset asthma, airway obstruction, bronchial hyperresponsiveness, and exacerbations was identified.[13] Obesity may have an effect on the pattern of asthma inflammation; obesity in patients with difficult-to-treat asthma inversely correlated with sputum eosinophils and fractional exhaled nitric oxide (FeNO),[21] as indicated in the Netherlands cohort. This paradigm shows the close relationship between clinical and pathobiologic phenotypes of severe asthma.

Pathology/Pathophysiology Phenotypes

From a pathologic point of view, at least two phenotypes of severe asthma have been proposed, each associated with distinct clinical and pathophysiologic characteristics. These subtypes include the persistent eosinophilic and noneosinophilic forms of severe asthma.[43] These phenotypes are becoming increasingly associated with distinct clinical and physiologic inflammatory and repair processes.[44] Usually, inflammatory cells are present and activated in the airways of patients with severe asthma and persist despite treatment, but their relevance to control and severity of the disease is largely unknown. These cells include not only eosinophils and neutrophils but also T lymphocytes, mast cells, and macrophages. Structural cells are also involved in the inflammatory reaction and remodeling in asthma.

Eosinophilic severe asthma is the best-studied pathologic phenotype. Eosinophilic phenotypes have traditionally been identified using induced sputum or endobronchial biopsy analysis.[43,45] Additionally, exhaled nitric oxide concentration has been proposed as a less-invasive tool.[46] Eosinophils may be an important biomarker of some key features of severe asthma. Persistent eosinophilic phenotype in severe asthma is often associated with adult-onset disease and fixed airway obstruction.[18] Patients with eosinophilic inflammation frequently have more symptoms, worse disease control, and a greater risk of

exacerbations than those with asthma of other pathologic phenotypes.[22] In the ENFUMOSA study,[3] the persistence of eosinophils in induced sputum and the presence of increased urinary leukotriene E_4 (LTE$_4$) and eosinophil protein X (EPX), despite inhaled and oral corticosteroid treatment, shows that the inflammatory response in severe asthma may be inadequately controlled. Whether eosinophilia is a permanent phenotype or one dependent on current treatment and level of disease control remains to be clarified.

Severe asthma may also be associated with neutrophilic inflammation, as indicated in the ENFUMOSA cohort,[3] but the precise role of neutrophils remains to be determined. This phenotype seems to be less responsive to corticosteroid therapy than eosinophilic asthma.[10] However, many patients with neutrophilic inflammation can have concomitant eosinophilic inflammation. These features combined identified patients with asthma with the lowest lung function, worse asthma control, and increased symptoms in the SARP cohort.[12]

The patterns of airway remodeling can also distinguish different subtypes of severe asthma. Remodeling is associated with more severe airflow obstruction and airway hyperresponsiveness; however, the clinical significance of this is still under debate.[47] Small airway inflammation is another interesting field in the phenotyping of patients with severe asthma. In the study by Balzar and colleagues,[48] small airways in patients with severe asthma had significantly higher numbers of inflammatory cells than medium or large airways. This increased inflammation of distal airways can contribute to the air trapping/airway closure that characterizes a subgroup of patients with severe asthma.[30] In a substudy in the SARP cohort,[4] quantitative CT-determined air trapping in patients with asthma identifies a group of individuals at high risk for severe disease, with poor asthma control and frequent exacerbations.

Airway smooth muscle (ASM) greatly affects airway caliber, and ASM dysfunction contributes to the pathophysiology of severe asthma.[49] In an Australian postmortem study of fatal (n = 107) and nonfatal asthma (n = 37), thickness of the ASM layer correlated with severity but not duration of asthma.[50] A recent study from Canada[51] further emphasizes the role of ASM in airway remodeling. In this study, patients with severe asthma with chronic persistent obstruction have increased ASM with ongoing T-helper types 1 and 2 inflammatory responses. Neither airway imaging nor sputum analysis was able to identify these patients. Therefore, it is important to recognize this ASM-prodominant phenotype of severe asthma, because a novel treatment focusing on this feature of remodeling, bronchial thermoplasty, was introduced recently with good results.[52]

Treatment

The current pharmacologic approach to the treatment of difficult asthma is similar to that used for the treatment of patients with milder forms of the disease. Most patients with difficult asthma meet the GINA[53] or NAEPP guidelines[54] criteria for steps 4 and 5, severe, uncontrolled asthma, and require high-dose ICS, long-acting inhaled β_2-agonists, and additional medications, such as theophylline, oral steroids, leukotriene antagonists, and omalizumab. To date, ICS and bronchodilators are the mainstay of severe persistent asthma treatment,[55,56] but most patients remain uncontrolled on high medication doses, with high future risk and poor quality of life.[5] Oral steroids are often used, although many questions remain to be answered, such as when to initiate regular oral treatment and whether steroid-refractory asthma really exists or is a matter of compliance. A study by Elisabeth Bel's group[19] showed that patients with refractory asthma uncontrolled on oral steroids fared better with parenteral treatment. Parenteral steroids reduced sputum eosinophils and increased forced expiratory volume in the first second of expiration (FEV_1). The study raises the question of whether this is an issue of refractoriness to particular steroid preparations or simply a matter of compliance. Cochrane reviews have shown that steroid-sparing drugs, such as methotrexate and cyclosporine A, do not have a beneficial risk effect ratio and do not seem to provide an alternative.[57,58]

A newer medication used in severe asthma is omalizumab, a monoclonal anti-IgE antibody.[59] This medication should be used in patients with documented sensitization to an aeroallergen and IgE detected in their serum. In selected patients, omalizumab improves quality of life and reduces the doses of inhaled steroids.[60] Good phenotypic characterization is required, because the medication does not improve all patients and the cost of the drug is high. A recent study from the United States examined the costs and consequences of omalizumab from a payer perspective, and suggested that the addition of omalizumab to usual care may improve asthma control but at a significant increase in direct medical costs.[61]

Newer medications are currently being tested, such as anti–tumor necrosis factor (TNF), anti–interleukin (IL)-5, and a soluble IL-2 receptor. Anti-TNF is used in the treatment of rheumatoid arthritis with good results and has been tested in severe asthma, but the study was discontinued because no good risk-effect ratio was shown.[62] Anti–IL-5 treatment was also tested and these studies provide a good example of the importance of phenotyping in asthma.[63] In the initial anti–IL-5 studies, inclusion of patients was not based on specific phenotypes, and the studies were negative.[64,65] However, later studies showed that the medication was beneficial in eosinophilic asthma.[66,67] Therefore, the successful outcome depends on the phenotype of the selected patients. However, preliminary data support that patients with neutrophilic asthma may benefit from treatment with CXCR2,[68] but again, larger studies are needed. Daclizumab, a soluble receptor of IL-2 currently used as an immunosuppressor in organ transplantation, has been shown to improve pulmonary function and asthma control in patients with moderate to severe chronic asthma inadequately controlled on ICS.[69] For patients with smooth muscle hyperplasia, bronchial thermoplasty may prove beneficial because it has been shown to improve control in severe asthma.[70,71] All of these studies examine a small number of patients who were not meticulously phenotyped and the results are not clear.

Research into newer compounds is clearly necessary and should be supported. Studies should involve adequate cohorts of well-characterized patients and be long-term. However, because the outcome is very important but refers to a small number of patients, and no financial gain is expected, these studies would be better supported if severe asthma was considered an orphan disease.

RARE DISEASES AND ORPHAN DRUGS

No single, satisfactory, worldwide-accepted definition for rare or orphan diseases exists. The United States and Europe have a different set of rules and definitions regarding orphan diseases, whereas country-specific regulations also exist. Most definitions for orphan diseases usually involve the number of people affected by the disease and other factors, such as the lack of available treatments or the severity of the disease.

In the United States, orphan diseases are defined by the Rare Diseases Act[72] of 2002. According to this Act, rare diseases and disorders are those affecting small patient populations, typically populations smaller than 200,000 in the United States. In the European Union (EU), rare diseases are defined by the European Medicines Agency as "life-threatening or chronically debilitating diseases which are of such low prevalence that special combined efforts are needed to address them."[73]

Drugs, biologics, medical devices, and foods intended for the safe and effective treatment, diagnosis, or prevention of rare diseases are termed "orphan drugs," because the pharmaceutical industry has little interest in developing and marketing products intended for only a small number of patients with rare conditions. Orphan drug status is provided according to the U.S. Orphan Drug Act[74] (ODA), which ensures a 7-year marketing exclusivity to sponsors of approved orphan products, a tax credit of 50% of the cost of conducting human clinical testing, and research grants for clinical testing of new therapies to treat orphan diseases. Before this legislation, private industry had little incentive to invest money in the development of treatments for small patient populations, because the drugs were expected to be unprofitable.

Similar to the ODA, in the EU orphan drug designation is done according to the Orphan Medicinal Products Regulation of 2000, accompanied by a 10-year marketing exclusivity and tax reductions that depend on the Member State. In addition to the United States and EU, similar legislation has been implemented in Japan, Singapore, and Australia offering subsidies and other incentives to encourage the development of drugs to treat orphan diseases.[75,76]

According to the EU definition, a disease should be life-threatening, chronically debilitating, and inadequately treated, not just statistically rare, to be considered orphan. Severe asthma is indeed life-threatening, debilitating, inadequately treated, and rare.

SUMMARY

Is severe asthma, then, an orphan disease? Should severe asthma be disassociated from asthma that responds to treatment? Is it a different disease? And should resources be allocated into research for severe asthma drugs under the orphan drug act? Clearly, a group of patients with severe asthma fits this orphan disease description. They are few, experience symptoms and debilitating restrictions to their daily activities, often experience life-threatening attacks, have asthma that does not respond to currently available medications or responds partially to very high doses of medications, and face unacceptable side effects and very high long-term risk. This severe spectrum of the disease probably fits the definition of a rare or orphan disease.

REFERENCE

1. Moore WC, Bleecker ER, Curran-Everett D, et al. Characterization of the severe asthma phenotype by the National Heart, Lung, and Blood Institute's Severe Asthma Research Program. J Allergy Clin Immunol 2007;119(2):405–13.
2. Wenzel SE, Busse WW. Severe asthma: lessons from the Severe Asthma Research Program. J Allergy Clin Immunol 2007;119(1):14–21.
3. The ENFUMOSA cross-sectional European multi-centre study of the clinical phenotype of chronic severe asthma. European Network for Understanding Mechanisms of Severe Asthma. Eur Respir J 2003;22(3):470–7.
4. Busacker A, Newell JD Jr, Keefe T, et al. A multivariate analysis of risk factors for the air-trapping asthmatic phenotype as measured by quantitative CT analysis. Chest 2009;135(1):48–56.
5. Campbell JD, Borish L, Haselkorn T, et al. The response to combination therapy treatment regimens in severe/difficult-to-treat asthma. Eur Respir J 2008;32(5):1237–42.
6. Contoli M, Baraldo S, Marku B, et al. Fixed airflow obstruction due to asthma or chronic obstructive pulmonary disease: 5-year follow-up. J Allergy Clin Immunol 2010;125(4):830–7.
7. Dolan CM, Fraher KE, Bleecker ER, et al. Design and baseline characteristics of the epidemiology and natural history of asthma: outcomes and treatment regimens (TENOR) study: a large cohort of patients with severe or difficult-to-treat asthma. Ann Allergy Asthma Immunol 2004;92(1):32–9.
8. Fabbri LM, Romagnoli M, Corbetta L, et al. Differences in airway inflammation in patients with fixed airflow obstruction due to asthma or chronic obstructive pulmonary disease. Am J Respir Crit Care Med 2003;167(3):418–24.
9. Gaga M, Papageorgiou N, Yiourgioti G, et al. Risk factors and characteristics associated with severe and difficult to treat asthma phenotype: an analysis of the ENFUMOSA group of patients based on the ECRHS questionnaire. Clin Exp Allergy 2005;35(7):954–9.
10. Green RH, Brightling CE, Woltmann G, et al. Analysis of induced sputum in adults with asthma: identification of subgroup with isolated sputum neutrophilia and poor response to inhaled corticosteroids. Thorax 2002;57(10):875–9.
11. Haselkorn T, Fish JE, Zeiger RS, et al. Consistently very poorly controlled asthma, as defined by the impairment domain of the Expert Panel Report 3 guidelines, increases risk for future severe asthma exacerbations in The Epidemiology and Natural History of Asthma: outcomes and treatment regimens (TENOR) study. J Allergy Clin Immunol 2009;124(5):805–902.

12. Hastie AT, Moore WC, Meyers DA, et al. Analyses of asthma severity phenotypes and inflammatory proteins in subjects stratified by sputum granulocytes. J Allergy Clin Immunol 2010;125(5):1028–36.

13. Holguin F, Bleecker ER, Busse WW, et al. Obesity and asthma: an association modified by age of asthma onset. J Allergy Clin Immunol 2011;127(6): 1486–93.

14. Miller MK, Lee JH, Blanc PD, et al. TENOR risk score predicts healthcare in adults with severe or difficult-to-treat asthma. Eur Respir J 2006;28(6): 1145–55.

15. Moore WC, Meyers DA, Wenzel SE, et al. Identification of asthma phenotypes using cluster analysis in the Severe Asthma Research Program. Am J Respir Crit Care Med 2010;181(4):315–23.

16. Ponte EV, Souza-Machado A, Souza-Machado C, et al. Clinical characteristics and prognosis in near-fatal asthma patients in Salvador, Brazil. J Bras Pneumol 2011;37(4):431–7.

17. Romagnoli M, Caramori G, Braccioni F, et al. Near-fatal asthma phenotype in the ENFUMOSA Cohort. Clin Exp Allergy 2007;37(4):552–7.

18. ten Brinke A, Zwinderman AH, Sterk PJ, et al. Factors associated with persistent airflow limitation in severe asthma. Am J Respir Crit Care Med 2001;164(5):744–8.

19. ten Brinke A, Zwinderman AH, Sterk PJ, et al. "Refractory" eosinophilic airway inflammation in severe asthma: effect of parenteral corticosteroids. Am J Respir Crit Care Med 2004;170(6):601–5.

20. ten Brinke A, Sterk PJ, Masclee AA, et al. Risk factors of frequent exacerbations in difficult-to-treat asthma. Eur Respir J 2005;26(5):812–8.

21. van Veen IH, ten Brinke A, Sterk PJ, et al. Airway inflammation in obese and nonobese patients with difficult-to-treat asthma. Allergy 2008;63(5):570–4.

22. Haldar P, Pavord ID, Shaw DE, et al. Cluster analysis and clinical asthma phenotypes. Am J Respir Crit Care Med 2008;178(3):218–24.

23. National Asthma Education and Prevention Program Expert Panel Report 2. Guidelines for the diagnosis and management of asthma. Bethesda (MD): National Heart, Lung, and Blood Institute; 1997.

24. Global Initiative for Asthma. Asthma management and prevention. NIH Publication number 95-3659A. Bethesda (MD): National Institutes of Health; 1995.

25. Bousquet J, Mantzouranis E, Cruz AA, et al. Uniform definition of asthma severity, control, and exacerbations: document presented for the World Health Organization Consultation on Severe Asthma. J Allergy Clin Immunol 2010;126(5):926–38.

26. Chung KF, Godard P, Adelroth E, et al. Difficult/therapy-resistant asthma: the need for an integrated approach to define clinical phenotypes, evaluate risk factors, understand pathophysiology and find novel therapies. ERS Task Force on Difficult/

27. Therapy-Resistant Asthma. European Respiratory Society. Eur Respir J 1999;13(5):1198–208.

27. Proceedings of the ATS workshop on refractory asthma: current understanding, recommendations, and unanswered questions. American Thoracic Society. Am J Respir Crit Care Med 2000;162(6):2341–51.

28. Chanez P, Wenzel SE, Anderson GP, et al. Severe asthma in adults: what are the important questions? J Allergy Clin Immunol 2007;119(6):1337–48.

29. Bel EH, Sousa A, Fleming L, et al. Diagnosis and definition of severe refractory asthma: an international consensus statement from the Innovative Medicine Initiative (IMI). Thorax 2011;66(10):910–7.

30. Sorkness RL, Bleecker ER, Busse WW, et al. Lung function in adults with stable but severe asthma: air trapping and incomplete reversal of obstruction with bronchodilation. J Appl Physiol 2008;104(2): 394–403.

31. Bel E, ten Brinke A. A rational approach to the management of severe refractory asthma. Treat Respir Med 2005;4(6):365–79.

32. Wenzel SE. Asthma: defining of the persistent adult phenotypes. Lancet 2006;368(9537):804–13.

33. Boulet LP, Boulay ME. Asthma-related comorbidities. Expert Rev Respir Med 2011;5(3):377–93.

34. Apter AJ, Wang X, Bogen DK, et al. Problem solving to improve adherence and asthma outcomes in urban adults with moderate or severe asthma: a randomized controlled trial. J Allergy Clin Immunol 2011;128(3):516–23.

35. de MR, Marcon A, Jarvis D, et al. Prognostic factors of asthma severity: a 9-year international prospective cohort study. J Allergy Clin Immunol 2006; 117(6):1249–56.

36. Bai TR, Vonk JM, Postma DS, et al. Severe exacerbations predict excess lung function decline in asthma. Eur Respir J 2007;30(3):452–6.

37. Covar RA, Spahn JD, Murphy JR, et al. Progression of asthma measured by lung function in the childhood asthma management program. Am J Respir Crit Care Med 2004;170(3):234–41.

38. Simpson A, Tan VY, Winn J, et al. Beyond atopy: multiple patterns of sensitization in relation to asthma in a birth cohort study. Am J Respir Crit Care Med 2010;181(11):1200–6.

39. Bresciani M, Paradis L, Des RA, et al. Rhinosinusitis in severe asthma. J Allergy Clin Immunol 2001; 107(1):73–80.

40. Liou A, Grubb JR, Schechtman KB, et al. Causative and contributive factors to asthma severity and patterns of medication use in patients seeking specialized asthma care. Chest 2003;124(5):1781–8.

41. Teodorescu M, Polomis DA, Hall SV, et al. Association of obstructive sleep apnea risk with asthma control in adults. Chest 2010;138(3):543–50.

42. Grammer LC, Weiss KB, Pedicano JB, et al. Obesity and asthma morbidity in a community-based adult

cohort in a large urban area: the Chicago Initiative to Raise Asthma Health Equity (CHIRAH). J Asthma 2010;47(5):491–5.

43. Wenzel SE, Schwartz LB, Langmack EL, et al. Evidence that severe asthma can be divided pathologically into two inflammatory subtypes with distinct physiologic and clinical characteristics. Am J Respir Crit Care Med 1999;160(3):1001–8.

44. Gaga M, Zervas E, Chanez P. Update on severe asthma: what we know and what we need. Eur Respir Rev 2009;18(112):58–65.

45. Lemiere C, Ernst P, Olivenstein R, et al. Airway inflammation assessed by invasive and noninvasive means in severe asthma: eosinophilic and noneosinophilic phenotypes. J Allergy Clin Immunol 2006; 118(5):1033–9.

46. Silkoff PE, Lent AM, Busacker AA, et al. Exhaled nitric oxide identifies the persistent eosinophilic phenotype in severe refractory asthma. J Allergy Clin Immunol 2005;116(6):1249–55.

47. Bergeron C, Tulic MK, Hamid Q. Tools used to measure airway remodelling in research. Eur Respir J 2007;29(3):596–604.

48. Balzar S, Wenzel SE, Chu HW. Transbronchial biopsy as a tool to evaluate small airways in asthma. Eur Respir J 2002;20(2):254–9.

49. An SS, Bai TR, Bates JH, et al. Airway smooth muscle dynamics: a common pathway of airway obstruction in asthma. Eur Respir J 2007;29(5):834–60.

50. James AL, Bai TR, Mauad T, et al. Airway smooth muscle thickness in asthma is related to severity but not duration of asthma. Eur Respir J 2009; 34(5):1040–5.

51. Kaminska M, Foley S, Maghni K, et al. Airway remodeling in subjects with severe asthma with or without chronic persistent airflow obstruction. J Allergy Clin Immunol 2009;124(1):45–51.

52. Wahidi MM, Kraft M. Bronchial Thermoplasty for Severe Asthma. Am J Respir Crit Care Med 2012; 185(7):709–14.

53. From the Global Strategy for Asthma Management and Prevention, Global Initiative for Asthma (GINA). 2010. Available at: http://www.ginasthma.org/. Assessed March 15, 2012.

54. National Asthma Education and Prevention Program Expert Panel Report 3. Guidelines for the diagnosis and management of asthma. Bethesda (MD): National Heart, Lung, and Blood Institute; 2007.

55. Strek ME. Difficult asthma. Proc Am Thorac Soc 2006;3(1):116–23.

56. Peters SP, Ferguson G, Deniz Y, et al. Uncontrolled asthma: a review of the prevalence, disease burden and options for treatment. Respir Med 2006;100(7): 1139–51.

57. Davies H, Olson L, Gibson P. Methotrexate as a steroid sparing agent for asthma in adults. Cochrane Database Syst Rev 2000;2:CD000391.

58. Evans DJ, Cullinan P, Geddes DM. Cyclosporin as an oral corticosteroid sparing agent in stable asthma. Cochrane Database Syst Rev 2001;2:CD002993.

59. Busse W, Corren J, Lanier BQ, et al. Omalizumab, anti-IgE recombinant humanized monoclonal antibody, for the treatment of severe allergic asthma. J Allergy Clin Immunol 2001;108(2):184–90.

60. Walker S, Monteil M, Phelan K, et al. Anti-IgE for chronic asthma in adults and children. Cochrane Database Syst Rev 2006;2:CD003559.

61. Campbell JD, Spackman DE, Sullivan SD. The costs and consequences of omalizumab in uncontrolled asthma from a USA payer perspective. Allergy 2010;65(9):1141–8.

62. Wenzel SE, Barnes PJ, Bleecker ER, et al. A randomized, double-blind, placebo-controlled study of tumor necrosis factor-alpha blockade in severe persistent asthma. Am J Respir Crit Care Med 2009;179(7):549–58.

63. Samitas K, Radinger M, Bossios A. Current update on eosinophilic lung diseases and anti-IL-5 treatment. Recent Pat Antiinfect Drug Discov 2011;6(3): 189–205.

64. Flood-Page PT, Menzies-Gow AN, Kay AB, et al. Eosinophil's role remains uncertain as anti-interleukin-5 only partially depletes numbers in asthmatic airway. Am J Respir Crit Care Med 2003;167(2): 199–204.

65. Flood-Page P, Swenson C, Faiferman I, et al. A study to evaluate safety and efficacy of mepolizumab in patients with moderate persistent asthma. Am J Respir Crit Care Med 2007;176(11):1062–71.

66. Nair P, Pizzichini MM, Kjarsgaard M, et al. Mepolizumab for prednisone-dependent asthma with sputum eosinophilia. N Engl J Med 2009;360(10): 985–93.

67. Haldar P, Brightling CE, Hargadon B, et al. Mepolizumab and exacerbations of refractory eosinophilic asthma. N Engl J Med 2009;360(10):973–84.

68. Gaga M, Nair P, Hargreave FE, et al. SCH527123, a novel treatment option for severe neutrophilic asthma. Am J Respir Crit Care Med 2010;181: A6763.

69. Busse WW, Israel E, Nelson HS, et al. Daclizumab improves asthma control in patients with moderate to severe persistent asthma: a randomized, controlled trial. Am J Respir Crit Care Med 2008; 178(10):1002–8.

70. Castro M, Rubin AS, Laviolette M, et al. Effectiveness and safety of bronchial thermoplasty in the treatment of severe asthma: a multicenter, randomized, double-blind, sham-controlled clinical trial. Am J Respir Crit Care Med 2010;181(2):116–24.

71. Thomson NC, Rubin AS, Niven RM, et al. Long-term (5 year) safety of bronchial thermoplasty: Asthma Intervention Research (AIR) trial. BMC Pulm Med 2011;11:8

72. Rare Diseases Act of 2002. Available at: http://history.nih.gov/research/downloads/PL107-280.pdf. Accessed March 15, 2012.

73. Public Consultation Rare Diseases: Europe's Challenges. Available at: http://ec.europa.eu/health/rare_diseases/policy/legal/index_en.htm. Accessed March 15, 2012.

74. US Food and Drug Administration. The Orphan Drug Act (as amended). Available at: http://www.fda.gov/RegulatoryInformation/Legislation/FederalFoodDrugandCosmeticActFDCAct/SignificantAmendmentstotheFDCAct/OrphanDrugAct/default.htm. Accessed March 15, 2012.

75. Lavandeira A. Orphan drugs: legal aspects, current situation. Haemophilia 2002;8(3):194–8.

76. Haffner ME, Torrent-Farnell J, Maher PD. Does orphan drug legislation really answer the needs of patients? Lancet 2008;371(9629):2041–4.

Immunologic Therapeutic Interventions in Asthma
Impact on Natural History

Arnaud Bourdin, MD, PhD[a,b,*], Marc Humbert, MD, PhD[c], Pascal Chanez, MD, PhD[d]

KEYWORDS

- Asthma • Immunology • Therapeutic intervention

KEY POINTS

- Whether immunologic interventions will really affect the natural history of asthma is a source of debate.
- Strong efforts are required to personalize and accurately describe the predominant process involved in treatment failures.
- Biologic properties of the subtle regulation of the immune system in the airways balanced between tolerance and more or less well-orientated inflammatory response in highly specialized epithelium are new areas of interest but also of concern.

NATURAL HISTORY OF ASTHMA

Asthma is a chronic inflammatory disorder of the airways that leads to acute episodes of wheezing; exacerbations; and for a small part of the population, fatal or near-fatal exacerbations. The chronicity of the disease hallmarked by recurrent episodes of bronchoconstriction[1] and potentially sustained inflammatory infiltration of the airways is suspected to account for the future risk of asthma.[2] These risks include an accelerated decline in lung function[3] in a so-called remodeling process associated with structural modifications of the airways[4] but also treatment side effects, disability, and poor quality of life. Nearly 5% of the whole asthma population responds to these criteria but are accounting for more than half of the costs engaged.[5]

Despite these potential issues, all patients with asthma will fortunately not follow this hectic natural history.[6,7] For the last 30 years, inhaled corticosteroids (ICS) demonstrated their ability to improve asthma control and save lives.[8] According to the largest clinical trials, currently available treatments (namely combination of ICS and long-acting beta-2 agonists [LABA]) are likely to positively influence about 85% of patients with asthma.[9] One year after the initiation of this therapy, about 35% are still uncontrolled.[10] In the real world, asthma control rates are disappointingly low, closer to 1 out of 2 patients with asthma.[11,12] Both adherence and

[a] Department of Respiratory Disease, Hôpital Arnaud de Villeneuve, CHU Montpellier, Montpellier, France; [b] INSERM U1046 Physiologie et Médecine expérimentale du coeur et des muscles, Université Montpellier 1 et 2, CHU Arnaud de Villeneuve, Montpellier, France; [c] INSERM U999, Pulmonary Hypertension: Pathophysiology and Novel Therapies, Service de Pneumologie et Réanimation Respiratoire, Centre National de Référence de l'Hypertension Pulmonaire Sévère, Hôpital Antoine Béclère Assistance Publique Hôpitaux de Paris, Université Paris-Sud 11, 157, rue de la Porte de Trivaux, Clamart 92140, France; [d] Département des Maladies Respiratoires, AP-HM, Laboratoire d'immunologie INSERM CNRS U 1067, UMR7733, Aix Marseille Université, Marseille, France
* Corresponding author. Service des Maladies Respiratoires, Hôpital Arnaud de Villeneuve, CHU Montpellier, Montpellier, France.
E-mail address: a-bourdin@chu-montpellier.fr

Clin Chest Med 33 (2012) 585–597
http://dx.doi.org/10.1016/j.ccm.2012.06.004
0272-5231/12/$ – see front matter © 2012 Elsevier Inc. All rights reserved

environment are classical triggers involved in this gap between clinical trial and real life but are not to discount the reality of severe asthma in other patients.[13,14] Patients with mild asthma are still accounting for most of the emergency department visits and intensive care unit (ICU) admissions because of low levels of ICS exposure,[15] low symptoms perception, and long periods of remission.[16–18] Therapeutic adherence and environmental control, including requirement of cautious behavior when exposed to different life events and particularly occupational exposure, represent an unacceptable burden even for patients with the mildest asthma.

Patients unable to achieve and sustain control despite receiving optimal management should be referred to a tertiary center specialized in difficult-to-treat asthma.[14,19] An accurate clinical approach will address the critical questions of diagnostic consolidation, comorbidity assessment, environmental inventory, and therapeutic adherence.[20] Once insufficient responsiveness to currently available treatment is positively documented on a long-term basis, better understanding of the pathologic and immunologic pathways involved will open the avenue to different interventions.

Although understanding mild asthma opens the way for long-term strategies to cure it, in severe asthma, which still represents a challenge for science and treatments, the ambition will remain to control the disease and anticipate future risks.

In patients with severe asthma, when current asthma treatment has been optimized and reassessed on a long-term basis, few strategies remain possible:

- First, anti–immunoglobulin E (IgE) (omalizumab) in eligible patients, (in Europe, patients with uncontrolled severe allergies)
- Second, long-term minimal required dose of oral corticosteroids
- Last, an inclusion in a clinical trial for an innovative therapy

One of the main criticisms that can be raised against currently conducted and published clinical trials in these patient populations is their relative short-term basis, usually 6 to 12 months. So they did not allow addressing adequately the question of the impact of the new drug to interfere on the natural history of the disease. The ideal term for assessment is unknown because important fluctuations are features of asthma.[21,22] To date, ICS are the only medication that reached this certainty with a high degree of confidence.[8,23] The outcomes related to the natural history of the disease are summarized in **Box 1**.

Box 1
Outcomes related to the natural history of asthma

Physician-related outcomes, ideal term for assessment is unknown

- Control, including short acting beta2-agonist consumption
- ICS dose to obtain and maintain control
- Exacerbation/emergency department visit/hospitalization/ICU requirement
- Death
- Level of bronchial hyperresponsiveness
- Lung function variability and loss of reversibility
- Accelerated lung function decline
- Air trapping, distension, hyperinflation
- Inacceptable therapeutic side effects (oral corticosteroids)
- Costs

Patient-related outcomes; ideal term for assessment is unknown

- Absenteeism
- Quality of Life
- Costs
- Symptoms, including anxiety
- Disability
- Side effects, including psychological consequences

THE NEED FOR PHENOTYPING: TOWARD A PERSONALIZED MEDICINE

The absence of a therapeutic response to current pharmacologic management (ICS+LABA) supports the scientific hypothesis that some complex and significant biologic pathway abnormalities may contribute to the severity of the disease. These pathways remain untouched or resistant to the current strategy.

Severe asthma is a heterogeneous disease as illustrated by the possibility to respond to one medication but not to another. Clinicians are now more familiar with the phenotyping exercise. It consists of identifying asthma traits associated with the disease. Historically, phenotyping deserved insights into disease nosology and common biologic pathways and shared prognosis.[24] The most common features of asthma history included in efforts of phenotyping are summarized in **Box 2**.

Two key studies attempted to gather all of the asthma features of patients followed in specialized eosinophils concentration in the induced sputum[27] allowed to conduct trials whereby monitoring this count was greater than a classical management in reducing the exacerbation rate.[28]

The future of asthma management will probably follow these study designs by integrating longitudinal data.[22] These investigations will improve our understanding of the natural history of the disease, and have the potential of adding an in-depth analysis of the main biologic pathways at play, to develop targeted therapies.

FROM INFLAMMATION TO STRUCTURAL CHANGES IN THE AIRWAYS: NEW CONCEPTS AND TARGETS

At present, innovative immunologic interventions in asthma are supported by the common inflammatory type 2 T-helper cells (TH2) paradigm[29–31] and downstream key cytokines (**Fig. 1**).

Using this approach, a potential biomarker has been tested to recognize patients that will respond to a monoclonal antibody against interleukin 13 (IL-13).[32]

New antiinflammatory treatments were not always successful. The remodeling of the airways paradigm raised interest in new interventions directed toward bronchial epithelium and smooth muscle cells.[33–35] Epithelial cells are suspected as a potential culprit of an enhanced bronchial

centers and used a cluster analysis to identify consistent phenotypes.[25,26]

Basically, both studies identified different phenotypes that efficiently discriminated among patients' groups when considering cross-sectional data but they failed to identify different biologic phenotypes.

In one of these studies, a subgroup follow-up study demonstrated the efficiency of a management based on the monitoring of eosinophils count in the induced sputum (less exacerbations, lower doses of ICS) in patients belonging to the eosinophilic phenotype. Accordingly, decreasing the daily dose of ICS in patients of the noneosinophilic phenotype (so-called disproportionate symptoms) was safe (no more exacerbation, no decline in lung function) and not less efficient (same level of control).[25] This study enrolled a small number of patients. Identifying eosinophilic asthma by the

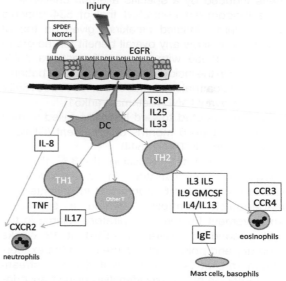

Fig. 1. Immunologic interventions in asthma. CC, chemokine receptor; CXC chemokine receptor; DC, dendritic cells; EGFR, epidermal growth factor receptor; GMCSF, granulocyte-macrophage colony-stimulating factor; IL, interleukin; SPDEF, SAM pointed domain-containing ETS transcription factor; TNF, tumor necrosis factor; TSLP, thymic stromal lymphopoietin.

triggering of asthma mechanisms (see **Fig. 1**).[36] Acting as a mechanical barrier, the bronchial epithelium also encompasses properties of innate immunity by secreting bioactive peptides (antimicrobial, antiinflammatory, linking pollutants, promoting the resolution of the inflammation)[37–39] and crosstalking with submucosal dendritic cells (DCs).[40]

MODULATION OF THE TH2 PATHWAY

IL-4 and IL-13 share one of their receptor subunits (IL-4R alpha) to activate the target cells (**Table 1**).[41] Accordingly, blocking one cytokine will be sufficient to avoid the risk of redundancy and potentially a subsequent clinical failure.[42,43] IL-4 and IL-13 are thought to play distinct important roles in B-cell commutation to IgE production, mast cell expression of the IgE receptor (fragment crystallizable [Fc] epsilon R [FcεRI]), and eosinophil recruitment.[44–46]

Clinical trials using monoclonal antibodies (mAbs) directed toward IL-4 and IL-4R failed to demonstrate a clinical impact on asthma outcomes.[47–49] In patients with moderate persistent asthma, nebulization of altrakincept (a soluble form of the alpha subunit of the IL-4 receptor) prevented asthma worsening despite a reduction in the daily dose of ICS. But a larger phase II trial failed to demonstrate a sufficient benefit. Inhaled pitrakinra, which blocked both IL-4 and IL-13, significantly prevented airway hyperresponsiveness induced by a specific allergen challenge.[50] In a randomized controlled trial of 534 patients with asthma, inhaled pitrakinra given on top of ICS did not show any overall benefit for the group except in those with eosinophilic asthma (37% reduction in the incidence of asthma exacerbations) (http://clinicaltrials.gov/ct2/show/NCT00801853? term5Aerovant1AND1asthma&rank51).

A mAb directed toward IL-4 also failed in mild asthma despite 6 months of treatment (ClinicalTrials.gov Id: NCT00024544).

In a clinical trial blocking IL-13,[32] the investigators demonstrated in a double-blind placebo-controlled 6-month trial in patients with inadequately controlled asthma a significant improvement for forced expiratory volume in the first second of expiration (FEV_1) at 12 weeks (primary end point) and a decrease in the exacerbation rate at 24 weeks. An IL-13 downstream key molecule previously identified using transcriptomic analysis, periostin, assessed in the blood at the beginning of the trial, was shown as a potentially efficient biomarker.[51] The level of periostin was associated with a better response in terms of FEV_1 improvement and a trend toward a reduction in severe exacerbation episodes ($P = .08$).

Even though daily symptoms did not improve, the satisfactory safety profile and the possibility to predict a positive clinical response deserve 2 comments. First, this is one of the first trials whereby a biomarker consistent with the therapeutic intervention is identified. Second, the gap between the absence of a benefit in symptoms measured by the Asthma Control Questionnaire (ACQ) despite improved lung function suggests the importance of identifying specific symptoms associated with this phenotype. Namely, given the importance of IL-13 in mucin secretion[52,53] and fibrotic changes,[54,55] it might be worth assessing to what extent cough and sputum production and computed tomography scan airway obstruction and thickening are affected by the treatment. Other anti–IL-13 mAbs are currently under investigation. IMA-638 binds to a different IL-13 epitope. In mild atopic asthma, this treatment decreased both the early and late asthmatic responses after provocation but did not affect the level of airway hyperresponsiveness.[56]

EOSINOPHILS AND ANTI–IL-5 REVIVAL

By the 1990s, eosinophils were considered the key effectors of asthma loss of control and chronicity.[57,58] Further investigations identified IL-5 as the main mediator for eosinophil activation, recruitment, bone marrow proliferation, and bronchial survival.[59–62] The first large clinical trials in asthma provided disappointing negative results in terms of symptoms and lung function and bronchial hyperreactivity improvement despite a spectacular decrease of systemic and local eosinophilia.[63,64] Again, phenotyping was considered the obligatory requirement to deserve further clinical trials.[57] Identifying patients with asthma with evidence of persistent eosinophilic inflammation (systemic or local) successfully led to better results.[65–67] Monitoring airway eosinophilia in the induced sputum[28] or by the indirect exhaled nitric oxide levels[68] was shown to be effective in reducing asthma exacerbations.

Mepolizumab is a humanized mAb available by subcutaneous or intravenous routes. It has been used in the hypereosinophilic essential syndrome[69–71] with more than 5 years of safety experience in that population, mepolizumab is now entering a large pivotal phase III trial supported by 2 previous proof-of-concept studies, one in patients with refractory eosinophilic asthma (patients treated with a high dose of inhaled steroids)[67] and the other in patients with eosinophilic prednisone-dependent asthma identified by a greater than 3% eosinophil count in the induced sputum.[66] In those studies, a decreased rate of exacerbation

Table 1
Main immunologic interventions directed toward TH2 cytokines and downstream key molecules

Biologic Target	Dci	Asthma Phenotype	Route of Administration	Phase of Development	Main Criteria Outcome	Remarks
IgE	Omalizumab	Atopic IgE 50–700 KUI	SC	IV	Exacerbation	On the market worldwide
IL-5	Mepolizumab Reslizumab	Refractory eosinophilic (>3% IS despite steroids)	SC or iv	III	Exacerbation	New interest in specific eos patients
IL-5R	Benralizumab	—	SC	II	—	Ongoing
IL-13	Lebrikizumab Tralokinumab	Periostin high	SC	III	FEV_1	—
IL-9	MEDI-528	—	—	II	—	—
IL-17	—	Neutrophilic	—	—	—	—
IL-4R	Altrakincept	Moderate to severe	Nebulized	III	ACQ	Negative
IL-4	Pascolizumab	ICS naive	—	II	ACQ	Negative
IL-4 and IL-13	Pitrakinra	Eosinophilic subgroup	—	III	Exacerbation	Positive only in hypereosinophilic
CCR4	Mogamulizumab	?	—	II	—	—
CCR3	From GSK	Hypereosinophilic	oral	II	Eosinophils in induced sputum	—

Abbreviations: ACQ, asthma control questionnaire; CCR, CC type chemokine receptor; DCI, denomination commune internationale; eos, eosinophils; FEV1, forced expiratory volume in the first second of expiration; GSK, Glaxo SmithKline; IL, interleukin; IS, induced sputum; SC, subcutaneous.

and improvements in lung function were observed. Safety issues were satisfactorily addressed.

Other important question to address is the relevance of adherence and the threshold above which eosinophilia is considered refractory to steroid therapy.[72] A few years ago, ten Brinke and colleagues challenged the concept of steroid resistance.[73] They demonstrated that in patients with a persistent eosinophilia despite high doses of steroids, that all improved their lung function in response to a supervised systemic administration of triamcinolone in a placebo controlled study.

Reslizumab, another mAb directed against IL-5, is now entering phase III of its development in 4 different trials. Previous trials suggested a positive effect on the control of asthma assessed using the ACQ score even though the statistical significance was not reached at week 15 in patients with uncontrolled, steroid-treated, but still eosinophilic asthma. Those with nasal polyps tended to respond better, an effect expected from previous data.[74,75] The effect in hypereosinophilic syndrome is also demonstrated.[76]

Another interesting molecule directed toward IL-5R alpha, benralizumab,[77] is now in clinical development because of a good safety profile.[78] Potentially overtaking biologic effects offered by IL-5–blocking mAbs,[79] this interesting molecule is proposed in a large, multicenter, double-blind phase II trial involving patients with uncontrolled asthma not selected by their eosinophilia.

TH2-CYTOKINE IL-9 BLOCKADE IN UNCONTROLLED ASTHMA

In animal models of asthma,[80,81] IL-9 plays an important role in mast cell recruitment and proliferation in the airways.[82,83] This role is associated with features of asthma, including airway hyperresponsiveness, inflammation, and structural modifications.[83] Mast cells are known to play a crucial role in promoting not only bronchoconstriction but also perpetuating bronchial inflammation.[84] Targeting the IL-9 pathway may provide a new therapeutic modality for asthma.[85] Small clinical studies with a humanized anti–IL-9 mAb, MEDI-528, in patients with asthma[86] reported no particular safety issues and a small signal of efficacy. Of note, mast cells can be targeted by tyrosine kinase inhibitors, such as masitinib or imatinib, which focus the stem cell factor receptor c-kit.[87]

THE CCR3 PATHWAY

The recruitment of inflammatory cells in the airways requires the expression of chemokines on which C-C chemokine receptor type 3 (CCR3) was shown as one of the most important to drive the local TH2 response.[88–90] Using an antisense oligonucleotide directed against CCR3 but also beta chains of the TH2 cytokines involved into mast cells and eosinophils activation and recruitment (IL-3, IL-5, and granulocyte-macrophage colony-stimulating factor),[91,92] Gauvreau and colleagues[92] reported a significant reduction in the early asthmatic response to an allergenic challenge observed in 17 patients in a crossover study and a trend toward a significant reduction also in the late asthma response observed. Eosinophils and total inflammatory cell counts were blunted in the induced sputum of treated patients. To date, blocking the CCR3 chemokine is still under investigation in one trial with an orally active compound (http://clinicaltrials.gov/ct2/show/NCT01160224).

IS OMALIZUMAB AFFECTING THE NATURAL HISTORY OF ASTHMA?

Conceptually, blocking IgE was considered an attractive therapy targeting one of the end products of the TH2 pathway. Omalizumab followed a program of development that led to its commercialization worldwide since the mid 2000s. The pivotal Investigation of Omalizumab in Severe Asthma Treatment (INNOVATE) trial included 419 patients in a double-blind placebo-controlled design for 28 weeks.[93] The most important findings were severe exacerbation reduction, lower rate of emergency visits, reduced dose of oral steroids requirement, and improved patient-related outcomes. Targeting IgE initiated the concept of phenotyping because only patients with ongoing evidences of atopy (ie, positive skin prick test or documented specific IgE for a perennial allergen) and in-the-range levels of total IgE concentrations were, and are, eligible. But still no one can predict the magnitude of response to omalizumab therapy.[94] Successful effects were also denoted in rhinosinusitis symptoms[95,96] (probably > initially thought[97]) and urticaria.[96] The treatment cost and the need for a long-term safety evaluation in a real-life setting deserve further evaluations balancing the cost-effectiveness of this treatment.[98–100] Omalizumab therapy interruption remains a pivotal question to address because no one can tell whether this treatment sustains its effect on the natural history of the disease on a long-term basis. In young inner-city patients with asthma, the benefit of omalizumab was demonstrated again over a 60-week period by a reduction in the number of days with asthma symptoms and the proportion of the participants who had at least one exacerbation. Those who had the better response had sensitization and exposure to allergens, such as cockroach and house dust mites. The most interesting observation from this trial was the absence of an effect of the virus nasal carriage during and out of an asthma exacerbation while seasonal variations were dampened, suggesting a highly efficient symptomatic effect rather than an interaction with the natural history of the disease.[101]

Although the reemergence of symptoms are related to free IgE levels after omalizumab withdraw,[102] it was reported in a small group of patients that the positive effects observed with omalizumab could be sustained 3 years after withdrawal, with features of mild to moderate asthma.[103] Even though these findings are difficult to explain by a simple pharmacologic effect, this observation deserves more investigation.[104] Nopp[103] has shown a sustained decrease in basophil reactivity (basophil allergen threshold sensitivity) and hypothesized that this accounted for this sustained response. More potent anti-IgE antibodies are currently in development and will potentially address the unsolved question of the factors associated with unresponsiveness to omalizumab.[105]

Similar to atopic asthma, bronchial biopsies from nonatopic asthma show an enhanced expression of TH2-type cytokines (IL-4, IL-5, and IL-13)[106–108] and FcεRI[109] compared with controls. It has been shown that it is only in patients with asthma, regardless of atopic status, that bronchial mucosal class switching to IgE occurs, and local IgE seemed to be related with cellular inflammation, lung function, and clinical outcomes in asthma.[110–112] These findings suggest that there are more similarities than differences in the atopic and nonatopic forms of the disease and that there might be local IgE production directed against unidentified antigens in this important form of the disease.[113] Of note, recent studies have indicated that some IgE-mediated responses to common perennial aeroallergens, such as *Dermatophagoides* pteronyssinus, may occur in the airways of patients with so-called nonatopic asthma.[114] It is, therefore, likely that patients with severe nonatopic asthma might also benefit from omalizumab, and a few case reports of favorable outcomes using this approach have supported this hypothesis, which remains to be tested properly.

WIDE T CELLS TARGETING USING IMMUNOSUPPRESSANT

Cyclosporin and tacrolimus are inhibiting purine metabolism and should be highly effective in T-cell–dependent diseases.[115] A beneficial effect on asthma symptoms was shown in an open study of children treated by tacrolimus for atopic

dermatitis.[116] Moreover, aspirin-triggered asthma was shown to potentially benefit from this drug,[117] which is a controversial result.[118] Inhaled tacrolimus formulation trials in asthma are currently tested. Three trials only looked at cyclosporin as a steroid-sparing agent[119–122] but side effects are potentially precluding its use in routine practice, although some beneficial effects were observed.[123] A meta-analysis of methotrexate add-on therapy in patients with steroid-dependent asthma concluded that there is a small and insufficient benefit.[124]

Future Direction

IL-25 and IL-33 are novel cytokines able to expand a new T-cell subtype called nuocytes that are potentially critical in type-2 immunity.[125] Targeting these TH2 promoting cytokines might be interesting in asthma.

STRATEGIES DIRECTED TOWARD NON-TH2 PATHWAYS

Deeper insights into asthma phenotypes raised the concept of neutrophilic and paucigranulocytic asthma. Namely, these patients with severe asthma were found with no eosinophils in their induced sputum while investigated under their current medications.

Strategies that aimed to focus on neutrophils and on targets not directly related to inflammation were then developed.

TUMOR NECROSIS FACTOR ALPHA BLOCKADE

In patients with noneosinophilic severe asthma, tumor necrosis factor (TNF) alpha levels were found to be elevated both at the protein and mRNA level in the bronchoalveolar lavage fluid.[126] Subsequently, open-label studies using off-label anti-TNF alpha were conducted and reported impressive clinical results. Infliximab was tested in 2006.[127] Lung function, symptoms, and level of airway hyperresponsiveness were significantly improved after 12 weeks in 17 patients with etanercept.[128] The first placebo-controlled trial conducted in 10 patients with severe asthma provided similar results.[129] Unfortunately, these hopes were not confirmed in a larger trial when unacceptable safety issues appeared in front of no real evidences for clinical efficacy.[130] A small subgroup of patients tended to have a positive response, but the anti–TNF alpha adventure in asthma is considered over at the moment.[131]

NEUTROPHILS
Anti-CXCR2

CXC chemokine receptor type 2 (CXCR2) is one of the receptors for IL-8. It is mainly expressed by neutrophils and structural cells on which it acts as a potent chemokine receptor to drive the neutrophilic influx into airway tissue. By consequence, blocking the CXCR2 will make the neutrophils blind to IL-8 overexpression classically observed in severe asthma.[132] CXCR2 blockers seem to be a potential therapeutic avenue, especially in patients with evidence of neutrophilic inflammation. In asthma, the CXCR2 antagonist SCH527123 has been shown to inhibit either blood and airway neutrophilia (but not bone marrow neutrophilia).[133] Clinical results are shortly expected.

TH17 AND IL-17

Cumulative evidence demonstrated the importance of IL-17 in the inflammatory process observed in asthma. IL-17–secreting T cells, so-called TH17, are insensitive to steroids and add a piece of complexity in the TH1/TH2 classical paradigm.[134] IL-17 is reported as one of the key cytokines for neutrophil recruitment, structural modifications, and clinical manifestations of chronicity in asthma.[135] Nonetheless, no clinical data are available at the moment.

DESCRIBING AND DISRUPTING THE LINK BETWEEN STRUCTURE AND INFLAMMATION

The all-inflammation strategy might then be regarded as a potential mistake because a significant proportion of patients will remain uncontrolled despite optimal antiinflammatory management. New biologic findings are supporting an important role played by the epithelium, the smooth muscle, and mucus secretion in severe asthma.

SEVERE ASTHMA IS AN EPITHELIAL DISEASE

By modulating the DC function and cytokine production in the microenvironment, the epithelium is playing a critical role in airway homeostasis. The renewal of the epithelium and the plasticity of the epithelial phenotype can lead to clinical manifestations associated with severe asthma, including chronic airflow obstruction, excessive mucus production, and poor steroid responsiveness. Antimicrobial and immunomodulatory properties of the mucus content are essential in the innate immunity. Indeed, strategies aiming to interfere in the epithelium-DC, epithelium-epithelium, and epithelium-mesenchymal crosstalks are mainly based on the recent description of the key molecules, thymic stromal lymphopoietin (TSLP), SAM pointed domain-containing ETS transcription factor (SPDEF), and epidermal growth factor receptor, respectively.[136] TSLP polymorphism has been frequently reported as a candidate asthma gene in genome-wide association studies[36,137,138] and is currently investigated as a potential noninvasive biomarker. Specific humanized antibodies are currently developed and future exciting results are expected. SPDEF is a downstream molecule of the defective Notch pathway observed in asthma[38] and it represents a candidate for a future therapeutic axis. TLR7-agonists are inducing an acute and sustained protection against TH2 inflammation in a mouse model of asthma by modulating the pattern of interferon response.[139]

SUMMARY

Whether immunologic interventions will really affect the natural history of asthma is a fantastic source of debate. The heterogeneity of the disease and the multidimensional approach required to manage severe asthma are both arguments to oppose to targeted strategies reviewed here. Strong efforts are required to personalize and accurately describe the predominant process involved in treatment failures. Biologic properties of the subtle regulation of the immune system in the airways balanced between tolerance and a more or less well-orientated inflammatory response in highly specialized epithelium are sources of new areas of interest but also of concern. The ideal duration of targeted therapies and worth time of introduction (ie, at disease onset vs only in severe, during exacerbation vs at stable state, etc) are 2 main issues that have to be perfectly addressed before rendering any clinical conclusion.

REFERENCES

1. Grainge CL, Lau LC, Ward JA, et al. Effect of bronchoconstriction on airway remodeling in asthma. N Engl J Med 2011;364(21):2006–15.
2. Thamrin C, Zindel J, Nydegger R, et al. Predicting future risk of asthma exacerbations using individual conditional probabilities. J Allergy Clin Immunol 2011;127(6):1494–1502, e3.
3. Lange P, Parner J, Vestbo J, et al. A 15-year follow-up study of ventilatory function in adults with asthma. N Engl J Med 1998;339(17):1194–200.
4. Vignola AM, Chanez P, Bonsignore G, et al. Structural consequences of airway inflammation in asthma. J Allergy Clin Immunol 2000;105(2 Pt 2):S514–7.
5. Godard P, Chanez P, Siraudin L, et al. Costs of asthma are correlated with severity: a 1-yr prospective study. Eur Respir J 2002;19(1):61–7.

6. Strachan DP, Griffiths JM, Johnston ID, et al. Ventilatory function in British adults after asthma or wheezing illness at ages 0-35. Am J Respir Crit Care Med 1996;154(6 Pt 1):1629–35.

7. Roorda RJ, Gerritsen J, van Aalderen WM, et al. Follow-up of asthma from childhood to adulthood: influence of potential childhood risk factors on the outcome of pulmonary function and bronchial responsiveness in adulthood. J Allergy Clin Immunol 1994;93(3):575–84.

8. Suissa S, Ernst P, Benayoun S, et al. Low-dose inhaled corticosteroids and the prevention of death from asthma. N Engl J Med 2000;343(5):332–6.

9. Bateman ED, Boushey HA, Bousquet J, et al. Can guideline-defined asthma control be achieved? The Gaining Optimal Asthma Control study. Am J Respir Crit Care Med 2004;170(8):836–44.

10. Bateman ED, Bousquet J, Busse WW, et al. Stability of asthma control with regular treatment: an analysis of the Gaining Optimal Asthma Control (GOAL) study. Allergy 2008;63(7):932–8.

11. Rabe KF, Vermeire PA, Soriano JB, et al. Clinical management of asthma in 1999: the Asthma Insights and Reality in Europe (AIRE) study. Eur Respir J 2000;16(5):802–7.

12. Godard P, Huas D, Sohier B, et al. Asthma control in general practice: a cross-sectional survey of 16,580 patients. Presse Med 2005;34(19 Pt 1): 1351–7 [in French].

13. Chanez P, Godard P. Is difficult asthma still clinically meaningful? Eur Respir J 2006;28(5):897–9.

14. Chanez P, Wenzel SE, Anderson GP, et al. Severe asthma in adults: what are the important questions? J Allergy Clin Immunol 2007;119(6):1337–48.

15. Salmeron S, Liard R, Elkharrat D, et al. Asthma severity and adequacy of management in accident and emergency departments in France: a prospective study. Lancet 2001;358(9282):629–35.

16. van der Merwe L, de Klerk A, Kidd M, et al. Case-control study of severe life threatening asthma (SLTA) in a developing community. Thorax 2006; 61(9):756–60.

17. Lanes SF, Lanza LL, Wentworth CE 3rd. Risk of emergency care, hospitalization, and ICU stays for acute asthma among recipients of salmeterol. Am J Respir Crit Care Med 1998;158(3):857–61.

18. Turner MO, Noertjojo K, Vedal S, et al. Risk factors for near-fatal asthma. A case-control study in hospitalized patients with asthma. Am J Respir Crit Care Med 1998;157(6 Pt 1):1804–9.

19. Chung KF, Godard P, Adelroth E, et al. Difficult/therapy-resistant asthma: the need for an integrated approach to define clinical phenotypes, evaluate risk factors, understand pathophysiology and find novel therapies. ERS task force on difficult/therapy-resistant asthma. European Respiratory Society. Eur Respir J 1999;13(5):1198–208.

20. Bel EH, Sousa A, Fleming L, et al. Diagnosis and definition of severe refractory asthma: an international consensus statement from the Innovative Medicine Initiative (IMI). Thorax 2011;66(10): 910–7.

21. Frey U, Maksym G, Suki B. Temporal complexity in clinical manifestations of lung disease. J Appl Physiol 2011;110(6):1723–31.

22. Stern G, de Jongste J, van der Valk R, et al. Fluctuation phenotyping based on daily fraction of exhaled nitric oxide values in asthmatic children. J Allergy Clin Immunol 2011;128(2):293–300.

23. Ernst P. Inhaled corticosteroids moderate lung function decline in adults with asthma. Thorax 2006;61(2):93–4.

24. Heaney LG, Robinson DS. Severe asthma treatment: need for characterising patients. Lancet 2005;365(9463):974–6.

25. Haldar P, Pavord ID, Shaw DE, et al. Cluster analysis and clinical asthma phenotypes. Am J Respir Crit Care Med 2008;178(3):218–24.

26. Moore WC, Meyers DA, Wenzel SE, et al. Identification of asthma phenotypes using cluster analysis in the Severe Asthma Research Program. Am J Respir Crit Care Med 2010;181(4):315–23.

27. Lemiere C, Ernst P, Olivenstein R, et al. Airway inflammation assessed by invasive and noninvasive means in severe asthma: eosinophilic and noneosinophilic phenotypes. J Allergy Clin Immunol 2006;118(5):1033–9.

28. Green RH, Brightling CE, McKenna S, et al. Asthma exacerbations and sputum eosinophil counts: a randomised controlled trial. Lancet 2002; 360(9347):1715–21.

29. Colavita AM, Reinach AJ, Peters SP. Contributing factors to the pathobiology of asthma. The Th1/Th2 paradigm. Clin Chest Med 2000;21(2):263–77.

30. Magnan AO, Mely LG, Camilla CA, et al. Assessment of the Th1/Th2 paradigm in whole blood in atopy and asthma. Increased IFN-gamma-producing CD8(+) T cells in asthma. Am J Respir Crit Care Med 2000;161(6):1790–6.

31. Holt PG, Macaubas C, Stumbles PA, et al. The role of allergy in the development of asthma. Nature 1999;402(Suppl 6760):B12–7.

32. Corren J, Lemanske RF, Hanania NA, et al. Lebrikizumab treatment in adults with asthma. N Engl J Med 2008;365(12):1088–98.

33. Zhou B, Comeau MR, De Smedt T, et al. Thymic stromal lymphopoietin as a key initiator of allergic airway inflammation in mice. Nat Immunol 2005; 6(10):1047–53.

34. Allakhverdi Z, Comeau MR, Jessup HK, et al. Thymic stromal lymphopoietin is released by human epithelial cells in response to microbes, trauma, or inflammation and potently activates mast cells. J Exp Med 2007;204(2):253–8.

35. Seshasayee D, Lee WP, Zhou M, et al. In vivo blockade of OX40 ligand inhibits thymic stromal lymphopoietin driven atopic inflammation. J Clin Invest 2007;117(12):3868–78.

36. Ziegler SF, Artis D. Sensing the outside world: TSLP regulates barrier immunity. Nat Immunol 2010; 11(4):289–93.

37. Xiao C, Puddicombe SM, Field S, et al. Defective epithelial barrier function in asthma. J Allergy Clin Immunol 2011;128(3):549–556.e1–12.

38. Maeda Y, Chen G, Xu Y, et al. Airway epithelial transcription factor NK2 homeobox 1 inhibits mucous cell metaplasia and Th2 inflammation. Am J Respir Crit Care Med 2011;184(4):421–9.

39. Chanez P. Severe asthma is an epithelial disease. Eur Respir J 2005;25(6):945–6.

40. Siracusa MC, Saenz SA, Hill DA, et al. TSLP promotes interleukin-3-independent basophil haematopoiesis and type 2 inflammation. Nature 2011;477(7363):229–33.

41. Munitz A, Brandt EB, Mingler M, et al. Distinct roles for IL-13 and IL-4 via IL-13 receptor alpha1 and the type II IL-4 receptor in asthma pathogenesis. Proc Natl Acad Sci U S A 2008;105(20):7240–5.

42. Corry DB, Kheradmand F. Biology and therapeutic potential of the interleukin-4/interleukin-13 signaling pathway in asthma. Am J Respir Med 2002;1(3): 185–93.

43. Holgate ST. Pathophysiology of asthma: what has our current understanding taught us about new therapeutic approaches? J Allergy Clin Immunol 2011;128(3):495–505.

44. Barnes PJ. Cytokine-directed therapies for asthma. J Allergy Clin Immunol 2001;108(Suppl 2):S72–6.

45. Jiang H, Harris MB, Rothman P. IL-4/IL-13 signaling beyond JAK/STAT. J Allergy Clin Immunol 2000; 105(6 Pt 1):1063–70.

46. Corry DB, Kheradmand F. Induction and regulation of the IgE response. Nature 1999;402(Suppl 6760): B18–23.

47. Borish LC, Nelson HS, Corren J, et al. Efficacy of soluble IL-4 receptor for the treatment of adults with asthma. J Allergy Clin Immunol 2001;107(6):963–70.

48. Borish LC, Nelson HS, Lanz MJ, et al. Interleukin-4 receptor in moderate atopic asthma. A phase I/II randomized, placebo-controlled trial. Am J Respir Crit Care Med 1999;160(6):1816–23.

49. Hart TK, Blackburn MN, Brigham-Burke M, et al. Preclinical efficacy and safety of pascolizumab (SB 240683): a humanized anti-interleukin-4 antibody with therapeutic potential in asthma. Clin Exp Immunol 2002;130(1):93–100.

50. Wenzel S, Wilbraham D, Fuller R, et al. Effect of an interleukin-4 variant on late phase asthmatic response to allergen challenge in asthmatic patients: results of two phase 2a studies. Lancet 2007;370(9596):1422–31.

51. Woodruff PG, Boushey HA, Dolganov GM, et al. Genome-wide profiling identifies epithelial cell genes associated with asthma and with treatment response to corticosteroids. Proc Natl Acad Sci U S A 2007;104(40):15858–63.

52. Wynn TA. IL-13 effector functions. Annu Rev Immunol 2003;21:425–56.

53. Kuperman DA, Huang X, Koth LL, et al. Direct effects of interleukin-13 on epithelial cells cause airway hyperreactivity and mucus overproduction in asthma. Nat Med 2002;8(8):885–9.

54. Grunig G. IL-13 and adenosine: partners in a molecular dance? J Clin Invest 2003;112(3):329–31.

55. Zhu Z, Homer RJ, Wang Z, et al. Pulmonary expression of interleukin-13 causes inflammation, mucus hypersecretion, subepithelial fibrosis, physiologic abnormalities, and eotaxin production. J Clin Invest 1999;103(6):779–88.

56. Gauvreau GM, Boulet LP, Cockcroft DW, et al. Effects of interleukin-13 blockade on allergen-induced airway responses in mild atopic asthma. Am J Respir Crit Care Med 2011;183(8):1007–14.

57. Busse WW, Ring J, Huss-Marp J, et al. A review of treatment with mepolizumab, an anti-IL-5 mAb, in hypereosinophilic syndromes and asthma. J Allergy Clin Immunol 2010;125(4):803–13.

58. Bousquet J, Chanez P, Lacoste JY, et al. Eosinophilic inflammation in asthma. N Engl J Med 1990;323(15):1033–9.

59. Flood-Page PT, Menzies-Gow AN, Kay AB, et al. Eosinophil's role remains uncertain as anti-interleukin-5 only partially depletes numbers in asthmatic airway. Am J Respir Crit Care Med 2003;167(2):199–204.

60. Flood-Page P, Menzies-Gow A, Phipps S, et al. Anti-IL-5 treatment reduces deposition of ECM proteins in the bronchial subepithelial basement membrane of mild atopic asthmatics. J Clin Invest 2003;112(7):1029–36.

61. Menzies-Gow AN, Flood-Page PT, Robinson DS, et al. Effect of inhaled interleukin-5 on eosinophil progenitors in the bronchi and bone marrow of asthmatic and non-asthmatic volunteers. Clin Exp Allergy 2007;37(7):1023–32.

62. Romagnoli M, Vachier I, Tarodo de la Fuente P, et al. Eosinophilic inflammation in sputum of poorly controlled asthmatics. Eur Respir J 2002;20(6): 1370–7.

63. Flood-Page P, Swenson C, Faiferman I, et al. A study to evaluate safety and efficacy of mepolizumab in patients with moderate persistent asthma. Am J Respir Crit Care Med 2007;176(11):1062–71.

64. O'Byrne PM. The demise of anti IL-5 for asthma, or not. Am J Respir Crit Care Med 2007;176(11):1059–60.

65. Wenzel SE. Eosinophils in asthma–closing the loop or opening the door? N Engl J Med 2009;360(10): 1026–8,

66. Nair P, Pizzichini MM, Kjarsgaard M, et al. Mepolizumab for prednisone-dependent asthma with sputum eosinophilia. N Engl J Med 2009;360(10):985–93.

67. Haldar P, Brightling CE, Hargadon B, et al. Mepolizumab and exacerbations of refractory eosinophilic asthma. N Engl J Med 2009;360(10):973–84.

68. Smith AD, Cowan JO, Brassett KP, et al. Use of exhaled nitric oxide measurements to guide treatment in chronic asthma. N Engl J Med 2005; 352(21):2163–73.

69. Roufosse F, de Lavareille A, Schandene L, et al. Mepolizumab as a corticosteroid-sparing agent in lymphocytic variant hypereosinophilic syndrome. J Allergy Clin Immunol 2010;126(4):828–835.e3.

70. Boulware DR, Stauffer WM 3rd, Walker PF. Hypereosinophilic syndrome and mepolizumab. N Engl J Med 2008;358(26):2839.

71. Rothenberg ME, Klion AD, Roufosse FE, et al. Treatment of patients with the hypereosinophilic syndrome with mepolizumab. N Engl J Med 2008; 358(12):1215–28.

72. ten Brinke A, Zwinderman AH, Sterk PJ, et al. Factors associated with persistent airflow limitation in severe asthma. Am J Respir Crit Care Med 2001; 164(5):744–8.

73. ten Brinke A, Zwinderman AH, Sterk PJ, et al. "Refractory" eosinophilic airway inflammation in severe asthma: effect of parenteral corticosteroids. Am J Respir Crit Care Med 2004;170(6):601–5.

74. Castro M, Mathur S, Hargreave F, et al. Reslizumab for poorly controlled, eosinophilic asthma: a randomized, placebo-controlled study. Am J Respir Crit Care Med 2011;184(10):1125–32.

75. Gevaert P, Lang-Loidolt D, Lackner A, et al. Nasal IL-5 levels determine the response to anti-IL-5 treatment in patients with nasal polyps. J Allergy Clin Immunol 2006;118(5):1133–41.

76. Ogbogu PU, Bochner BS, Butterfield JH, et al. Hypereosinophilic syndrome: a multicenter, retrospective analysis of clinical characteristics and response to therapy. J Allergy Clin Immunol 2009; 124(6):1319–1325.e3.

77. Seale JP. European Respiratory Society (ERS) - 20th Annual Congress. IDrugs 2010;13(11):762–4.

78. Busse WW, Katial R, Gossage D, et al. Safety profile, pharmacokinetics, and biologic activity of MEDI-563, an anti-IL-5 receptor alpha antibody, in a phase I study of subjects with mild asthma. J Allergy Clin Immunol 2010;125(6):1237–1244.e2.

79. Kolbeck R, Kozhich A, Koike M, et al. MEDI-563, a humanized anti-IL-5 receptor alpha mAb with enhanced antibody-dependent cell-mediated cytotoxicity function. J Allergy Clin Immunol 2010; 125(6):1344–1353.e2.

80. Nicolaides NC, Holroyd KJ, Ewart SL, et al. Interleukin 9: a candidate gene for asthma. Proc Natl Acad Sci U S A 1997;94(24):13175–80.

81. Longphre M, Li D, Gallup M, et al. Allergen-induced IL-9 directly stimulates mucin transcription in respiratory epithelial cells. J Clin Invest 1999; 104(10):1375–82.

82. Cheng G, Arima M, Honda K, et al. Anti-interleukin-9 antibody treatment inhibits airway inflammation and hyperreactivity in mouse asthma model. Am J Respir Crit Care Med 2002;166(3):409–16.

83. Kearley J, Erjefalt JS, Andersson C, et al. IL-9 governs allergen-induced mast cell numbers in the lung and chronic remodeling of the airways. Am J Respir Crit Care Med 2011;183(7):865–75.

84. Tunon-de-Lara JM, Berger P, Marthan R. Chymase-positive mast cells: a double-edged sword in asthma? Am J Respir Crit Care Med 2005;172(5):647–8.

85. Antoniu SA. MEDI-528, an anti-IL-9 humanized antibody for the treatment of asthma. Curr Opin Mol Ther 2010;12(2):233–9.

86. Parker JM, Oh CK, LaForce C, et al. Safety profile and clinical activity of multiple subcutaneous doses of MEDI-528, a humanized anti-interleukin-9 monoclonal antibody, in two randomized phase 2a studies in subjects with asthma. BMC Pulm Med 2011;11:14.

87. Humbert M, de Blay F, Garcia G, et al. Masitinib, a c-kit/PDGF receptor tyrosine kinase inhibitor, improves disease control in severe corticosteroid-dependent asthmatics. Allergy 2009;64(8): 1194–201.

88. Kitaura M, Nakajima T, Imai T, et al. Molecular cloning of human eotaxin, an eosinophil-selective CC chemokine, and identification of a specific eosinophil eotaxin receptor, CC chemokine receptor 3. J Biol Chem 1996;271(13):7725–30.

89. Ochi H, Hirani WM, Yuan Q, et al. T helper cell type 2 cytokine-mediated comitogenic responses and CCR3 expression during differentiation of human mast cells in vitro. J Exp Med 1999; 190(2):267–80.

90. Humbles AA, Lu B, Friend DS, et al. The murine CCR3 receptor regulates both the role of eosinophils and mast cells in allergen-induced airway inflammation and hyperresponsiveness. Proc Natl Acad Sci U S A 2002;99(3):1479–84.

91. Allakhverdi Z, Allam M, Guimond A, et al. Multitargeted approach using antisense oligonucleotides for the treatment of asthma. Ann N Y Acad Sci 2006;1082:62–73.

92. Gauvreau GM, Boulet LP, Cockcroft DW, et al. Antisense therapy against CCR3 and the common beta chain attenuates allergen-induced eosinophilic responses. Am J Respir Crit Care Med 2008;177(9): 952–8.

93. Humbert M, Beasley R, Ayres J, et al. Benefits of omalizumab as add-on therapy in patients with severe persistent asthma who are inadequately controlled despite best available therapy (GINA

2002 step 4 treatment): INNOVATE. Allergy 2005; 60(3):309–16.

94. Wahn U, Martin C, Freeman P, et al. Relationship between pretreatment specific IgE and the response to omalizumab therapy. Allergy 2009;64(12):1780–7.

95. Grundmann SA, Hemfort PB, Luger TA, et al. Anti-IgE (omalizumab): a new therapeutic approach for chronic rhinosinusitis. J Allergy Clin Immunol 2008; 121(1):257–8.

96. Saini S, Rosen KE, Hsieh HJ, et al. A randomized, placebo-controlled, dose-ranging study of single-dose omalizumab in patients with H1-antihistamine-refractory chronic idiopathic urticaria. J Allergy Clin Immunol 2011;128(3):567–573.e1.

97. Pinto JM, Mehta N, DiTineo M, et al. A randomized, double-blind, placebo-controlled trial of anti-IgE for chronic rhinosinusitis. Rhinology 2010;48(3):318–24.

98. Campbell JD, Spackman DE, Sullivan SD. The costs and consequences of omalizumab in uncontrolled asthma from a USA payer perspective. Allergy 2010;65(9):1141–8.

99. Sullivan SD, Turk F. An evaluation of the cost-effectiveness of omalizumab for the treatment of severe allergic asthma. Allergy 2008;63(6):670–84.

100. Revicki D, Brown R, Dale P. Questioning the economic evaluation of omalizumab. J Allergy Clin Immunol 2008;121(6):1514.

101. Busse WW, Morgan WJ, Gergen PJ, et al. Randomized trial of omalizumab (anti-IgE) for asthma in inner-city children. N Engl J Med 2011;364(11): 1005–15.

102. Slavin RG, Ferioli C, Tannenbaum SJ, et al. Asthma symptom re-emergence after omalizumab withdrawal correlates well with increasing IgE and decreasing pharmacokinetic concentrations. J Allergy Clin Immunol 2009;123(1):107–113.e3.

103. Nopp A, Johansson SG, Adedoyin J, et al. After 6 years with Xolair; a 3-year withdrawal follow-up. Allergy 2010;65(1):56–60.

104. Walker S, Monteil M, Phelan K, et al. Anti-IgE for chronic asthma in adults and children. Cochrane Database Syst Rev 2006;2:CD003559.

105. Bousquet J, Wenzel S, Holgate S, et al. Predicting response to omalizumab, an anti-IgE antibody, in patients with allergic asthma. Chest 2004;125(4): 1378–86.

106. Humbert M, Durham SR, Ying S, et al. IL-4 and IL-5 mRNA and protein in bronchial biopsies from patients with atopic and nonatopic asthma: evidence against "intrinsic" asthma being a distinct immunopathologic entity. Am J Respir Crit Care Med 1996;154(5):1497–504.

107. Humbert M, Durham SR, Kimmitt P, et al. Elevated expression of messenger ribonucleic acid encoding IL-13 in the bronchial mucosa of atopic and nonatopic subjects with asthma. J Allergy Clin Immunol 1997;99(5):657–65.

108. Ying S, Humbert M, Barkans J, et al. Expression of IL-4 and IL-5 mRNA and protein product by CD4+ and CD8+ T cells, eosinophils, and mast cells in bronchial biopsies obtained from atopic and nonatopic (intrinsic) asthmatics. J Immunol 1997;158(7): 3539–44.

109. Humbert M, Corrigan CJ, Kimmitt P, et al. Relationship between IL-4 and IL-5 mRNA expression and disease severity in atopic asthma. Am J Respir Crit Care Med 1997;156(3 Pt 1):704–8.

110. Ying S, Humbert M, Meng Q, et al. Local expression of epsilon germline gene transcripts and RNA for the epsilon heavy chain of IgE in the bronchial mucosa in atopic and nonatopic asthma. J Allergy Clin Immunol 2001;107(4):686–92.

111. Takhar P, Corrigan CJ, Smurthwaite L, et al. Class switch recombination to IgE in the bronchial mucosa of atopic and nonatopic patients with asthma. J Allergy Clin Immunol 2007;119(1):213–8.

112. Balzar S, Strand M, Rhodes D, et al. IgE expression pattern in lung: relation to systemic IgE and asthma phenotypes. J Allergy Clin Immunol 2007;119(4): 855–62.

113. Humbert M, Menz G, Ying S, et al. The immunopathology of extrinsic (atopic) and intrinsic (nonatopic) asthma: more similarities than differences. Immunol Today 1999;20(11):528–33.

114. Mouthuy J, Detry B, Sohy C, et al. Presence in sputum of functional dust mite-specific IgE antibodies in intrinsic asthma. Am J Respir Crit Care Med 2011;184(2):206–14.

115. Corrigan CJ. Asthma refractory to glucocorticoids: the role of newer immunosuppressants. Am J Respir Med 2002;1(1):47–54.

116. Virtanen H, Remitz A, Malmberg P, et al. Topical tacrolimus in the treatment of atopic dermatitis–does it benefit the airways? A 4-year open follow-up. J Allergy Clin Immunol 2007;120(6):1464–6.

117. Kawano T, Matsuse H, Kondo Y, et al. Tacrolimus reduces urinary excretion of leukotriene E(4) and inhibits aspirin-induced asthma to threshold dose of aspirin. J Allergy Clin Immunol 2004;114(6):1278–81.

118. Stevenson DD, Mehra PK, White AA, et al. Failure of tacrolimus to prevent aspirin-induced respiratory reactions in patients with aspirin-exacerbated respiratory disease. J Allergy Clin Immunol 2005; 116(4):755–60.

119. Lock SH, Kay AB, Barnes NC. Double-blind, placebo-controlled study of cyclosporin A as a corticosteroid-sparing agent in corticosteroid-dependent asthma. Am J Respir Crit Care Med 1996;153(2):509–14.

120. Nizankowska E, Soja J, Pinis G, et al. Treatment of steroid-dependent bronchial asthma with cyclosporin. Eur Respir J 1995;8(7):1091–9.

121. Alexander AG, Barnes NC, Kay AB, et al. Clinical response to cyclosporin in chronic severe asthma

is associated with reduction in serum soluble interleukin-2 receptor concentrations. Eur Respir J 1995;8(4):574–8.

122. Alexander AG, Barnes NC, Kay AB. Trial of cyclosporin in corticosteroid-dependent chronic severe asthma. Lancet 1992;339(8789):324–8.

123. Evans DJ, Cullinan P, Geddes DM. Cyclosporin as an oral corticosteroid sparing agent in stable asthma. Cochrane Database Syst Rev 2001;2: CD002993.

124. Marin MG. Low-dose methotrexate spares steroid usage in steroid-dependent asthmatic patients: a meta-analysis. Chest 1997;112(1):29–33.

125. Neill DR, Wong SH, Bellosi A, et al. Nuocytes represent a new innate effector leukocyte that mediates type-2 immunity. Nature 2010;464(7293): 1367–70.

126. Howarth PH, Babu KS, Arshad HS, et al. Tumour necrosis factor (TNFalpha) as a novel therapeutic target in symptomatic corticosteroid dependent asthma. Thorax 2005;60(12):1012–8.

127. Erin EM, Leaker BR, Nicholson GC, et al. The effects of a monoclonal antibody directed against tumor necrosis factor-alpha in asthma. Am J Respir Crit Care Med 2006;174(7):753–62.

128. Morjaria JB, Chauhan AJ, Babu KS, et al. The role of a soluble TNFalpha receptor fusion protein (etanercept) in corticosteroid refractory asthma: a double blind, randomised, placebo controlled trial. Thorax 2008;63(7):584–91.

129. Berry MA, Hargadon B, Shelley M, et al. Evidence of a role of tumor necrosis factor alpha in refractory asthma. N Engl J Med 2006;354(7):697–708.

130. Holgate ST, Noonan M, Chanez P, et al. Efficacy and safety of etanercept in moderate-to-severe asthma: a randomised, controlled trial. Eur Respir J 2011;37(6):1352–9.

131. Wenzel SE, Barnes PJ, Bleecker ER, et al. A randomized, double-blind, placebo-controlled study of tumor necrosis factor-alpha blockade in severe persistent asthma. Am J Respir Crit Care Med 2009;179(7):549–58.

132. Pignatti P, Moscato G, Casarini S, et al. Downmodulation of CXCL8/IL-8 receptors on neutrophils after recruitment in the airways. J Allergy Clin Immunol 2005;115(1):88–94.

133. Todd CM, Murphy DM, Watson RM, et al. Treatment with the CXCR2 antagonist SCH527123 reduced neutrophil levels in blood and airways but not bone marrow in mild asthmatic subjects. Am J Respir Crit Care Med 2010;181:A4237.

134. McKinley L, Alcorn JF, Peterson A, et al. TH17 cells mediate steroid-resistant airway inflammation and airway hyperresponsiveness in mice. J Immunol 2008;181(6):4089–97.

135. Kawaguchi M, Adachi M, Oda N, et al. IL-17 cytokine family. J Allergy Clin Immunol 2004;114(6): 1265–73 [quiz: 1274].

136. Park KS, Korfhagen TR, Bruno MD, et al. SPDEF regulates goblet cell hyperplasia in the airway epithelium. J Clin Invest 2007;117(4):978–88.

137. Hirota T, Takahashi A, Kubo M, et al. Genome-wide association study identifies three new susceptibility loci for adult asthma in the Japanese population. Nat Genet 2011;43(9):893–6.

138. Torgerson DG, Ampleford EJ, Chiu GY, et al. Meta-analysis of genome-wide association studies of asthma in ethnically diverse North American populations. Nat Genet 2011;43(9):887–92.

139. Xirakia C, Koltsida O, Stavropoulos A, et al. Toll-like receptor 7-triggered immune response in the lung mediates acute and long-lasting suppression of experimental asthma. Am J Respir Crit Care Med 2010;181(11):1207–16.

Index

Note: Page numbers of article titles are in **boldface** type.

Clin Chest Med 33 (2012) 599–604
http://dx.doi.org/10.1016/S0272-5231(12)00086-X
0272-5231/12/$ – see front matter © 2012 Elsevier Inc. All rights reserved

Printed and bound by CPI Group (UK) Ltd, Croydon, CR0 4YY

03/10/2024

01040348-0002